Microcurrent Electro-Acupuncture

Bio-Electric Principles, Evaluation and Treatment

by

Darren Starwynn, O.M.D., Dipl. Ac.

Desert Heart Press
Tiburon, California

Copyright © August, 2002
by Darren Starwynn, O.M.D.

First Printing September, 2002

Second Edition December, 2017

All rights reserved.

No parts of this book may be reproduced or transmitted in any form or by any means, mechanical or electronic, including photocopying, recording or by any information storage and retrieval system, without permission in writing from the author, except short excerpts for review purposes.

ISBN: 978-1981972715

Published by *Desert Heart Press*
4 Circle Drive, Suite D, Tiburon, CA 94920
E-Mail: info@DrStarwynn.com

Cover artwork by Jack Crompton/Applied Creativity Studios
jscrompton@qwest.net

Proofreading and table formatting: Jan Allen, Lic. Ac.

Library of Congress Control Number: 2002112502

Printed in the United States of America

CONTENTS

Acknowledgements

Disclaimer & Contraindications

Forward I by Jan Allen, L.Ac.

Forward II by John Stebbins, O.M.D.

Preface

SECTION I - ELECTROMEDICAL PRINCIPLES

CHAPTER 1- INTRODUCTION ... 19
Conventional Electotherapy ... 20
The Electrical Nature of Life ... 21
Electromagnetic Pollution ... 23
Medicine of the Future ... 24

CHAPTER 2 – ELECTROPHYSIOLOGY AND THE ACUPUNCTURE SYSTEMS ... 27
Introduction ... 27
Electrical Parameters of the Human Body ... 29
Microcurrents and the Meridian System ... 31
Electrical Effects of Acupuncture Needling ... 32
Semiconduction and Piezoelectricity ... 34
What are Meridians? ... 36
Non-needle Acupuncture ... 36
Combining Needling and Microcurrents ... 38

CHAPTER 3 – UNIVERSAL LAWS OF ENERGY MEDICINE ... 42
Universal Law #1 - The Law of Resonance ... 43
Universal Law #2 - The Law of Polarity ... 44
Universal Law #3 - The Law of Economy ... 47
Universal Law #4 - The Law of Biasology ... 48
Accommodation ... 48
Kinesiology ... 50

CHAPTER 4 – A BRIEF PRIMER IN ELECTRICAL TERMINOLOGY AND THEORY ... 51
Electro-therapeutic Treatment Parameters ... 54
Treatment Presets ... 58

CHAPTER 5 – PRINCIPLES OF PAIN MANAGEMENT EAST AND WEST ... 59
Western Pain Electro-physiology ... 60
Western Pain Treatments ... 61
Traditional Chinese Medicine Pain Theory and Practice ... 62
Etiology of Pain According to TCM ... 63
The Liver and Pain Management ... 65
Chinese Medical Diagnosis ... 66
Root and Branch ... 68

SECTION II - MICROCURRENT ELECTRO-ACUPUNCTURE TREATMENT TECHNIQUES

INTRODUCTION 73

CHAPTER 6 – SHORTCOMINGS OF MODERN ELECTRO-THERAPY, AND SOLUTIONS 77
Shortcoming #1: Overemphasis on Local Stimulation 78
Shortcoming #2: Use of "Overkill" Stimulation Currents That Inhibit Healing and Carry-over of Relief ... 79
Shortcoming #4: Incorrect Choice of Electrode Polarities Leading to Inappropriate Treatment of Extremities and Radiculopathies 80
Shortcoming #5: Passive Electro-stimulation 81
Summary 83

CHAPTER 7 – MICROCURRENT TREATMENT – PROBE TECHNIQUES 85
User Interface 86
Search and Treat Modes 86
How to Search With A Microcurrent Device 87
A Brief Discussion Of Myofascial Trigger Points 89

Probe Techniques:

Circling the Dragon 91
Dermatome and Distal 93
Acute Probe Treatment 97
Gentle/Chronic Probe Treatment 99
Specific Muscle Treatments 100
Nerve Root Stimulation 103
Microcurrent Mu-Shu method 108
Micro-Macro Technique 112

CHAPTER 8 – TREATMENT OF GREAT LOOPS 115
General principles 115
Step-by-step Great Loops treatment 120
Combining microcurrent and needle stimulation 122
Summary 122

CHAPTER 9 – ELECTRO-THERAPEUTIC PAD TREATMENTS 125
Electro-Therapy Devices 125
Therapeutic Effects Of Electrical Pad Stimulation 127
Pad electrodes 127
Electro-therapeutic pad techiques 128
Milliamp pad techniques 128
Microamp pad techniques 131
Microcurrent Interferential 132
Kinetic Electro-Therapeutics 133

SECTION III - FOUR-STEP PROTOCOL

CHAPTER 10 – FOUR-STEP TREATMENT INTRODUCTION 135

CHAPTER 11 – STEP ONE – BALANCING THE MERIDIAN SYSTEM 143
Step-By-Step Overview 145

MANAKA MERIDIAN BALANCING METHOD 147
More on Choosing Treatment Meridians and Points 148
Treatment Laterality 150
Master Points and Polarity 151
Other Step One Treatments 152
The Five Elements in Step One Treatments 155
Emotional Balancing with the Five Elements 156
Other Meridian Relationships 158
Extraordinary Vessel Symptomatology and Points 158

CHAPTER 12 – STEP TWO – YANG MERIDIAN TREATMENTS 161
Revisiting Yin and Yang 161
Back Shu Points 162
Kyutoshin Treatment Technique 162
Back Shu Point Selection 163
Other Step Two Treatment Points 165
Microcurrent Mu-Shu Technique 166

CHAPTER 13 – STEP THREE – MICROCURRENTS, BODYWORK AND MANIPULATION 169
Overview 169
Microcurrents, Exercise and Proprioception 170
Step Three Treatment Techniques 172
Sotai 173
Electro-massage 174
Interferential electro-massage 174
Step Three for Chiropractors and Bodyworkers 177

CHAPTER 14 – STEP FOUR – SYMPTOMATIC AND TAKE-HOME TREATMENTS 179
The Priorities of Treatment and Techniques 181
Home Treatments 185

SECTION IV - MERIDIAN DIAGNOSTICS

INTRODUCTION 191

CHAPTER 15 – ALARM POINT KINESIOLOGY DIAGNOSIS 195
O Ring Kinesiology Instructions 196
Arm Raise Kinesiology 199
Alarm Point Kinesiology 199

CHAPTER 16 – ELECTRONIC MERIDIAN TESTING 205
Introduction 205
Is Electronic Meridian Testing For Real? 206
Ryodoraku 208
Electroacupuncture According to Voll (EAV) 208
Distal Meridian Point Balancing 209
Quadrant Measurement and Balancing 210
Choice of EMT Test Points 211
Electronic Meridian Testing Instructions 213
Instructions for performing BFD test 214
Interpreting Electronic Meridian Testing Patterns 215
Common EMT Patterns 219
More EMT patterns from Nakatani 220

CHAPTER 17- POLAR MERIDIAN PAIRS AND GASTROCNEMIUS DIAGNOSIS 223
  Introduction 223
  Micro-systems and the Gastrocnemius 224
  Palpation Points Location and Method 225
  Treatment points 226

SECTION V. TREATMENT FORMULARIES

TREATMENT FORMULARY SECTION I – BY BODY AREA 229
  Head Region 232
  Neck Region 236
  Shoulder Region 240
  Elbow 246
  Forearms, Wrist and Hands 248
  Abdominal Region 250
  Low Back Region 252
  Hips and Knee 256
  Legs, Ankles and Feet 258

TREATMENT FORMULARY SECTION II – OTHER SPECIFIC CONDITIONS 263
  Acne 264
  Allergies 266
  Arthritis 266
  Asthma 268
  Addiction Release 268
  Acceleration of Wound Healing 270
  Bell's Palsy 272
  Brachial Neuralgia, "Pinched Nerve Syndrome" 272
  Back/Vertebral Disk Injuries 272
  Cancer Pain 274
  Chronic Pain and Depression 276
  Edema 277
  Eye Diseases 278
  Fibromyalgia/Chronic Fatigue Syndrome 280
  Lymph Drainage 282
  Peripheral Neuropathy, Nerve Regeneration 282
  Reflex Sympathetic Dystrophy 284
  Restless Leg Syndrome 284
  Scar and Adhesions Treatments 285
  Shingles or Other Rib Pain 286
  Stroke, Paralysis and Major Head Injury 286
  Tendinitis 288
  Thoracic Outlet Syndrome 288
  Whiplash 288

TREATMENT FORMULARY SECTION III – EAV TREATMENT PROTOCOLS .... 290 - 305

BIBLIOGRAPHY
RESOURCES
INDEX
INTAKE FORM

Acknowledgements

Microcurrent electro-acupuncture, as presented in this book, is a system of patient evaluation and treatment that includes many diverse principles and techniques. My best contribution here is not to "invent" something new, but rather to clearly and practically integrate many valuable aspects of theory and practice. I express my appreciation and thanks here to all the dedicated researchers, practitioners and supporters whose contributions were vital in making this book possible. Thanks to:

Charles McWilliams, my first teacher of electromedicine, who taught me the importance of non-needle electronic acupuncture, introduced me to the work of Reinhold Voll, and showed me how to impact groups of practitioners. Thanks also for his permission to reproduce some of his EAV point diagrams.

My acupuncture teachers who generously shared their knowledge and experience- Steve Miller, James Pinkman, Bill Berlin, Mark Seem, Steven Birch, Kiko Matsumoto, Stuart Watts and others.

Richard Tan, from whom I have learned a lot, and who gave me permission to include some of his distal acu-point suggestions in my writing.

Richard Niemtzow, editor of journal <u>Medical Acupuncture</u>, for his permission to re-use material from my article <u>Electrophysiology and the Acupuncture Systems</u> which appeared in the Volume 13, Number One edition of the journal in 2001, in Chapter Two of this book.

Thomas Wing, Daniel Kirsch and other pioneers whose work helped establish the art of microcurrent therapy in the United States

Nguyen Van Nghi, who mentored me in the ways of French energetic acupuncture.

Yoshio Manaka, whose dedicated practice and research was a major inspiration to the creation of this book.

Reinhold Voll, one of the most innovative practitioners of the 20th century, whose awesome contributions have not yet been fully acknowledged.

Margaret McReynolds, who shared her front-line treatments of many challenging neuropathic pain conditions with me.

John Stebbins, a fellow adventurer on the microcurrent highway, for his contribution about sports medicine and trigger points.

Devra West and Kathleen Loek, brilliant lights upon my path, for their spiritual support and teachings about the Universal Laws of Energy.

Collette Taaffe, Shasta Richards and others who gave permission for their pictures to be used in this book's illustrations.

Jack Crompton for a great cover art design.

The engineers at Datran and KWM Electronics, for hanging in there with me through the challenging birthing of my Acutron devices.

Christina, Christine, Kathy, Marlene, Teri and Ahmad, the team that has at different times in recent years supported me with their positive energy and hard work, without which I never would have had the time to write this book.

Alejandro Katz and Richard Niemtzow, advanced acupuncturists I have had the pleasure to teach with, for sharing their valuable experiences that have influenced some of the treatment protocols in this book. Appreciation also to Herman Vega and Susan Mitchell, for offering their clinical wisdom at some of my seminars.

William and Wilkins, publisher, for their permission to reproduce some trigger point diagrams from their publication <u>Travel and Williams Trigger Point Flip Charts</u>.

My sister, Laura Davis, for her example as a successful writer in inspiring me to go for it myself. My parents Abe and Temme, for always encouraging my explorations of life and truth without dogma.

Maharaji, who more than anyone else taught me the meaning of Within.

And greatest acknowledgment to the Great Universal Spirit, known by so many names, for being my foundation and giving me life breath, loving inspiration and empowerment to be a teacher, enjoy my life and fulfill my potential.

Disclaimer

Please read carefully before using the information contained in this book
The information contained in this book is intended to provide valuable techniques, treatment plans, acupuncture point formulas and electro-therapeutic parameters for educational purposes. It is made available with the understanding that the author and publisher are not engaged in rendering medical, health, psychological, or any other kind of personal professional services in this book. The information should not be considered complete and does not cover all diseases, ailments, physical conditions or their treatment. It should not be used in place of a call or visit to a medical, health or other competent professional, who should be consulted before adopting any of the suggestions in this book or drawing inferences from it.

It is the sole responsibility of the reader of this book to individually evaluate and diagnose each patient or client, and to determine suitable, safe and effective treatment. It is also the responsibility of the reader to know his or her limitations, and to refer patients with potentially dangerous medical conditions to a suitable physician for diagnosis and/or treatment of any underlying disease processes prior to performing the electro-therapeutic techniques detailed in this book.

Darren Starwynn and all concerned with the publishing of this book specifically disclaim all responsibility for any liability, loss or risk, personal or otherwise, which is incurred as a consequence, directly or indirectly, of the use and application of any of the material in this book or any associated seminars, websites, verbal discussions or other forms of communication.

Contraindications

Electro-therapeutic devices are regulated by the United States Food and Drug Administration in the United States. All manufacturers of such devices are required by the FDA to publish the following contraindications concerning the use of electro-therapeutic devices. These contraindications are based on use of milli-amperage devices such as TENS units. *In the case of microcurrent electro-therapies, which utilize much lower treatment current intensities, all of the following contraindications may not be fully relevent.* Yet it remains the sole responsibility of the practitioner to make the determination of applicability of any treatment for any individual patient. The term "TENS" is used in the following to indicate any electro-therapeutic pain management device.

- The safety of TENS devices for use during pregnancy or delivery has not been established.
- TENS is not effective for pain stemming from the central nervous system. (This includes headache)
- TENS devices have no curative power.
- TENS is a symptomatic treatment that suppresses the sensation of pain that would otherwise serve as a protective mechanism.

- Keep out of reach of children.
- Electronic monitoring equipment (such as ECG monitors and ECG alarms) may not operate properly when TENS stimulation in use.
- Possibility of adverse reactions such as skin burns or irritation in subjects with sensitive skin, especially in long term application.
- Effectiveness is dependant on patient selection.
- Electrical current greater than a charge per pulse of 20 µC (microculombs) must not flow through the thorax because it may cause cardiac arrhythmia!
- TENS devices should be used only under the continued supervision of a physician.

FDA CONTRAINDICATIONS FOR USE:

- Any electrode placement that applies current to the carotid sinus on the neck.
- Any use of TENS on patients with demand-type cardiac pacemakers.
- Any electrode placement that causes current to flow through head.
- The use of TENS whenever pain syndromes are undiagnosed, until etiology is established.
- Use on broken or ulcerated skin.

ADDITIONAL CAUTIONS FROM THE AUTHOR:

Do not place any electrical stimulation on the head or neck of persons with epilepsy or other convulsive disorders, as it may trigger a seizure. It is vital to screen for these conditions in your initial intake process.

Do not apply extended electrical stimulation through pad electrodes over cancerous tumors, or in those with metastatic cancer conditions. Until research reveals more about this, the effects of electrical stimulation on cancer is unpredictable, and may cause the tumor to grow. Brief microcurrent probe treatment of applicable local and distal acu-points to treat pain in cancer patients is unlikely to have this risk, and can be quite beneficial.

Do not use milliamperage currents, or local stimulation of painful zones with microcurrents, as primary treatment for highly sensitive and delicate patients. Even with the use of gentle microcurrent this may aggravate their pain. It is better to use a whole-body treatment strategy as taught in this book for best results with such patients.

Pregnant women often require pain relief, and microcurrent electro-acupuncture can be very helpful. It is again the sole responsibility of the practitioner to decide when it is safe to treat. Some guidelines:

A. The risk of a treatment- caused miscarriage is much higher during the first trimester of pregnancy.

B. The risk of a treatment-caused miscarriage is much higher in women with "unstable blood" who are prone to miscarriage.

C. It is best to avoid stimulation of the so-called "forbidden points" of pregnancy with needles or electrical stimulation. A partial list of such points: Sp 6, UB 67, abdomen-zigong and other abdominal acu-points, and strong stimulation of St 36, LI 4, Ling Ku or GB 21.

D. It is safer to use a distal point strategy for pregnant women, utilizing gentle technique and stimulation.

Foreward I

By Jan Allen, L.Ac., Dipl. Ac.

I first met Dr. Darren Starwynn several years ago at a training seminar he was conducting in Hawaii on "Microcurrent Electroacupuncture". As a student of Traditional Oriental Medicine (TCM), I had a broad educational background in the physical sciences, Western and Oriental medical theory, acupuncture, herbal medicine and much more. However, I had almost no exposure, either in my training or private practice, to the field of electromedicine and I was completely unfamiliar with microcurrent technology. What Dr. Starwynn shared at the seminar and the experiences that followed changed my view of the importance of electromedicine in the art and science of healing. Today, microcurrent electroacupuncture is an indispensable tool and a cornerstone of my acupuncture practice.

At the Lani'aina Wellness Center for Energetic and Herbal Medicine, I use the Acutron Mentor -- a highly advanced microcurrent device developed by Dr. Starwynn, as an integral part of nearly every diagnostic and therapeutic protocol. Many of my patients seek treatment for acute and chronic pain, so I began using microcurrent as an adjunct to acupuncture for individuals experiencing all types of painful conditions, including joint pain, headache, backache, TMJ, traumatic injury and peripheral neuropathy. The results were so profound and dramatic that I soon began using microcurrent as a stand-alone modality, and in conjunction with acupuncture, in the treatment of internal disease and mental-emotional conditions ranging from sinusitis to cancer pain to anxiety and depression with similar beneficial outcomes. Virtually every acupuncture patient can benefit from the safe, painless, effective and rapid treatment possible with microcurrent electroacupuncture. I also routinely use electronic meridian testing (EMT) as a key element in differential diagnostic methods to evaluate the condition of the body's Qi energy. Observation of electrical response at specific acupoints on the body, such as the Source, Alarm and Associated points, is also a rapid and effective way to evaluate the condition of internal organs.

Today, microcurrent technology plays a crucial role in all aspects of my practice, including diagnosis, treatment and evaluation. In the future, as practitioners of traditional and complementary medicine awaken to the tremendous healing potential of electromedicine, microcurrent electroacupuncture will become an indispensable adjunct to their healing practices. Microcurrent electroacupuncture is a valuable modality for anyone dedicated to helping others heal -- chiropractors, physical therapists, bodyworkers, energy workers, allopathic physicians, and acupuncturists.

In this comphrensive and enlightening book, Dr. Starwynn has compiled information from leaders in the fields of Oriental Medicine, electromedicine and science, such as Manaka, Voll, Nakatani and others. He has shared with us, in an understandable and useful way, a synthesis of his many years of research in electromedicine, combined with his extensive personal experiences in using this technology, to help his patients to regain balance and to heal. Whether helping to relieve pain, treating internal disease, assisting a patient in harmonizing and balancing emotions, or enhancing a woman's appearance through facial rejuvenation, microcurrent therapy is a painless way of re-balancing the flow of vital life energy to the body and mind.

Thank you, Dr. Starwynn.

Jan Kaleinani Allen, M.S., L.Ac., Dipl. Ac. (NCCAOM)
Founder, Lani'aina Wellness Center for Energetic and Herbal Medicine
Redondo Beach, California

Forward II

by John Stebbins, O.M.D..

Electroacupuncture has gone through quite a transformation over the last few decades.

Electricity has been applied to acupuncture points in some way, shape, or form, since the 1860s. Starting with crude applications involving leyden jars, techniques have evolved into sophisticated computerized equipment which no longer even requires acupuncture needling.

As an intern in Chinese medicine school I remember often connecting the acupuncture needles to an electrical stimulator. We would turn the stimulation up until the patient said it was strong and 'that was that'. We were operating under the assumption that the electrical stimulation would enhance the treatment, yet no further information was provided. My western medical background provoked me to ask "What is it that we are actually doing through the electrical stimulation?" There was no information readily available at that time, so I began my own odyssey to find out how electricity actually assisted acupuncture. Several years later I attended a seminar in California on 'Electrical Acupuncture'. I was the only acupuncturist present among a group of chiropractors, dentists, and podiatrists. At this time I was introduced to the concept of using microcurrents to stimulate acupuncture points *without needles*. Skeptical at first, I listened to different practitioners touting the benefits of this 'new' therapy. I purchased a simple microcurrent device, modified my own connectors for acupuncture needles, and have used microcurrent electro-therapy ever since. There are many therapies and techniques we learn about in school and in seminars. Some we find useful, while others we reject. If I were limited to only one or two therapies to use in conjunction with acupuncture, microcurrents would most definitely be included.

I have used microcurrent-assisted acupuncture extensively in the treatment of musculo-skeletal conditions, particularly in the area of sports medicine. I use microcurrent probe treatments for effective release of painful myofascial trigger points and local-distal acupuncture point combinations. I have also well utilized interferential pad treatments with simultaneous exercise as a mainstay for accelerating rehabilitation of injured players. These methods, and much more, are clearly taught in this book. It is clear that this approach is getting injured athletes and workers back to their vocations considerably faster than would be possible with conventional rehab methods.

One of the main lessons regarding the body and electricity is that 'less is often more'. We really can't force the body to heal itself. While strong therapies are sometimes necessary, 'soft' therapies (i.e. Japanese needling techniques, microcurrent electrical stimulation, homeopathy, qi gong) can actually enhance healing while minimizing injury to the body. The cornerstone of life has been shown to be based upon the underlying forces of subtle electricity and magnetism. We already use this information diagnostically in EEGs, EKGs, and MRIs. Now, medical therapies are growing in their use and understanding of subtle electromagnetism.

In 1993, I was speaking about microcurrents at a seminar in New Mexico. Darren Starwynn was also speaking on the subject. Since then we have shared a kindred spirit through our mutual pursuit of microcurrent therapy and Oriental medicine. Darren has taken his interest a step further by designing and developing the Acutron Multiwave, and subsequently the Acutron Mentor microcurrent devices. Of all the machines I have investigated, this has been my favorite. Most teachers of electro-therapies do not have a background in traditional Chinese medicine. But the two complement each other very well. Darren has impressed me with his expertise and his ability to teach electronics as well as Oriental medicine in a clear and concise way. His love and respect for the subject matter are apparent. Additionally, Darren has a strong spiritual emphasis upon his approach to medicine, which is refreshing and all too often lacking.

Most practitioners have an inadequate understanding of how electrical stimulation can enhance their treatments. It is no longer acceptable to simply hook-up acupuncture needles, or place pads on the patient and turn on some machine. We need to be much more cognizant of what we're actually doing. This is where Darren's book can be invaluable. It is the first publication to adequately cover the theoretical and clinical application of microcurrents. So, read on. You will not be disappointed.

John Stebbins, OMD
Co-Founder – National Sports Acupuncture Association
Instructor – Colorado School of Traditional Chinese Medicine

Preface

By Darren Starwynn, O.M.D.

This book fills the need for a clear, practical text about microcurrent electro-acupuncture. I have been teaching seminars about this subject for well over a decade. After hearing students repeatedly ask me where they can get a good book about electro-acupuncture, and having to keep telling them that it doesn't exist, it dawned on me in 1999 that I would have to write one myself. Since then I have devoted a considerable amount of time and research toward the creation of this book. It is intended to offer health care professionals a thorough grounding in the principles, techniques and specifics of using low-level electrical currents for the evaluation and treatment of the human energy systems, with a focus on pain management and rehabilitation. I have drawn on my extensive teaching experience to organize and write the book in the manner I have found it easiest for students to understand and practically apply. It is structured in two ways- as a book that can be read all the way through as well as a reference manual. It offers an extensive Table of Contents and Index to make it easy to quickly find the information you need.

I believe this book will help you make sense of the often confusing and incomplete information that most of us have had to contend with around the subject of electrical stimulation and electro-acupuncture. The book can also be of interest to lay people who want to understand the emerging field of electrical energy medicine.

As a clinical practitioner for close to 20 years, and teacher of this subject and designer of microcurrent devices over the last 14 years, I have personally communicated with many hundreds of pain management professionals, including medical doctors, osteopaths, chiropractors, physical therapists, acupuncturists, nurses, massage therapists, veterinarians, podiatrists, dentists, and more. During my years of teaching, researching and communicating, I have discovered much of what really works and what does not. I have also evolved a highly effective teaching method for empowering professionals to understand the principles of electro-therapeutic pain management and start getting impressive results quickly. This book contains the refined fruits of this experience.

Most of the literature previously available on the subject of electro-acupuncture and microcurrent therapies was provided by manufacturers of electro-therapy devices, and has generally been very limited and incomplete. While some useful manuals and articles have been written about this subject, few deal with much more than symptomatic techniques of application with little or no explanation of the underlying energetic principles. In the opinion of the author, a few pages of guiding principles are worth far more than hundreds of pages of "cookbook" application techniques. There is an old saying that goes like this- give a man a meal and he will be fed for a day and hungry tomorrow. Teach him how to grow his own food, and he will be fed for the rest of his life. In the spirit of this saying, it is similarly true that a basic understanding of the electrical nature of the human body, and how to work in harmony with it, will go far in a clinical practice.

Section One of this book gives an overview of electrical energy medicine and explains the vital energetic principles that must be understood and applied for clinical success. Section Two details a wide range of treatment techniques, using probe and pad electrode interfaces. Each technique has significant value, and familiarity with all of them gives you a "tool belt" from which you can draw precisely what is needed in each patient encounter. Section Three is about the Four-Step Protocol. This is a most effective and elegant clinical approach to pain management and treatment of internal conditions. It is a structure within which a treatment plan can be erected that embraces treatment of the causative factor (Root), overall energetic balancing, direct myofascial adjustment of the physical body, and symptomatic relief. The Four-Step method was originated by Yoshio Manaka of Japan, whose distinguished career as a practitioner and researcher in the acupuncture field is unsurpassed. I have adapted his method for use with microcurrent electro-acupuncture and other modern clinical tools.

Section Four of this book is about diagnosis, and covers three valuable methods that are not commonly taught – Alarm Point Kinesiology, Electronic Meridian Testing (EMT) and Gastrocnemius testing.

When the writing of all these sections of the book was finished in the summer of 2001, I realized that, as complete as it already was, readers would also want more protocols and techniques for specific medical conditions. I then added the three-part Treatment Formulary that you will find at the end of the book.

Those of us choosing a career in the energy-based healing arts usually do so, at least in part, due to an inner calling to serve others in a fundamental and more Root level than is offered in traditional medicine. I believe that the practice of skilled and effective energy medicine is a major growth industry, and that demand for this service will increase over the coming years. It is my hope that this text will help empower you to expand your clinical skills and energetic sphere of influence, for the benefit of yourself and those you serve.

A Note About Microcurrent Devices

Most of the treatment methods taught in this book require the use of a clinical microcurrent stimulator. There are several companies that manufacture or distribute such devices, which are available in a wide range of designs, pricing and quality. I have not included a comparison of devices in this book, but rather have given generic instructions and device settings that can be applied to most quality clinical microcurrent stimulators.

I am an inventor and device designer, and have created the Acutron Mentor electromedical device, which is highly versatile and includes extensive microcurrent capabilities. It offers pre-set treatment protocols to speed set-up. Because I am aware that large numbers of practitioners and students that use this device will be reading this book, I have included frequent references to help guide them in selection of Acutron Mentor treatment pre-sets for the techniques and conditions described. The information taught herein is by no means limited to this device, however.

While even small, inexpensive microcurrent devices can be used to perform many of the techniques taught in this book, a unit with the following features is required to fully utilize this information and obtain maximum results:

Microcurrent outputs with adjustable intensity

Dual probe electrodes with treatment activation trigger switch

Pad electrodes, preferably with interferential capabilities

Switchable polarity: positive, negative and biphasic (this is a vitally important feature that several microcurrent devices on the market lack)

Adjustable frequency

Conductivity meter display with numerical scale from 0 – 100 for skin resistance testing (galvanic skin resistance, or GSR)

Timer relay system

Milliamp and microamp capabilities (not required for microcurrent protocols, but very useful for pain clinic and rehabilitation work)

Section I

ELECTROMEDICAL PRINCIPLES

Chapter 1
INTRODUCTION

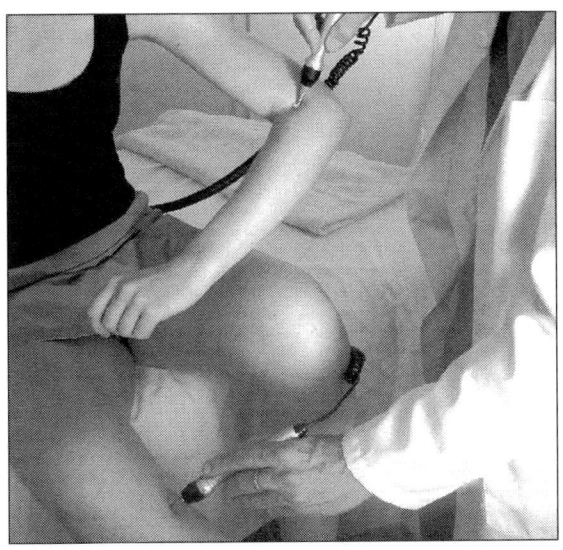

This book is about the electrical nature of acupuncture and the electrical nature of life itself. It is a practical guide and reference text containing many valuable evaluation and treatment methods for bio-electric[1] therapy and healing, and the principles and theory underlying these treatments. This subject is vital, enormous, and closer to home than most of us realize. The relationship between the human body and electrical energy is so intertwined that all life processes, and virtually all health care interventions, deal with this relationship in some way. In health care, this relationship runs the gamut from acupuncture needling, osseous manipulation, bodywork and physical therapies to even herb and drug treatments and psychological counseling. All of these interventions "work" because, on some level, because they induce adjustments in the bio-electric field and flows of the body.

The rapidly growing field of *energy medicine* encompasses many disciplines whose common thread is the recognition that all disturbances in the physical body and emotions are directly linked to imbalances of vital energy in the organism. *Electro-medicine*, an aspect of energy medicine, deals specifically with the utilization of electro-magnetic energies for diagnosis and healing. There are established treatments or promising research in the use of electro-medicine for chronic pain, cancer, AIDS and other viral infections, parasite overgrowth, eye diseases, addiction, stress management and much more.

Electro-acupuncture is an aspect of electro-medicine that deals with the applications of electrical energy in diagnosing and treating the acupuncture meridian system. *Microcurrent electro-acupuncture*, which in my opinion is the most powerful and effective electro-therapeutic treatment, uses gentle, often sub-sensational electrical currents applied through acupuncture points. The primary focus of this book is the use of microcurrent electro-acupuncture for pain management and rehabilitation.

Microcurrents are gentle electrical currents delivered in the millionths of amps range. Microcurrents are more harmonious with the body's innate bioelectric activity than the high-intensity milliamp currents used in traditional electro-acupuncture and electro-therapy.

---

[1] The electrical nature of life processes

While our modern culture often propagates the view that "more and bigger is better", in the field of energy medicine the reverse is usually true: "less is more." The remarkable effectiveness of this system is based on four far-reaching universal laws- the Laws of Resonance, Polarity, Economy and Biasology. These are explained in Chapter 2. The result is a holistic[2] intervention that can be far more effective than traditional electro-acupuncture for long-term pain relief and support of homeostasis[3].

Traditional allopathic medicine has largely dealt with the relationships between function, structure and biochemistry. This has led to a reliance on drug and surgical interventions for pain and disease. Yet, an overwhelming amount of recent research confirming the effects of electrical characteristics of life processes has shown us that function, structure and biochemistry are all intimately linked with electro-magnetic fields. As stated in the excellent book Vibrational Medicine[4], this would yield the equation:

$$\text{STRUCTURE} \leftrightarrow \text{FUNCTION} \leftrightarrow \text{BIOCHEMISTRY} \leftrightarrow \text{ELECTRO-MAGNETIC ENERGY FIELDS}$$

In the forward to Vibrational Medicine, Dr. Tilley goes on say this equation should be extended to interplay with subtle etheric[5] energy fields.

On the spectrum of healing methods, microcurrent electro-acupuncture falls about midway between the biochemical and structural interventions of Western medicine and subtle etheric energy healing methods such as laying-on-of-hands and homeopathy. Therefore, it is an excellent and appropriate discipline for bridging between these paradigms.

Conventional Electro-therapy

Electro-therapy is a broad field that includes the application of many types of electrical devices to the body. Traditionally, this has been for relieving pain, muscle tension, edema, and other symptoms. Electro-therapy has been utilized since ancient times, and its modern acceptance started in earnest with the development of Transcutaneous Electric Nerve Stimulator (TENS) units in the 1960's. Electro-therapeutic devices in common use today include TENS units, electric muscle stimulators, interferential units, high volt pulsed galvanic, iontophoresis, microcurrent stimulators and others.

Few professionals with experience in traditional electro-therapy are highly excited about it, however. The clinical results derived from these practices have been quite inconsistent and often disappointing. Yet, those who have applied the principles and practices of microcurrent electro-acupuncture have reported many significant, impressive results with a high percentage of effectiveness. In addition, they have long lists of excited patients eager to tell their friends and family about their results. What is the difference?

Most of the theory and practice of electro-therapy taught in health care schools is based on information provided by manufacturers, which is woefully inadequate in addressing the laws and vital principles of energy medicine that lead to clinical success. In my seminars, I refer to most of what is being currently taught as "stone-age electro-therapy" (with no insult intended to our pre-civilized ancestors!) because it often runs counter to actual principles required to evoke a positive clinical response. For example, in treatment of lateral epicondylitis, or "tennis elbow", most electro-therapy manuals advocate an application of sandwiching the elbow

---

[2] A system dealing with the whole rather than focusing on the parts
[3] A relative balance of physiological functions that promotes good health
[4] Richard Gerber, M.D., Vibrational Medicine, Bear and Company, 1988
[5] Many volumes have already been written about subtle energy healing methods, and some references are in the bibliography.

between two or four electrode pads, usually using high-intensity milliamp currents. Rarely have I or the professionals with whom I have communicated found this method to give very good results. Either it is totally ineffective, provides only short-lived relief, or the patient may even feel worse after the therapy. Yet, when using polarized microcurrent probe electrodes, with the positively charged probe on the painful elbow, and the negatively charged electrode on a corresponding acu-point on the opposite knee[6], we have frequently seen complete relief of pain. It is common for these results to last for a long time, sometimes after a single treatment. Choosing the proper polarity and effective points involves simple, clear principles that can be easily learned.

> **A WORD ABOUT CONVENTIONAL ELECTRO-ACUPUNCTURE**
>
> The term "electro-acupuncture" is commonly used to describe the technique of attaching a high–intensity milliamp stimulator directly to acupuncture needles via alligator clips to produce analgesia for surgery or acute pain conditions. This can be quite effective in creating a nerve block for temporary pain control or surgical anesthesia; however, it is an invasive procedure using currents that are far in excess of what is required to support circulation and balance of the acupuncture meridian system. This technique also has potential negative side effects, such as burning of the tissues, broken needles, toxic metal deposits through electrolysis and profound dispersion of Qi.[7]

The Electrical Nature of Life

<u>The Body Electric</u>[8], the title of the landmark book by Robert Becker, M.D., is quite insightful. Indeed, all of our life functions are directly or indirectly associated with electrical activity. It is important to examine the root of why electrical energy is so intimately tied to the human body. This goes back to Albert Einstein's famous equation $E=mc^2$. This equation states that all matter is equivalent to energy, at a much slower rate of vibration. In essence, our physical bodies, and all matter, are made of frozen light. Just before his death, Einstein, considered one of the most brilliant scientists of our time, stated his recognition of the mysterious Spirit essence that motivates the entire Universe. His view is well summed up by Richard Gerber, M.D.:

> "The spiritual dimension is the energetic basis of all life, because it is the energy of spirit which animates the physical framework. *The unseen connection between the physical body and the subtle forces of spirit holds the key to understanding the inner relationship between matter and energy.* When scientists begin to comprehend the true relationship between matter and energy, they will come closer to understanding the relationship between humanity and God.... The evolving field of science which will bring humankind to this new level of understanding is vibrational medicine."[9]

---

[6] Or other local/distal placements are described in this book
[7] The energetic substance that is a basis for all life and the manifested and unmanifested Universe
[8] Robert Becker and Gary Selden, <u>The Body Electric</u>, Quill/Morrow, 1985
[9] <u>Vibrational Medicine</u>, Ch 1

Any agent can only affect our bodies is if there is a receptor site, or vibrational resonance, for it. This holds true for a pharmaceutical drug, a hormone, a nutrient, acupuncture stimulation, an electrical current, or even a kiss! A substance for which there is no receptor site or resonance is considered inert. Electricity, or any other manifestation of energy, can only affect the body because it is already "wired" for it. Have you ever thought about all the ways our bodies are electrical organisms? Here are some of them:

- *Heartbeat* - The steady beat of our hearts, which sustains our life and powers the entire circulatory system, is regulated by an electrical pacemaker nerve bundle. This pacemaker functions largely independently from the brain. When this internal pacemaker fails, doctors can now replace it with an artificial one.

- *Nervous system* - The action potentials that drive all sensing and motor actions are electrical events which consist of rapid polarization and depolarization of nerve cells to propagate a signal in a given direction.

- *Brain, consciousness* - Although scientists don't understand exactly how electricity interacts with consciousness, measuring electrical brain waves is the primary diagnostic tool for the brain. Devices for this practice are called electroencephalograms (EEG). Epilepsy, a disease characterized by attacks of bodily shaking and convulsions, is associated with bursts of excess electrical activity in the brain.[10] Microcurrent stimulation applied to the brain has shown some promise in preventing epileptic seizures.[11]

- *Wound healing* - Healing is an electrical activity. The mitochondria, the powerhouses of the cell, store electrically charged particles of ATP (adenosine triphosphate). ATP acts as the energy currency of the cell, and is necessary for healing, growth and regular cellular functions. It has also been determined that charged calcium ions must migrate into the cells through active transport via electrically sensitive ion channels in order to facilitate the healing process. Dr. Robert Becker used sensitive instruments to measure the electrical potentials around wounds and showed that electrical polarity shifts can be measured during periods of intense regeneration in the healing process.[12] There has been research with so called Qigong[13] masters in China to scientifically measure the electrical discharge from their hands while doing healing work. A highly trained Qigong master can create effects of tissue healing and anesthesia in patients just by directing energy from their hands. Studies have shown that the energy emanations from their hands are much different from non-trained individuals.

- *Muscular movement* - For any action or movement of the body to take place, muscle cells must be electrically stimulated by the nervous system to initiate patterns of contractions. Diseases affecting the muscles such as polio, myasthenia gravis and hemiplegia are associated with reduced or blocked electrical energy in the affected areas.

- *Fascia* - Fascia are the thin, elastic sheaths of connective tissue that wraps around muscles, bone, organs and other tissues of the body. Because fascia is so abundant, it produces a continuous network that interconnects all parts of the body. Pain and injuries that involve muscles and connective tissues are classified as myofascial.[14] Fascia, like

---

[10] For this reason it is contraindicated to apply any electrical stimulation to the head and neck of an epileptic. Make sure a question about epilepsy is on your patient intake form.
[11] Comparative Effects of MicrocurrentStimulation on EEG Spectrum and Correlation Data by M. Heffernan, *Integrative Physiological and Behavioral Science*, July-Sept. 1996
[12] *Ibid.*, Ref 8
[13] Ancient Chinese art of Qi cultivation in the human body
[14] Pertaining to the muscles and fascia of the body

bone, possesses piezoelectric properties. Piezoelectric tissues or objects are those that release an electrical charge when mechanically stretched or deformed. Therefore, all movements of the body cause our fascia to stretch and continually release subtle electrical charges. It is the view of some Japanese acupuncture researchers that the acupuncture meridian system actually exists in the fascial network of the body.[15] Most effective approaches to pain management and rehabilitation include some method to release myofascial constrictions and imbalances.

- *Bone* - Bone is a tissue with piezoelectric properties. The stresses on bone caused by gravity and movement cause it to release subtle electric charges that support fracture healing and ongoing migration of calcium into the bone matrix. Loss of bone calcium through osteoporosis was a great concern for astronauts traveling through space where there is no gravity. I believe osteoporosis is more common in people with more sedentary lifestyles. In The Body Electric, Dr. Becker goes further to explain the entire electrically orchestrated process of de-differentiation and reconstitution of bone cells that underlies fracture healing.[16]

- *Glandular system* - Our endocrine glands are vital links in the regulation of our electrical and subtle energy systems. For example, the pituitary hormone prolactin, which stimulates milk production in nursing mothers, also seems to make cells more electrically sensitive as part of the process of healing and regeneration.[17] Acupuncture stimulation of the Extraordinary Meridian system[18] can also have direct healing and regulatory effects on the endocrine glands. Many systems of Yoga and Qigong as part of the process of spiritual growth act to energize and activate the electrical charge of these glands.

Electromagnetic Pollution

Of course, anything with such profound power to support and heal has the potential to harm. Certain currents and frequencies of electricity are supportive of the health of the human body, while other frequencies can provoke stress reactions leading to fatigue, mental illness, immune system weakening, cancer and other diseases. Becker's books The Body Electric and Cross Currents offer excellent explanations and a thorough listing of research studies concerning these effects. Electromagnetic pollution is produced by power lines, handheld appliances such as hair dryers and cellular phones, computers, microwave transmissions for communication purposes, televisions and so much more.

---

[15] Matsumoto and Birch, Hara Diagnosis, Reflections of the Sea, Paradigm Publications, Ch. 7 and 8
[16] The Body Electric, Ch 6
[17] The Body Electric, p. 183
[18] Deep energetic functions that distribute Source Kidney Qi and regulate the principal meridians

> **HIGHER FREQUENCIES AND ELECTROMAGNETIC POLLUTION**
>
> One fascinating fact is that the very low frequency range of 0 – 35 Hz is more or less supportive of the health of the human body, while frequencies above 100 Hz are only harmful when we are exposed to them intensely and for long periods of time. This is probably because life developed amid the electromagnetic field of the Earth, which geophysicists have measured at about 7 – 10 Hz. It is the midrange of 35 – 100 Hz that appear to be the most harmful, with the most severe immunological damage and stress induction. Is it a coincidence that all of our household and industrial electrical power is supplied at 60 Hz, probably one of the most harmful frequencies for our health?[19]

Medicine of the Future

Those of us who have watched "Star Trek" and "Star Wars" have seen the use of energy-based healing devices that diagnose and heal serious wounds and diseases quickly and powerfully. The technology for these inventions is not so fanciful, however. Many energy medicine devices in use are not so different from those used in "Star Trek." There is an electrical basis for most, if not all, injuries and disease, and healing is an electrically orchestrated event. Much of the essence of healing is to introduce or induce an energy vibration to the body that supports its normal functioning, or in effect cancels out negative pain and disease vibrations.

Therefore, there are two vital elements to advanced energy healing. The first is to scan or measure the energy fields of the affected area to determine its vibratory rate. The second is to introduce a resonant vibration to neutralize or harmonize the negative energy and bring about homeostasis. Several notable healing systems have already been developed based on these principles.

One of the oldest in modern times is homeopathy developed by Samuel Hahnemann in the 1700's. In this healing art, remedies made of herbs, animals, minerals and medicines are potentized to vibratory rates that match disease conditions, and are given to the patient. Using the homeopathic Materia Medica, Homeopathic doctors select the correct vibratory substance through a lengthy process of interviewing the patient to determine which "remedy picture" that matches the patient's signs and symptoms. If the remedy is well selected (that is, its vibratory rate resonates favorably with the problem condition), then a cure is effected.

Another fascinating system was that developed by Royal Rife, an American scientist who worked with resonance-based energy medicine in California in the early part of the 20th century. Rife discovered that specific radio frequencies resonated with pathogenic bacteria, viruses and cancer cells in the body to destroy them without harming the healthy surrounding tissues. He developed charts of resonant frequencies, each of which destroys a specific pathogen. Rife developed a very powerful microscope to view the pathogens and confirm at which frequency they were destroyed. This aspect of the Law of Resonance is the same as that which allows an opera singer with a powerful voice to shatter a wine glass. Rife's work inspired a great deal of interest among the California medical community in the 1930's until it was suppressed and much of it discredited by the medical associations. We can imagine

---

[19] The Body Electric, p. 292

without too much difficulty why this happened. Both homeopathy and Rife frequency generation are practiced today with growing interest, although with some legal obstacles.

Modern electronics now offers more accurate methods of detecting and generating resonant frequencies for healing purposes. In the 1960's, Dr. Reinhold Voll of Germany and his research associates developed an electronic method of measuring and treating the acupuncture meridian system with microcurrents. A parallel development occurred in Japan in the 1950's with the development by Dr. Yosio Nakatani of the Ryodoraku system. Both systems use a tiny test current through an ohmmeter to measure the electrical resistance of specific acu-points that reflect the condition of an entire meridian. Once these meridian imbalances are determined and graphed, an energetic diagnosis can be made. The pattern of imbalance can be corrected with either electrical stimulation of acupuncture points to tonify or sedate the affected meridians, or with potentized homeopathic remedies.

More recent innovations include devices such as the Mora, Bicom and others that claim to take negative vibrations out of the body, balance and correct them without any diagnosis required by the practitioner, and send them back into the body.

It is clear that the medicine of the future will move more toward such energy medicine devices as well as powerful mental, emotional and spiritual healing and clearing methods, and become less dependant on surgical and drug interventions. I envision a time not far off when each home will be equipped with a console that scans the energy systems of family members and corrects imbalances automatically. This could be a great addition to the morning cup of coffee! It is staggering to think how many diseases this procedure would prevent. The combination of these devices with changes in attitude toward greater individual empowerment and self-responsibility for health and dis-ease will bring about much more of a revolution in health.

Chapter 2

ELECTRO-PHYSIOLOGY AND THE ACUPUNCTURE SYSTEMS

Introduction

During the long history of Traditional Chinese Medicine (TCM) the results of needling acu-points has been described in both clinical and theoretical ways. The concepts of Qi, Blood, meridians and acu-points are critical to the understanding and application of TCM. Since its introduction into Western culture, there have been many experiments and writings to attempt to explain these concepts in Western scientific terms. Many early explanations were shallow and simplistic. For example, two explanations are that acupuncture is only placebo treatment and acupuncture is a primitive way to describe stimulation of the nervous system.

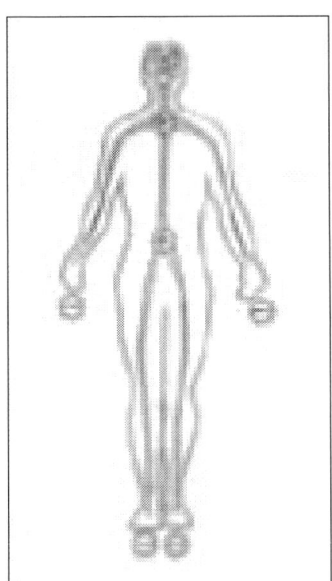

A growing number of insightful researchers have penetrated into the truths common to TCM and Western science. Their paths have led into the realms of electromagnetics and quantum physics. Bioelectro-magnetics (BEM) is a study of the relationships between electromagnetics and living systems. An entertaining and readable account of the history of research into this field in recent centuries can be found in the book <u>The Body Electric</u>[20]

Electromagnetic Fields and Life

In the early 20th century, there was a rush to embrace biochemical explanations for disease and healing as the modern pharmaceutical industry emerged with many impressive successes. Medical treatment became largely based on drug therapies and surgical interventions, and the 19th century boom of interest in electromagnetic healing methods was largely lost. In the midst of this, a few notable scientists published important discoveries in the field of bioelectromagnetics. Georges Lakhovsky wrote a valuable book in the 1920's called <u>The Secret of Life</u> in which he explained many interrelationships between high-frequency electromagnetic fields, including cosmic radiations, and living things. In the book's introduction he writes:

---

[20] Becker, R. and Seldon, G., *The Body Electric,* Morrow Publishing, 1985

> "What is life? It is the dynamic equilibrium of all cells, the harmony of multiple radiations that react upon one another. What is disease? It is the oscillatory disequilibrium of cells, originating from external causes." [21]

Lakhovsky explained that living things interrelate by receiving and giving off electromagnetic radiations. The radiatory energies of living cells described by Lakhovsky make direct energetic communication between life forms possible. The Russian scientist A.S. Pressman summed up three effects of such fields:[22]

- Allows living things to sense information about the environment
- Facilitates organization and control within the organism
- Used for communication between living things

F. A. Popp used the term "biophotons" to describe the energy communication medium between lifeforms, and explained how they regulate many physiological functions, including growth, maturation, cell differentiation, enzymatic activity and the immune system.[23] An American researcher, Emilio Del Giudice, expounded on a model of resonance and interaction between systems of particles bonded by electromagnetic fields, in which the particles move together harmoniously through field effects.[24]

Indeed, such particle communication has been demonstrated in the study of quantum physics. A basic principle of this science is that all parts of the Universe are connected to, and in communication with, all other parts. This communication is instantaneous, and freely available to those entities that can perceive it. Quantum theory was first advanced by Max Planck at the end of the 19th century, and was further refined by Niels Bohr. Bohr, who coined the term "quantum leap" in reference to the ability of electrons to instantaneously jump to different orbits through absorbing and dispersing energy, demonstrated that such movement happens at velocities faster than the speed of light.[25] Quantum physics has been described as a field of study in which modern scientific inquiry and measurements meet intuitive spiritual principles. The concept of a Universal data bank from quantum physics parallels the esoteric concept of the Akashic Records, which holds timeless records of all thoughts, words and events in history. The principle of the interrelatedness of all waves and particles in the Universe correlates with what has been described as God, Universal Mind, or Spirit.

The ancient Chinese descriptions of Qi and its pathways and accumulations in the body closely correlate with what is being discovered about subtle electromagnetic activity in life forms. The word "energy" is defined in the Webster's New World Dictionary (1984) as "force of expression or utterance, potential forces; inherent power; capacity for vigorous action, such forces or power, esp. in action." With a little clear thought, we can understand that energy exists in a continuum of power, subtlety and expression from cosmic source to the dense physical plane. The human organism is influenced by many levels of this continuum, from spiritual energies of unimaginable subtlety to those grossly apparent to our senses such as the "evils" of excessive cold, wind and heat spoken of by the ancient Chinese. The acupuncture systems are largely based on electromagnetic energies, which exist somewhere between these levels.

---

[21] Lachovsky, G., The Secret of Life, first published 1935, reprinted by Noontide Press, 1992
[22] Pressman, A.S., Electromagnetic Fields and Life, Plenum Press, NY 1970 (originally published in Russian)
[23] Popp, F.A, Becker, B, Electromagnetic Bioinformation ed 2. Urban and Schwarzengerg, Germany, 1988
[24] Del Giudice E, Coherence in condensed and living matter Pioneer Perspectives, 1993
[25] Royal, F.F., Understanding Homeopathy, Acupuncture and Electrodiagnosis: Clinical Applications of Quantum Mechanics, AJA, Vol 18, #1, 1990

What is the source of the energies the body processes through the acupuncture systems? A basic truth is that all living biological organisms are energy producing systems, even those that appear parasitic. All organisms are dependent on outside sources of energy as well, such as from food, air and the sun. In the human body, energy is produced on the cellular level by the Krebs (or citric acid) cycle, from the lung-heart connection, and the transformation of nutritive substances by the organs. According to TCM, the two Organs most responsible for production of energy are the Lungs and Spleen (Taiyin). The Triple Warmer function is the regulator of metabolism of the upper, middle and lower areas of the body. German acupuncturists have correlated the Triple Warmer to the endocrine gland system, which regulates metabolism and other life processes through hormonal control.

The energies produced by the body are electrical in nature, and produce an electrical field in and around the body. This field is analogous to the aura described by clairvoyants or the field of Qi built up by Qigong practitioners. According to such practitioners, dark or collapsed areas in the body's field are formed by disturbances or blocks in the body's energy production and flow. Using potentiometric measurements of the body's electrical potentials, Hartwig Schuldt, M.D., of Germany determined that the meridian system follows lines of condensation of the field force created by the body.[26] Becker stated that this field is inhomogeneous, and is determined by the underlying structures of the body, including tissue, fascia, muscles, bone, skin and proximity to organs. The field is also influenced by the relationship of these structures in terms of resistance, distance, interference, capacitance, polarity, and resonance. Acupuncture acts, in part, by interconnecting charges between these lines of force in the body[27].

According to Schuldt, some of the most severe physical symptoms, such as acute pain, spasm, tetany, and neuropathies are caused by distortions in the body's field due to damaged viscera. He stated that this is a much more significant factor in causing such symptoms than nerve injury and damage. His research showed that phantom limb pain, which is a prime example of pain due to field distortion, could be resolved through healing of the internal organs.

Electrical Parameters of the Human Body

Much of the early research into the electrical nature of acupuncture points dealt with the differences in skin resistance between acu-points and surrounding tissues. In the early 1950's, Yosio Nakatani found that some points on the body were more conductive than other points when a 12-volt current was applied to the skin. He called these low-resistance spots "good electro-permeable points" or Ryodoraku[28] in Japanese. Since then, many researchers have developed apparatuses to measure the electrical conductivity of acu-points in relation to non-points[29]. S. Krippner demonstrated in 1974 that the resistance of acu-points ranged from 100-200 k-ohms, while non-points had much higher resistances up to 1 mega-ohm. J.E.H. Niboyet used more sophisticated measurement devices to show that acu-points were about 50% more conductive than surrounding points. When electrodes were placed on points on the same meridian, electric currents passed more preferentially than if the electrodes were placed on different meridians.

---

[26] Schuldt, Hartwig From paper presented at the Third International Congress of Acupuncture in Berlin, 1976, published in AJA, Vol. 4, #4, Dec. 1976
[27] Mussat. M., Acupuncture Networks, Vol. II trans. by E. Serejski, 1997
[28] see Glossary of Terms
[29] Zhu Zong-xiang, Research Advances in the Electrical Specificity of Meridians and Acupuncture Points AJA, Vol 9, #3, 1981. All the references in this paragraph are quoted from this article

Capacitance is the ability of a substance to store and gradually release electrical charge. Electronic components called capacitors are used in most electronic equipment for this purpose. According to Dumitrescu[30], a Romanian researcher, acu-points store charge to a greater degree than surrounding tissues, as well as having lower resistance. He found that acu-points have capacitance readings of 0.02 – 0.5 µF (microfarads), while non-points were measured at less than 0.01 µF.

Polarity is another vital principle in the energetic workings of the human body and acupuncture treatment. Electrical potentials, which reveal polarity, were measured in the human body by Drs. Ionescu-Tirgoviste and Pruna in Romania using electroacupuncturogram (EAG) equipment.[31] In their studies they bilaterally connected distal acu-points GB 41 and TW 3 to an EAG device, which simultaneously measured the point's electrical potentials in millivolts in comparison to abdominal point CV 7, which was used as the ground. The EAG device itself did not significantly stimulate the points. These measurements were taken during various conditions, including acupuncture needle insertion, manipulation, and thermal and laser stimulation of points. The researchers found that, when the potential differences between the points was high, the patients reported energetic sensations ranging from gentle tingling to intense electric sensations as a result of the connections. When there was little potential differences, patients felt little or nothing. In this study, they observed that the distal acu-points could be positive or negative in relation to ground. The doctors concluded that meridians exist as canals in the interstitial spaces between the structures of the body along which endogenous electrical charges propagate. Blockages in the normal flow of these currents lead to high concentrations of positive or negative electrical charges. These high concentrations may cause pain and other symptoms of disease. This seems to indicate that imbalances of Yin and Yang (build-up of positive or negative ionic activity, respectively), when discharged through acupuncture stimulation, lead to the characteristic propagated sensations through the meridians and the "Te Chi"[32] phenomenon. Te Chi is the sensation of tingling, soreness, heaviness or throbbing that is the result of skillful needle insertion and manipulation of acu-points. It is different from the pain of hitting nerves, which is much more unpleasant. The greater the potential differences, the greater the Te Chi sensations. The meridians represent the charted "paths of least resistance" to the flow of endogenous ionic currents. Drs. Ionescu-Tirgoviste et al offered the following fascinating information.

---

[30] Dumitrescu I.F., Contribution to the Electro-Physiology of the Active Points, Int'l Acupuncture conference, Bucharest, Romania, 1977, as quoted in article Research Advances in the Electrical Specificity of Meridians and Acupuncture Points AJA Vol. 9 #3, 1981

[31] Ionescu-Tirgoviste and Pruna, The Acu-Point Potential, Electroreception and Bio-Electrical Homeostasis of the Human Body, AJA Vol. 18, #1 1990

[32] Te Chi is what an acupuncturist feels through her fingers when needling an active acupuncture point holding an ionic charge

FUNCTIONAL PARTICULARITIES OF THE SKIN AREAS USED IN ACUPUNCTURE

QUALITIES OF SUPERFICIAL ACUPUNCTURE POINTS	QUALITIES OF DEEP ACUPUNCTURE POINTS
High electric potentials (up to 300 mV)	Low deep perception threshold to an electric stimulus
High electric capacitance values (0.1 – 1 µF)	Capacitance (storage of electric charges)
Low electrical resistance	Electro-resonance with other acu-points
Increased skin respiration	High conductivity of isotopic tracers
High local temperature	
Spontaneous visible light emission from the Jing and Yuan points	
Sound signals at the acupuncture points (2-15 Hz, amplitude 0.5 – 1 mV, sharp or sine wave	

Figure 2.1: Functional Particularities of the Skin Areas Used in Acupuncture

From the research presented here, it can be deduced that acupuncture is probably most effective when the symptoms are associated with build-up of significant ionic imbalances that can be discharged through point stimulation.

Microcurrents and the Meridian System

In my extensive work with microcurrent electro-acupuncture, I have made measurements of skin resistance before and after brief 6-second bursts of microcurrent stimulation using the Acutron Mentor device. I have consistently observed that increases of skin electrical conductivity after such stimulation are far greater with patients who have actual pathologies than in healthy people. The study discussed above seems to corroborate this. Patients with pain and dysfunction have more of a build-up of electrical activity due to its impaired circulation. A microcurrent device, in reading out changes in skin resistance, can clearly show this change.

In explanation, the old "beaver dam" analogy is useful here. A free-flowing stream has an overall even energy. A device measuring its flow would not show many large fluctuations. Yet, if the beavers build a dam upstream from the measuring device, the flow rate will be greatly lessened. If the dam were suddenly knocked away, the device would then detect a major rush of increased water, which would then gradually settle back to more or less steady flow. This is exactly what we see when taking measurements with the Acutron Mentor device. When treating and measuring areas on the extremities in pain patients, with positive electrode proximal and negative electrode distal, it is common to see resistance changes between the points of as much as 60% after only 6 seconds of stimulation. I have observed that such large increases in conductivity usually correlate with rapid symptomatic relief of pain and improved range of motion. When, on the other hand, the conductivity readings do not change much after stimulation, symptomatic results have often been less clear-cut. This also supports the principle that large releases of built-up ionic imbalances in the electrical systems of the body are associated with good clinical results. The measurement circuit of the microcurrent device allows for instantaneous monitoring of changes in skin resistance after each stimulation period, and is therefore valuable in tracking this phenomenon.

Bjorn Nordenstrom M.D., an important Swedish medical researche, is best known in the medical field for his development of advanced catheters used in surgery. His contributions in energy medicine for cancer treatment are outstanding as well. He postulated the meridian systems as a vascular-interstitial closed circuit (VICC)[33]. According to Dr. Nordenstrom, this system allows for transfer of positive or negative ionic charges over long distances in the body, through the blood vessels and interstitial spaces. The system is powered by imbalances of positive and negative currents created by energy production of the organs, as well as "currents of injury" released by tissue damage and trauma. The most frequently utilized electrical channels form the meridians mapped out by Chinese medicine. According to Nordenstrom direct current flows in tissues, and high frequency alternating currents, as used in many clinical milliamp stimulators, are not effective for balancing the meridians systems. Therefore, microcurrents, which are generally used as a form of modulated direct current, are most useful for this purpose. High-frequency alternating currents, as used in classic interferential and other modalities, may be valuable, however, for grosser counter-irritation effects for acute pain, and possibly to destroy unhealthy tissues at high doses.

Dr. Yoshio Manaka's ion pumping cords also work on the principle of charge imbalance equalization in the body. By using the Master points[34] of the Extraordinary Vessels and principle meridians for ion pumping, this balancing is directed to the deepest energy layers of the body[35].

Dr. Nordenstrom's work with terminal cancer patients has been very impressive. Cancer cells are more sensitive to electrical energy than healthy cells and application of externally applied currents influence them strongly. He demonstrated direct microcurrent stimulation of tumors with implanted needle electrodes significantly blocked cancer pain for long periods, and in many cases caused the tumor to regress or disappear. The positive pole of the stimulator was placed in the tumor and the negative at some distance away. Dr. Nordenstrom's best explanation for this phenomenon was that the tumor would become dehydrated through electro-osmosis, which then blocked production of pain-causing substances in the tumor, such as histamine, substance-P and bradykinin. Research in the U.S. with high volt pulsed galvanic stimulators has also shown that the negative pole tends to be sclerolytic, or tissue softening, and the positive pole tends to be tissue hardening, probably associated with dehydration. It is sad that Nordenstrom's landmark work with cancer has not been carried forward in the United States. This is due more to political than scientific reasons.

Electrical Effects of Acupuncture Needling

Dr. Nordenstrom also studied the electrical effects of acupuncture needle stimulation. He made the following observations: The potential difference between the subcutis of the patient and the acupuncturist's fingers form a capacitive flow of current, eventually equalizing the charges. The charge may flow either way, depending on the relative strength of the acupuncturist's and patient's personal energy field. This confirms the importance of the practice of Qigong (and healthy living) by acupuncturists in order to keep their personal field stronger than that of the patients. Although plastic handled needles insulate the needle from direct contact with the acupuncturist's charge, the needle will still equalize the charges between the surface and deeper layers of the patient's tissues with which it is in contact.

Manipulation of the needle can also influence the flow of charge, depending on whether it is in a clockwise or counter-clockwise direction, or whether lifting or thrusting is done more forcefully. Anytime currents flow between metal and an electrolyte (body fluids), electrolysis

---

[33] Nordenstrom, B., An Electrophysiological View of Acupuncture: Role of Capacitive and Closed Circuit Currents And Their Clinical Effects in the Treatment of Cancer and Chronic Pain, AJA, Vol 17, #2, 1989
[34] see Glossary of Terms
[35] Manaka, Y., Chasing the Dragon's Tail Paradigm Publications, 1995

creates a build-up of deposits that eventually act as an insulator. Periodic manipulation and twirling of the needles can mechanically remove this coating, facilitating good continued electrical contact.

In another study by Ionescu-Tirgoviste[36], an EAG device was connected to acupuncture needles placed in the same points as indicated in the previously quoted study. The needles were manipulated in the following classical methods: clockwise twirling, counter-clockwise twirling, back-and-forth twirling, and lifting and thrusting (up and down) movement. The doctors found that the needles on the distal acu-points had a negative potential in comparison with the abdominal needle in all cases. However, the degree of potential varied between –25mV to –350mV according to the needling technique and the health of the patients. Healthy patients registered distal potentials between -150 to -250 mV, while those with diseases registered potentials above or below these levels. Needle manipulation changed the potentials, with counter-clockwise twirling and lifting and thrusting increasing the potentials the most. The healthy patients recovered their basal readings soon after manipulation, while unhealthy ones recovered more slowly or not at all, indicating some kind of energetic blockage. According to TCM theory, this is probably associated with impaired Liver function, as the Liver controls the function of spreading and circulation of Qi.

Perhaps the most detailed research into the electrical qualities of acupuncture needling has been done by Maurice Mussat, M.D., of France. He performed many experiments to measure the precise electrical activity generated by acupuncture needles of various metallic combinations.[37] His work conclusively demonstrated that acupuncture needling releases electrical energy into the body, and the acupuncture is the "original microcurrent therapy." Placing a metal needle into contact with body fluids, which act as an electrolyte, creates a simple battery. Generation of energy by such a battery is greatly increased by use of bi-metallic needles, such as those with handles made of a different metal than the shaft. Bi-metallic combinations that generate electrical energy when in contact with each other are known as thermocouples. Applying heat to the needle handles can greatly increase energy generation of the thermocouple.

In Mussat's early experiments, he found that acupuncture needles made of tungsten metal created the most powerful polarization and therapeutic effects when inserted into the body. Tungsten is used to make filaments in light bulbs because of its efficiency at converting electrical to light energy. Because these needles tended to lose their proper tip shaping rapidly due to brittleness and caused excessive pain, he searched for alternatives. He experimented with needles made out of the following metal combinations:

- Tungsten-silver
- Special stainless steel-copper
- Special stainless steel-cupron (nickel-copper alloy)
- Stainless steel-brass
- Stainless steel-brass with gold plating
- Chinese made needles of stainless steel and silver

Mussat used a micro-ammeter, a device that measures electrical activity, to measure the charge generated between the handle and tip of the needles. He found that the combinations

---

[36] Ionescu-Tirgoviste, Measurement of Acupuncture Injury Potential by Acupunctometry AJA, Vol 15, #3, 1987
[37] Mussat. M., Acupuncture Networks, Vol. II trans. by E. Serejski, 1997

creating the greatest discharge into the acu-points were tungsten-silver, copper-stainless steel and stainless steel-cupron with gold plating on the handles, with the last being the most efficient. Measurements of current generated by different kinds of needles ranged from 30 – 60 nanoamps (billionths of amps), with readings going as high as 20 μA when the needles were heated with a hot flame.

Steel needles with metal handles made of noble metals such as copper, brass or gold have a positive polarization of the tip in relation to the handle. In other words, the handle acts as the cathode and the tip the anode. The polarity reverses when the needle handle is heated to a temperature higher than the body region into which it is inserted.

As mentioned earlier, capacitance is the tendency of a substance to gradually discharge energy over time. Mussat also measured the capacitance of bi-metallic needles, and found that bi-metallic needles, again acting as mini-batteries, gradually discharge over time when in contact with a conductive medium (such as the human body.)

Mussat also measured electrical activity along meridians. In one experiment, he placed two needles along the trajectory of a single meridian with the two electrodes of the power source on the two needles. He then applied a few minutes of pulsed electrical stimulation of about one volt to the needles. After stopping the stimulation, he measured the charge between the needles and found it as high as 24 – 30 microamps. Yet, if he moved either needle slightly off the meridian pathway, the readings were much lower. This appears to indicate that the meridians also store electrical charges. This could be due to the electrical qualities of fascial connective tissue, which some Japanese researchers have identified as the physical substrate of the meridian system. The following discussion of semiconduction and piezoelectricity will expand on this subject.

Semiconduction and Piezoelectricity

Semiconduction and piezoelectricity are two electrical qualities of crystalline substances that, curiously enough, occur prolifically in the human body. Both are highly relevant to understanding the electrical qualities of the meridian system. There are three kinds of current conduction known to modern science- metallic conduction, ionic conduction and semiconduction. Metallic conduction only occurs in metal wires. Ionic conduction occurs through cell membranes, but is incapable of traversing more than minute distances in the body. Semiconduction is the only known mode of conduction outside of metal wires capable of transmitting very small currents over long distances. This is possible only in substances with very orderly molecular structures, such as crystals.

Albert Szent-Gyorgyi, an eastern European researcher, was the first to point out that the molecular structures of the human body are organized enough to support semiconduction through passing information along chains of protein molecules.[38] Robert Becker constructed many experiments to test this principle, and concluded that energy transmission and communication of the meridian system is based on semiconduction along the perineural glial cells that support the nervous system. These allow subtle currents to be transported over long distances without losing charge. He demonstrated that these semiconducted currents were completely different from electrical activity of the nerves themselves. Nerves transmit high-frequency electrical action potentials, while glial cells transmit slower, direct currents of much smaller amplitude. He postulated that such direct currents represented the more primitive aspect of our electro-physiology, which support healing and regeneration, and acupuncture

---
[38] Becker, R and Selden, G, The Body Electric, Morrow Publishing, 1985

points were in effect way stations that boosted the charge along the pathways.[39] Creatures with a greater preponderance of these DC systems than humans, such as lizards and salamanders, possess much greater powers of regeneration, and can re-grow amputated limbs and organs. Becker postulated, and demonstrated in preliminary ways, that use of correctly applied subtle direct currents may someday allow humans to do similar feats.

The body's semiconduction system as explained by Becker correlate well with the X-signal system theorized by Yoshio Manaka, M.D.[40]. According To Manaka, this system consists of extremely small charges in and around the body that ultimately regulate all life processes. While the X-signals cannot be measured with currently available tools, their effects can be clearly observed through changes in pressure pain on acu-points, pulse diagnosis and kinesiology (muscle testing). The X-signal system is exquisitely sensitive to polarity agents such as magnets, ion-pumping cords or polarized electrical probes. I am highly indebted to Manaka for this knowledge, and use polarized microcurrents through probe electrodes with excellent effect for rapidly balancing the meridian systems of my patients.

Piezoelectricity is another inherent electrical quality of the body. Piezoelectricity is the tendency of a crystalline structure, when deformed or struck, to release an electrical charge. The forces of movement and gravity on human and animal bodies are constantly triggering such charges. Becker measured such activity in bone, and showed that bone regeneration is turned on by endogenous charges generated by piezoelectricity. This phenomenon is not limited in the body to bone, however. In their excellent book Hara Diagnosis, Reflections on the Sea, Matsumoto and Birch offer explanations and many research citations about this subject. According to Matsumoto and Birch, connective tissues of many kinds possess piezoelectric properties that literally interconnect every part of the body with every other part.[41] Fascia can be compared to a complex, stretchy network that is constantly releasing and circulating subtle charges. Piezoelectric activity has been demonstrated in many kinds of connective tissues and blood vessels.[42]

James Oschman, as quoted in the book *Hara Diagnosis* states:

> "The (fascial) fabric is a semiconducting communication network that can convey the bioelectric signals between every part of the body and every other part. This communication network within the fascia in none other than the meridian system of traditional Oriental medicine, with its countless extensions into every part of the body... The mechanical, bioelectric and biomagnetic signals traveling through the connective tissue network, and through the space around the body, tell the various cells how to form and reform the tissue architecture in response to the tensions, compressions and movements we make."[43]

There are two main categories of fascia: subcutaneous fascia that underlies and supports the skin, muscles and skeleton and the subserous fascia that wraps around the internal organs and lines body cavities. There are also microscopic aspects of connective tissue through matrices within and surrounding cells, which include collagen and glycosaminoglycan fibers and microtubules. The connections between these networks and the fascial planes thus electrically connect every cell in the body with every other one[44].

---

[39] *Ibid.,.,* Reference 2, Ch. 13
[40] *Ibid.,.,* Reference 15 Ch. 2
[41] Matsumoto and Birch, Hara Diagnosis, Reflections On The Sea, Pardigm Publications, 1988
[42] *Ibid.,.,* Note #49, p. 440
[43] *Ibid.,.,* Reference 21, Ch.8
[44] According to sources quoted in the book Hara Diagnosis, any classical acupuncture texts from China and Japan expounded about the relationship of fascia and meridians. The Chinese terms *huang* and *gao* appear to refer to types of membranes, or connective tissues that are formed during embryological development, and which convey source energies through the Organs and meridians. There are several acu-points named after the *huang*, such as *huang shu* (K 16), *huangmen* (UB 47, lateral to UB 22,

These insights reveal that subtle electrical charges are being generated through piezo-electricity by all movement and the effects of gravity, and that these charges are semiconducted over long distances in the body. This gives great support to the healing and regenerative effects of hatha yoga, deep tissue massage, Rolfing, and exercise in general. All of these help to generate and circulate subtle energy throughout the body through stimulating piezoelectric activity and this is clearly associated with health and well-being.

What are Meridians?

It has been a common view among some Western physicians to simply ascribe the classically described acupuncture meridian system to a primitive way of describing the nervous system. Yet, a brief examination of these two systems quickly reveals that meridians rarely follow nerve pathways, and in some cases run perpendicular to them. While it is true that all peripheral nerves eventually have connections to the central switchboard of the brain, there are no direct nerve connections between many commonly treated local and distal acu-point combinations[45]. It has also been demonstrated that the propagation of sensations along a meridian that has been needled is between 5 and 1200 times slower than nerve conduction.[46]

There are many opinions and perspectives on what meridians are, some of which have been previously mentioned in this chapter. Some sources claim that acu-points were recognized earlier in history, and that meridians were theoretical constructs proposed to connect the points. Yet, some recent discoveries have shown that the existence of meridians was written about in earlier ancient Chinese texts than the ones mentioning acu-points[47]. The classic acupuncture texts *Nei Jing* and *Ling Shu* were the best known ancient texts to offer comprehensive information about meridians and acu-points, and this information continues to be used in modern acupuncture practice.

The perspective with the greatest historical support in Chinese medical classics is that the meridian system exists throughout the complex fascial network of the body. This perspective is in accordance with Becker's view that neuroglial cells conduct the meridian energies, as the glial cells are part of the body's connective tissue network.

Thus the classically described meridian, or *Jing-Luo* systems, are conductive pathways that link every part of the body with every other part. They primarily exist through the fascial network of the body, and have definite electrical qualities. The classically described maps of the meridians have stood the test of time, and have been studied and largely verified by modern researchers. These are likely to be preferential pathways for the transfer of ionic charges throughout the body. Electrical and needle stimulation through the meridian system apparently works through local effects as well as adjustment of the central and autonomic nervous systems and endocrine systems, which together regulate all bodily functions.

Non-needle Acupuncture

The preceding information confirms that traditional acupuncture is indeed working with the subtle electro-physiology of the body. It is of great significance that electrically conductive

---

the triple warner back shu), and *gaohuangshu* (UB 43, lateral to UB 13). These points apparently have significant energetic connections to the flow of source qi through the fascial network of the body. The Source points around the wrists and ankles, as well as the front-Mu and back-Shu point, all have very strong energetic attachments to the fascial network. This is probably why they offer such clear diagnostic properties for the meridian/Organ systems.

[45] Some meridians on the extremities do approximate parts of dermatome distributions, yet not consistently
[46] A. Bensoussan, The Vital Meridian, Churchill Livingstone 1991, p. 63
[47] Called the Han Ma-wang Burial Mound Silk Books

metals must be used for acupuncture needling to generate best results. We know that the ancient Chinese did not have modern electronic devices, and they worked with what was available. Nonetheless, are acupuncture needles necessary? The charts below summarizes the information in this chapter and my own research.

The table on the next page summarizes the advantages and limitations of needle and non-needle microcurrent techniques. A ♥ is placed in the column of the more advantageous technique.

COMPARISON OF NEEDLE AND NON-NEEDLE MICROCURRENT TECHNIQUES

CLINICAL CONSIDERATIONS	NEEDLES	NON-NEEDLE MICROCURRENT
Patient acceptance and comfort (especially children)		♥
Greater depth of penetration	♥	
Ability to correct imbalanced body polarities		♥
Ability to modulate energy input to body		♥
Resonance with of specific tissue frequencies		♥
Ability to stimulate multiple points simultaneously	♥	
Best effects for myofascial pain and constriction (*)	♥	♥
Best effects for visceral and blood treatment	♥	
Best effects for neuropathies		♥
Relaxation effect for tense or nervous patients	♥	
Shorter treatment time required for good results		♥

(*) Both methods can deliver outstanding results and combining them is often the most effective.

Figure 2.2: Comparison of Needle and Non-Needle Acupuncture Techniques

The next chart highlights some further comparisons between needle acupuncture and non-needle microcurrent techniques. The left column contains the aspect to be considered; the right column has a brief discussion of the relative advantages and disadvantages of the techniques.

BIO-ENERGY, ACUPUNCTURE AND MICROCURRENT STIMULATION

ENERGETIC CONSIDERATIONS OF ACUPUNCTURE	ACUPUNCTURE VS. NON-NEEDLE MICROCURRENT STIMULATION
EXTERNAL ENERGY AFFECTS MERIDIAN SYSTEM Externally applied energy strongly affects the meridian system for good or ill.	**MICROCURRENT EQUALIZES CHARGE WITHOUT AFFECTING PRACTITIONER** Needling can equalize charge in different levels of tissue, and can transmit charge from the practitioner to the patient (which can drain the practitioner!) Microcurrents use an external power source to accomplish the same without affecting the practitioner.
GENTLE CURRENTS INTERFACE WELL WITH MERIDIAN SYSTEM Gentle, slowly oscillating currents are best suited to interface with the meridian system. Most electro-therapy and electro-acupuncture devices do not produce such currents, and act more in a suppressive manner to control pain and muscle disorders.	**MICROCURRENT RESONATES WITH BODY BETTER THAN NEEDLES** Microcurrents are most commonly delivered as low frequency direct currents, which are harmonious with the natural frequencies of the body, which range from 0.1 – 10 Hz[48]. Such frequencies resonate positively with various tissue systems. Needles do not transmit such frequency information unless very accurately manipulated[49].
BEST RESULTS OCCUR WHEN POLARITY OF BODY IS MATCHED Energy stimulation is most effective when it matches the healthy polarities of the body.	**POLARIZED MICROCURRENT STIMULATION HAS POSITIVE EFFECTS** Needle insertions by themselves are not polarized. Manaka's ion-pumping cords must be attached to needles to create polarity effects. Proper use of positive and negative microcurrent stimulation can produce positive clinical effects without needles for extremity pain, peripheral neuropathies and many internal disorders
STIMULUS MODULATION ENHANCES TREATMENT EFFECTIVENESS Various forms of modulation of stimulation make treatment more effective with longer lasting effects. Modulation can be accomplished through needle manipulation techniques or electronic patterning of stimulation currents.	**MICROCURRENT DEVICES MODULATE CURRENT PAINLESSLY** Most American patients have little tolerance for extensive acupuncture needle manipulations. Advanced microcurrent devices create complex current modulations that can enhance energy balancing without any discomfort.
ACU-POINTS ARE ELECTRICALLY CONDUCTIVE Acupuncture and ah shi[50] points that require treatment are more electrically conductive than surrounding tissues.	**MICROCURRENT DEVICES ENHANCE DIAGNOSTIC AND TREATMENT EFFECTIVENESS** The increased conductance of open acu-points allows them to be detected and measured by electronic devices. This opens many valuable possibilities of diagnosis and precise administration of treatment.

Figure 2.3: Energy in the Body, Acupuncture and Microcurrent

These charts illustrate the significant value of microcurrent acupuncture treatment. Needle therapy is here to stay, however, as it still offers many advantages.

Combining Needling and Microcurrents

I often utilize a combination of needles and non-needle techniques to assist my most challenging patients, taking advantages of the strengths of each method. In most cases, I place needles in distal points effective for pain control of the affected area, and use

---

[49] Voll, R. Twenty Years of Electroacupuncture Therapy, AJA, Vol. 3, #4, October-Dec. 1975
[50] Ah shi points are spontaneously appearing acu-points in an injured or inflamed area

microcurrent probe stimulation of local and distal acu-points as well as pad applications to treat the local painful or injured area. For needle sites, I frequently use the distal acu-points described by Richard Tan in his excellent books.[51]

EXAMPLES OF COMBINATION OF ACUPUNCTURE AND MICROCURRENT THERAPIES

COMPLAINT	ACUPUNCTURE TREATMENT	MICROCURRENT TREATMENT
Sciatica	Ling Ku - contralateral UB 60 - ipsilateral K 3 - contralateral	Low back & buttocks - Microcurrent pad (+) Leg at distal location of radiating pain-, Microcurrent pad (-)
Frozen Shoulder	St 38 - contralateral GB 34 - contralateral Sp 9 or Sp 9a - contralateral	Shoulder (site of pain) - probe and interferential electro-massage
Migraine	Distal points on arms and legs according to distribution of pain	Head (site of pain) - , Microcurrent + probe; briefly touch distal needles.

Figure 2.3: Examples Of Combination of Acupuncture and Microcurrent Treatment

I do not often use or advocate the connection of needles with alligator clip wires directly to a milliamp stimulator, which is par for most electro-acupuncture practice. In my opinion the hazards and drawbacks outweigh the benefits, except when surgical or acute pain analgesia is called for. I have enjoyed excellent results by briefly touching + and – microcurrent probes to needles, metal to metal, for about 20 seconds per set of two needles. Microcurrent works so quickly that this has been sufficient to relieve pain and balance the meridian system. Dr. Alejandro Katz, an acupuncturist in Los Angeles who makes extensive use of microcurrent in his offices, applies pad electrodes directly over obliquely inserted needles in local pain areas with gratifying results. These methods offer the benefits of electro-acupuncture needle stimulation without the drawbacks.

Summary

The human body generates electrical energy through organic action, cellular respiration, currents of injury and piezoelectrical activity. These subtle currents form fields of force, the condensations of which form the charted meridian system. Researchers have placed the substrate of the meridians variously in the glial cells, fascial network, interstitial spaces and blood vessels. Subtle electrical charges can migrate long distances in the body through semiconduction, which passes tiny electrical charges through orderly molecular matrices. Variations in energy generation and currents of injury tend to form imbalances in ionic positive and negative charges in the body, which are associated with pain and disease. The therapeutic effects of acupuncture come from its ability to locally or distally discharge these potential differences, or otherwise help bring about optimal charge conditions of the body. Acupuncture points have greater electrical conductivity than surrounding tissues. Varieties of metals used together in manufacture of acupuncture needles create thermocouple effects for stronger stimulation of acu-points. The body's energy systems are polarized, with the trunk and head tending to be more electro-positive, and the extremities electro-negative.

---

[51] Tan, R., 12 and 12 in Acupuncture and 24 More in Acupuncture

Electro-stimulation that follows these natural polarities and significantly increases conductivity between the electrodes will tend to be more clinically effective. Non-needle microcurrent stimulation, especially when polarized to follow the body's natural polarization, can be a highly effective meridian balancing method. Non-needle microcurrent electro-acupuncture allows practitioners to work with the body's electro-physiology with greater precision and versatility than is possible with needles. Needle and non-needle acupuncture each offer advantages and limitations. Modern acupuncturists can provide the most effective service by understanding and utilizing the strengths of both methods.

Chapter 3
UNIVERSAL LAWS OF ENERGY MEDICINE

A philosophical foundation of traditional Chinese medicine is the following symbol:

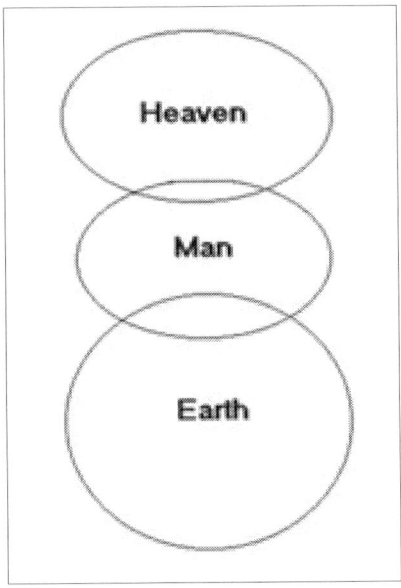

Figure 3.1: Heaven, Earth, Man

This diagram denotes the interrelationship between Heaven, Earth and Man. Heaven represents the male Universal Cosmic energy, the so-called Unified Field, which is the Void from which creation emanates. Earth is the feminine, solid, nurturing ground, the foundation and container for all that is physical and manifest. Man is the fruit of the marriage of Heaven and Earth. A fully realized human being has her consciousness open to the Cosmos, and yet is solidly grounded on Earth. Many aspects of acupuncture principles arise from this understanding of Heaven and Earth. Much of advanced Qigong and martial arts are based on this relationship.

Energy medicine is based on Universal laws that also apply to both the cosmic and earthly level. Some of these principles are introduced in this chapter to offer a larger context from which to understand how microcurrent electro-acupuncture works with the human body.

In this chapter will will examine four vital Universal Laws and some other principles of energy medicine. They are:

1) Law of Resonance
2) Law of Polarity
3) Law of Economy
4) Law of Biasology
5) Accommodation
6) Kinesiology

Universal Law #1 - The Law of Resonance

The Law of Resonance applies equally to Western scientific and energetic medicine. It has been summed up in the metaphysical phrase "as above, so below", and has been the basis for many esoteric systems of knowledge and healing, including astrology, homeopathy and magic. Any health care modality, treatment, herb or drug that has a therapeutic effect does so because of a positive vibrational resonance with the target tissues. The application of this principle has been called "digital biology" by Jacques Beneviste of France.[52] In the field of Chinese medicine, this law has manifested itself through elaborate systems of correspondence, as is found in the Five Element system of acupuncture. In this method, diagnosis and treatment are based on correspondences between bodily Organs, colors, sounds, foods, directions, seasons, flavors and much more.

Some of our most valuable medical devices work with the Law of Resonance. The Magnetic Resonance Imaging (MRI) machine is able to create detailed scans of the inside of the body. This works through a resonance between the specific frequency of a directed radio beam and the protons within the molecules of water inside the body, which are lined up by a powerful magnetic field. Doppler and ultrasound scans also work because of resonance effects between the sound waves and human tissue. Indeed, modern physics has determined that all interactions involve resonance.

A clear illustration of the Law of Resonance is a piano keyboard. Each musical note exists in 8 to 10 levels of pitch called octaves. The lowest C note is a related frequency to the upper C notes, yet it vibrates at a lower level, giving a deeper sound. Playing the low C is in direct resonance with the all C notes on the piano. Some classical Indian musical instruments such as the sitar have two sets of strings- one that is plucked by the musician, and another that is not plucked, but drone in resonance. This gives a fuller and more complex sound.

In the same manner as a piano keyboard, there are many octaves of energy that range from the Universal Cosmic level to those that can be directly felt and processed by an individual. Our bodies are not capable of withstanding direct contact with the highest octaves of energy, although meditation and spiritual development can increase our ability to do so. Yet we can directly experience the cosmos through "stepped down" octaves of these Universal energies. These graduations of the octaves of energy are reflected in our chakra[53] system, which steps down Universal energy to embrace aspects of our human functions and emotions.

Another easily grasped example of this stepping down process is our electrical power delivery system. Electrical generation systems such as dams and nuclear plants create currents that can supply entire cities with power. The currents generated by these plants would instantly

---

[52] For a fascinating example of this principle, look at website www.digibio.com
[53] Chakra, which means wheel in Sanskrit, are energy centers in and around the body that produce and regulate life functions and feelings through the transformation of Universal life force to various levels of human experience

burn out any electrical equipment or appliance if directly connected. Power stations in each region with huge transformers lower the voltage to levels that can supply individual businesses and houses with power. Breaker boxes in buildings further step down the current to levels that can power individual applications such as lights and other appliances and equipment. In this way it is necessary to step down the immense power of the main trunk lines several times before the electrical power can actually be used for practical applications.

The experience of resonance, or lack of it, is an everyday experience for all of us. What is often called "chemistry" between people is a positive energetic resonance. When a dog barks when certain people approach, it is feeling a disharmonious resonance. We are frequently making decisions and judgments in our business and personal lives based on the quality of resonance we feel with others.

The effectiveness of electro-acupuncture is also dependent on proper resonance. This is based on selection of proper frequency when setting up a device for treatment. Frequency, also called Hertz, is the number of pulses or waveforms that occur in each second of current output. Frequency may be adjusted on modern electro-stimulators, although little clear information about setting it is offered by most manufacturers.

German researchers have correlated low treatment frequencies with specific tissue systems in the body. The following chart illustrates some sample frequency resonances[54].

```
Some frequency examples from German EAV research:

2.5 Hz:  Contusions, edema, insomnia, sinusitis
3.3 Hz:  Arteriosclerosis
3.9 Hz:  Neuralgias
5.9 Hz:  Spastic paralysis
8.2 Hz:  Flaccid paralysis
9.2 Hz:  Ear problems, eczema, diastolic HBP, kidney weakness
9.4 Hz:  Bladder/prostate, circulatory disturbances, gouty arthritis
         paresthesias
9.5 Hz:  Laryngitis, migraine
9.7 Hz   Sciatica, rheumatism
10  Hz:  Phlebitis, varicose veins
```

Figure 3.2: EAV Hz Chart

Universal Law #2 - The Law of Polarity

The Law of Polarity is so far-reaching that it literally can be said to be the foundation for everything in the manifested universe! This is about the interplay of opposite poles of energy, and the dynamic tension this interaction produces. This law is about the dance of creation that creates all manifestation, growth, maturation, destruction, movement and transformation. The Chinese terms Yin and Yang are the purest descriptions available of these dynamic opposites. The famous

---

[54] Reinhold Voll, <u>Zwei Jahrzehnte Elecktroakupunktur – Forschung und Erfahrung in Diagnostik und Therapy</u>

Chinese oracle text the "I Ching", or "Book of Changes", describes the laws of change and transformation as they relate to human experience.

All matter has polarity properties, including molecules, the human body and the Earth. We see examples of this law around us every day, all the time: day and night, male and female, cold and hot, winter and summer, happy and sad, pleasure and pain, up and down, rich and poor, in and out, young and old. These pairs of opposites describe all aspects of our world. In fact, all businesses go through cycles of increased and decreased income. All human relationships go through highs and lows. A particularly dramatic example of the Law of Polarity in human relationships is marriage and divorce, such as couples who are blissfully "in love" for some time, then later hire divorce lawyers to battle their separation out to the last penny with bitterness and even hatred.

Most of us have played with magnets, and know that like poles repels and opposite poles attract. Those of us who have used jumper cables or other electrical connections should know (or sparks will fly!) that the negative and positive terminals must be properly connected.

Chinese Medicine and other traditional healing systems recognize that individual patients must be treated according to their physical constitution and unique presentation. The Eight Guiding Principles of Chinese medical diagnosis are completely based on the Law of Polarity. Those principles are as follows:

HOT	**COLD**
EXCESS	**DEFICIENCY**
EXTERNAL	**INTERNAL**
YANG	**YIN**

By classifying the patient's presentation according to these opposite polarities, the temperature, quality and location of the illness are understood in a way that leads to selection of herbal formulas and acupuncture treatment.

As mentioned in Chapter 2, Ionescu-Tirgoviste, Becker and other researchers have used simple electrical potential measurements to map the polarities of animals and humans. A clear pattern exists among all creatures. The head and central line of the body tend to be electro-positive, while the tail in primitive creatures and the extremities in people tend to be electro-negative. The following diagram shows the normal electrical polarities of humans as determined by Robert Becker[55] (see next page)

---

[55] The Body Electric, pp 94 - 99

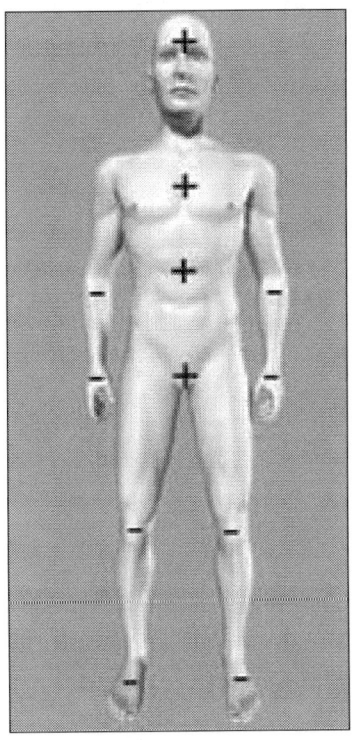

Figure 3.3: Normal Human Polarity

It is my view that many puzzling chronic pain conditions such as reflex sympathetic dystrophy (RSD) and some forms of peripheral neuropathy are associated with distortions and reversals of the normal human polarity patterns.

One fascinating experiment conducted by March and Beams in the 1950's involved passing polarized currents through flatworms. When a positive current was placed at the tail, and a negative current at the head, the worm's head actually changed into a tail, and the tail into a head![56]

An understanding of polarity patterns of the body directly leads to knowledge of correct electrode placements, especially for radiculopathies[57] and extremity disorders. See Chapters 7 and 9 for details of these techniques.

For this reason, the Law of Polarity is particularly vital in microcurrent electro-acupuncture. In my experience, the use of incorrect polarities is the factor that most commonly leads to disappointing clinical results. When we do not apply electrodes according to the natural polarities of the body, we are working *against* the body, not with it, and good results are unlikely. A striking example is sciatica, or painful radiation down the leg from a lower back or gluteal compression of the sciatic nerve. When the correct polarity pattern is followed, and a positive electrode is placed on the lower back and a negative electrode is placed on a painful area down the leg, pain is often reduced or eliminated. Yet, when in ignorance of this pattern, a negative or even biphasic[58] electrode is placed over the back and a positive or biphasic

---

[56] The Body Electric., p. 84

[58] Biphasic describes an electrical current that alternates polarity every few seconds. This is different than alternating current, which changes polarity with each pulse (as is found in standard house current).

electrode is placed down the leg, the most common reaction is poor results or even aggravation of the pain. Consider that most interferential and other stimulators used for treating sciatica only deliver biphasic current, and you will see why results with these devices are unreliable, and often make the patient feel worse. These devices are more successful, however, for pain that is localized only to the back without radiation down the leg, in which polarity is not as much of an issue.

Many Japanese acupuncture techniques utilize the Law of Polarity extensively using magnets or ion pumping cords[59]. Highly detailed techniques using north and south poles of magnets over Master acu-points have been developed for correcting structural and organic imbalances of the body[60].

> **POLARITY AND UNITY CONSCIOUSNESS**
>
> All aspects of our experience, mental, physical, emotional and energetic, are ruled by the ebbs and flows of polarity experience. It is the weariness of dealing with these constant ups and downs of experience that drives many of us to seek a spiritual path and look deeper within ourselves. The only experience available to us outside of polarity is Universal Love and deep meditation on the unchanging Source within. Touching on this experience is the fount of inner peace. An important essence of true healing is to facilitate the patient in understanding and shifting their identification as much as possible from polarity experiences to unity consciousness. This is what spiritual teachers have spoken of when they advised us to "Know Thyself".

Universal Law #3 - The Law of Economy

The Law of Economy is another vital way the Universe operates. Our bodies must also operate in harmony with this law to maintain life. Simply put, the Law of Economy is about obtaining the maximum result with the minimum expenditure of energy, or "getting more bang for your buck." It is this law that keeps the planets in their orbits, gives stability to matter, and allows life to flourish. The incredibly complex functioning of the human body requires tremendous energy. Homeostasis is defined as a state of balance within body functions that support health and well-being. Maintaining homeostasis requires a great deal of energy. Consider that it takes more energy (in the form of ATP) for a muscle to relax than to stay tense. Consider also the buffering systems in our bloodstream that maintain the narrow pH range of 7.35 – 7.45 necessary for survival. Complex feedback systems involving acid-base regulation, respiration and kidney excretion are required for this purpose. All require constant energy throughout our lifetimes. If our bodies did not operate according to the Law of Economy, we would all run out of energy frequently and our life systems would shut down.

The Law of Economy also rules subtle energy healing systems such as Toyo Hari acupuncture, homeopathy and network chiropractic. These systems recognize that a tiny amount of input can create a major amount of positive change. The X-signal system postulated by Dr. Yoshio Manaka,

---

[59] Ion pumping cords connect a set of two acupuncture needles, usually placed on Master points. They contain a diode which only allows one way flow of natural ionic current through the cord. Use of these cords greatly accelerates the energy balancing effect of these treatments. Polarized microcurrents can be used in a similar way without needles.
[60] A good example is <u>Extraordinary Vessels</u> by Matsumoto and Birch, Paradigm Publications

one of the inspirations of this book, is all about the human body's relationship with infinitesimal, immeasurable energy signals that have profound physiological and healing effects.

When the Law of Economy is not followed in the healing arts, the body has to contend with much more input than it can easily process. This puts a strain on the internal organs, primarily the liver and the kidneys. While unpleasant disease and pain symptoms may be relieved, through "overkill" drug and energy inputs, the excess stimulation or intervention often causes what are known as "side effects." Modern pharmacological medicine and surgery are full of side effects that range from annoying to life threatening. Homeopathic medicine was developed in the 1700's by Samuel Hahnemann as a reaction to heroic drug treatments that were killing and sickening many patients.

Microcurrents work through the Law of Economy in that such stimulation catalyzes the body to improve Qi and Blood circulation, and accelerate its cellular self-healing mechanisms with minimal energy input. Microcurrent electro-acupuncture is truly proof of the expression, "less is more."

Universal Law #4 - The Law of Biasology

A bias is a tendency held by a living system or being to repeatedly favor a particular direction or timing, which eventually manifests as a distortion of its structure. Biases can be physical, mental, emotional or energetic. Examples of physical biases would be the stronger right arm of a right-handed tennis player, or a forward-jutting head posture of a full time computer operator. Emotional or mental biases include prejudicial beliefs and attitudes such as "women are emotional", "acupuncture hurts" or "white men can't jump". Examples of energetic biases are adaptations our immune system makes in response to man-made electromagnetic fields around our cities, and the effect of the moon on women's menstrual cycles.

In order to correct a bias in the body, it is necessary to apply a counter-bias that balances it. Manaka made an extensive study of the biases in the human body that lead to pain and dysfunction, and formulated a system of counter-biases to correct them. He mainly used subtle energy polarity devices applied through the principal and Extraordinary meridian acu-points for this purpose. Extensive explanations and techniques for clinical applications of this principle are included in this book. To be an effective practitioner, it is vital to understand the biases that keep our patients in pain and structural imbalances, and how to correct them.

Biases can be addressed through meridian balancing, which is purely energetic, or through hands-on bodywork and manipulation. The use of both levels of input in a given treatment session can be expected to yield the most complete and long-lasting results. Again, according to the Law of Economy, we should use the minimum energy input necessary to correct biases, or side effects may be the result.

Accommodation

Accommodation, also called adaptation, is the tendency of any energy system to cease or reduce responsiveness after extended stimulation. This principle is also very important in electro-therapy and acupuncture. Recently, I dined with some friends at a restaurant in the Los Angeles area. At first, the loud rock music constantly blaring in the restaurant made communication difficult because my attention was drawn to it. After some time, however, I realized that I was much less aware of the background music and was engrossed in eating and conversation. My brain had accommodated to the ambience of the restaurant. Have you noticed the difference between a boring teacher and a captivating one? If you analyze their actions, you will see that the exciting teacher changes the tone and pitch of her voice frequently, and throws in anecdotes, jokes and practical examples. The boring teacher just directly delivers the information with less variation and interjection. In this case, the successful teacher is modulating her delivery, while the boring one is doing this much less. In the same way, a constant or repetitive energy stimulation of the body will quickly lose its ability to affect the target tissues or meridians. This is due to the body accommodating to the stimulation.

Modulation, then, is a way to re-pattern or interrupt delivery of energy in a way that prevents accommodation. This principle has been utilized in the field of acupuncture for thousands of years. Chinese acupuncture often utilizes complex needling manipulations that involve twisting, lifting, pausing and thrusting. Among other effects, these extend the effectiveness of the needling and prevent accommodation.

Modern electronics offer many methods of modulating therapeutic currents that can replace often uncomfortable needle manipulations. Even the simple and inexpensive WQ series of stimulators from China offers two knobs labeled F1 and F2 that allow two distinct alternating frequencies to be set. By attaching leads from this device to implanted needles on specific acu-points, long lasting surgical anesthesia can be induced. If a continuous frequency was used, this effect would not be as reliable, and the anesthesia would not last as long. This type of modulation, called Dense-Disperse, has been shown by modern research to activate two different pain control pathways in the body.[61] The higher frequency, set to above 100 Hz, activates dynorphins in the spinal cord and serotonin release in the brain. The lower frequency, in the 4 – 10 Hz range, stimulates release of endorphins and enkephalins through the bloodstream. This principle of modulation has been used in several modern electro-therapy devices. For example, here is a chart of the available modulations used in the Acutron Mentor device developed by the author. This device offers a wide range of valuable modulations:

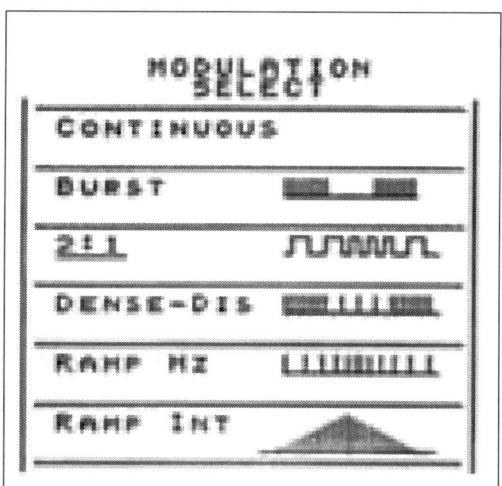

Figure 3.4: Acutron Mentor Device Modulations

Each type of modulation has a specific purpose in different preset protocols.

Another unique form of modulation offered by the Acutron Mentor is sequence combination treatments. In addition to the modulation patterns described above, effectiveness can be further extended by administering two-step treatments, with each step lasting from 5 – 10 minutes. Details on these protocols can be found in Chapter 9.

---

[61] American Journal of Acupuncture – Vol. 22, No. 1, 1994, pp. 47-54

The problem of accommodation is one of the major factors that have limited the usefulness of many energy devices, including electro-therapy devices and lasers. Creative uses of modulation have been found that counteract accommodation, thus extending the effectiveness of treatments.

Kinesiology

Kinesiology is the practice of testing the strength of a muscle or muscle group for diagnostic purposes. Much has been written and taught about this subject, including complex systems such as Applied Kinesiology and Touch for Health. Kinesiology is based on the principle that specific muscles correspond energetically to organs and systems, and certain muscle tests are accurate indicators for overall energy response. Thus, kinesiology offers a simple and reproducible way to get a "yes" or "no" answer from the body. This is quite useful for confirming in real time the appropriateness of any therapeutic technique, herb or medication. For example, if you wanted to know if a particular nutritional supplement would benefit a patient with chronic fatigue, the patient could hold the supplement while you tested an indicator muscle for overall body energy. If the muscle weakened, the supplement is of no value or harmful. If the muscle becomes strong, the supplement may be of value. For this type of testing to be accurate, however, the patient must first be cleared. [62]

Kinesiology has great value in an acupuncture practice. It can be used for accurate meridian/Organ diagnosis as well as choosing and confirming treatment points and techniques. Even with skillful Chinese medical diagnostic methods, there is still no precise indication of exactly how to treat the patient. There are many choices of acu-points, herbs or supplements for any diagnostic category. There are even more variables in the applications of microcurrent electro-acupuncture. We must choose appropriate frequencies, current intensities, polarity and much more. Selection of correct current parameters is even more important with highly sensitive chronic pain patients, as incorrect stimulation could easily aggravate their pain.

Manaka used a form of kinesiology called O Ring testing for meridian evaluation. This involves the patient touching diagnostic Alarm points with one hand while the practitioner uses the patient's other hand to test the strength of the indicator muscle. In this way, accurate readings of the energy levels of each meridian can be ascertained, and these readings can be compared with other evaluation methods such as pulse diagnosis and electronic meridian testing (EMT). Detailed instructions for O Ring testing and EMT can be found in Chapters 15 and 16.

In my practice, O Ring meridian diagnosis has been the first convincing proof of the reality of the energetic nature of their body for many of my patients. At first they often could not believe that their test hand went weak every time they touched a certain Alarm point, and then regained strength as soon as contact was broken with the point. Yet once they were convinced, their openness increased to exploring themselves as energetic beings, with non-physical causes of their pain or disease.

Summary

There are other principles of energy medicine, but those explained in this chapter are those most important for the purposes of this book. It is worth pondering these principles and observing their manifestations around you every day. As you come to understand the inevitability of the polarities of

---

[62] Clearing briefly establishes normal energy flow in the body so that results of energetic testing are accurate. This is necessary because many patients have emotional holding patterns in their bodies that can interfere with diagnosis. In a sense they are unconsciously holding back or hiding information.

your life, and become aware of positive and negative resonances in your relationships, you will become more sensitive to the responses of your patients. As you sense the oscillations of Yin and Yang and learn the polarity patterns of the human body, your ability to help them come into homeostasis and energetic balance will be greatly increased.

Chapter 4
A Brief Primer in Electrical Terminology and Theory

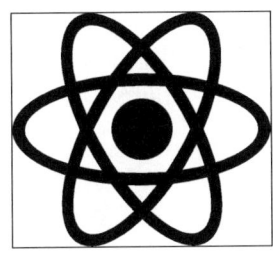

A basic understanding of electrical terms is essential for anyone utilizing microcurrent electro-acupuncture. In this chapter, you will learn how to speak intelligently about electricity and understand the electro-therapeutic parameters that make up a treatment protocol. Your first reaction may be to skip this chapter to avoid what may seem like boring, mind-numbing facts. Yet, I highly recommend taking a little time to grasp these concepts. This will greatly increase your clarity and confidence when setting up and modifying electrical therapies for your patients, and give you a peek into some of the most profound principles that govern our bodies and the Universe.

The following terms are most important in understanding electricity:

- *Atom* - the smallest unit of matter, which consists of atomic and sub-atomic particles in an electrical balance with each other. Atoms are also the smallest unit of each chemical element, such as oxygen, iron and plutonium. Although physicists have identified scores of atomic and sub-atomic particles, only two are immediately relevant to our study. Those are the electron, which is electrically negative, and the proton, which is electrically positive. Atoms differ depending on the amounts of electrons, protons and neutrons, which are electrically neutral. The electrons orbit the nucleus (composed of protons and neutrons) in discrete levels. When the outermost level of electrons is filled, and the number of electrons and protons is equal, then the unit is known as an atom, and is electrically neutral.

- *Ion* - an atom with an imbalance of either electrons or protons, making it either negatively or positively charged. Most living systems are based on ions, and energy production in a living organism is accomplished through electron transfer systems.

- *Electrical current* - the movement of electrons through a conductive medium. Electrical current is usually measured in electrical wires, but also exists in living tissues and the Earth. Currents can be harnessed to do work, such as lighting a room or running an air conditioner. Current flows from an area of greater concentration of electrons (negative pole, or cathode) to an area of lesser concentration (positive pole, or anode). Potential energy is the amount of current available for work, while kinetic energy is that current at work. When potential energy builds up to very high levels, there is often a spontaneous discharge, as in lightning or an epileptic having a seizure. Current is a measured in amperes. The output of therapeutic electromedical devices are measured in milliamps (1/1000th of an amp increments) or microamps (1/1,000,000th of an amp increments).

- *Circuit* - a medium with a positive and negative pole through which electrical currents flow. The positive pole is called the anode, and the negative pole is called the cathode. Current cannot flow through a circuit unless both poles are in contact with a conductive medium.

- *Electrical charge* - a fundamental property of matter. Biological and other substances are composed of molecules, which are made of atoms held together by electrical charges. The charge of an atom is determined by the relationship of its constituent particles, the most basic being neutrons with no charge, protons with a positive charge, and electrons with a negative charge. The ratio of electrons to protons determines the atom's charge. Electrons are much lighter than protons (1,836 times lighter) and orbit the nucleus, and so are more easily dislodged. The losing and gaining of electrons then changes the electrical charge of the atom. Electrical charge is measured in coulombs. Safety of electro-therapeutic devices is evaluated in part by the FDA[63] by the amount of micro-coulombs delivered in a given area of the body. A coulomb is defined as the charge of 6.25×10^{18} electrons.

- *Ampere (or Amp)* - a measurement unit of the amount of electrons. An ampere is defined as one coulomb of electrons moving past a fixed point in one second. When you adjust the intensity on an electro-therapeutic device, you are changing the amperage level. Therefore, intensity is the amount of milliamperes or microamperes the device is delivering to the patient.

- *Voltage* - the electromotive force, or pumping power in an electrical circuit. Frequently people confuse the terms "voltage" and "current." Put simply, *current* is the actual *amount of current* delivered in a set amount of time. *Voltage* is the *amount of force* pushing the current through the wires.

- *Resistance* - the quality of "drag" in a circuit that slows down the flow of current. The more resistance, the less current can flow. The human body is a resistor, and tends to slow the flow of electricity from electrodes. Good conductive mediums are required to minimize this effect. Resistance is measured in units called *ohms*.

- *Conductivity* - the inverse of resistance. An *ohmmeter* is a device that measures the amount of conductivity in a circuit. Devices that locate and electrically measure acu-points are or contain ohmmeters. Through the Law of Resonance, the conductivity measurements of acu-points on the skin surface reflect information about the meridians and Organs.

- *Ohm's Law* - the equation that defines the relationship between voltage, resistance and amperage. This is written as: CURRENT = VOLTAGE/RESISTANCE. This simply states that the amount of current, also called amperage, is equivalent to the voltage divided by the amount of resistance. This equation is the basis of the constant current systems used in quality electro-therapy devices. Constant current devices work by adjusting the voltage levels in accordance with changes in skin resistance, thereby keeping the current set by the user constant.

---

[63] United States Food and Drug Administration

> **OHM'S LAW AND THE HOT TUB**
>
> Your understanding of the above terms can be increased through the analogy to a hot tub spa, which may be more appealing to think of than these abstract terms alone. In a hot tub, one pipe brings heated water from the pump into the tub, while another takes water from the tub and returns it to the pump. The pipe bringing water in is analogous to the *negative pole* of an electrical circuit (cathode) that is *electron donating*. The pipe taking water out is analogous to the *positive pole* (anode) that is *electron receiving*. The pumping power of the pump motor corresponds to *voltage* in a circuit, while the diameter of the pipe creates *resistance*. The actual amount of water flowing past a fixed point in any pipe per second is equivalent to *current, or amperage*, while the total volume of water in the tub is equivalent to *coulombs*. Here's a hot tub analogy to Ohm's Law: If you make the input pipe a smaller diameter, that would create more resistance, and therefore, the pump would have to work harder (increase voltage) in order to keep the water (current) flowing into the hot tub at the same rate.

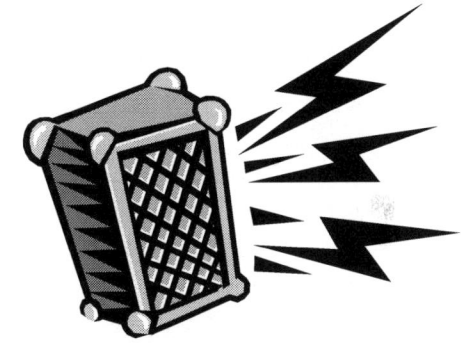

- *Capacitance* - the temporary storage and gradual discharge of electrons. This phenomenon is responsible for the ability of musical speakers to transmit sound, and is one of the ways the human body modifies or reduces electrical stimulation. According to German electro-acupuncture teachings, measurements of capacitance in the organs and tissues of the body can indicate organic degeneration and allergy conditions. For example, when measuring a test point for the Liver meridian, if the reading is in a normal range and is steady, the Liver is energetically healthy. If the reading drifts downward while the tester is maintaining steady pressure with the probe on the test point, then energy is leaking from the organ through capacitance, and there is likely to be a health problem. Chapter 16 contains more information about electronic meridian testing. Capacitors are electronic components used to create gradual discharges of current in electronic circuits to supply integrated circuit components (IC's) with their exact current requirements.

- *Frequency* - the oscillation of electrical current as it moves through a circuit. Frequency is measured in cycles per second (CPS), also known as Hertz (Hz). Correct frequency is essential to providing good clinical results for patients. According to the Law of Resonance, only a frequency that has resonance with a target tissue can affect it. German research has shown that the tissues and Organs of the body mainly resonate with very low frequencies in the 0.1 – 10 Hz range. Other American chiropractic and naturopathic research has determined specific frequencies that favorably affect pathology in joints, muscles and tendons. As mentioned in Chapter 2, Rife determined frequencies in the thousands of Hertz range that destroy pathogens while leaving healthy tissues unharmed. Fortunately, for those of us subscribing to the KISS formula[64], most microcurrent treatments can be successfully administered at the universal frequency of 10 Hz.

- *Magnetism* - electrical currents create electro-magnetic fields around itself, which have attractive and repulsive properties. Magnetism, which is measured in gauss, is used for healing purposes by some Japanese acupuncturists by placing north or south poles of magnets over specific acupoints. More general magnetic stimulation is also used through bracelets, pads and magnetic mattresses. Proponents of these treatments claim that modern civilization has cut people off from the natural magnetic fields of the Earth, creating a "magnetic deficiency syndrome." Other geophysical research has shown that the magnetic fields of the Earth have greatly decreased over the last thousands of years, leading to many chronic health problems. Research has also shown that tiny particles of magnetite or ferritin, magnetic iron containing substances, exist in the brains of animals and humans. These particles respond to the magnetic fields of the Earth, helping to guide migratory paths and offering an inner sense of direction.[65]

Electro-therapeutic Treatment Parameters

When setting up an electro-therapeutic device to treat a patient, it is necessary to select appropriate electronic treatment parameters. This is often a challenge for practitioners who consider themselves far less than a "whiz" when it comes to technical electronic terms. Some device manufacturers have reduced this stress by offering units with treatment presets. Presets allow the practitioner to set up complex treatments with a single button press. This input then instructs the microprocessor within the unit to use a set of parameters selected by the manufacturer or user to be effective for a particular disorder, such as acute low back pain or carpal tunnel syndrome.[66] Further explanations of specific presets follow later in this chapter.

To attain proficiency in pain management it is essential to have a rudimentary understanding of treatment parameters. While treatment presets greatly simplify set-up, it is sometimes necessary to modify the parameters of a preset, or create a new preset, to meet the needs of a patient or for a new protocol. The most important treatment parameters, and their effects on the body, are presented below. Some of these terms may have already been referenced previously, but they are included here for completeness.

- *Intensity* - the amount of electron current flow, measured in milli (thousandths) or micro (millionths) of an ampere. The "intensity" parameter must be adjusted frequently, and an intensity control is always easily available during treatment sessions. Microcurrent treatments are often subsensationsal, that is, "unfeelable", and so an intensity must be chosen on the basis of previous clinical experience or kinesiology[67]. Milliamp treatments must always be started at 0 intensity, and then gradually turned up to patient comfort or tolerance after starting the treatment.

    Very low currents of 10 – 50 µA offer healing acceleration effects with less immediate pain control. Relatively higher levels can control pain more directly, and may still have healing properties, although levels of 150 µA and higher may be uncomfortable to some very sensitive patients. I generally use 75 µA for most probe treatments, as this level offers rapid pain control with some degree of healing acceleration, and 50 – 100 µA for most microcurrent pad

---

[64] Keep It Simple, S--- (you fill in the last word)
[65] The Body Electric, pp .250-255
[66] The Acutron Mentor device designed by the author offers 19 pre-programmed presets and allows users to program 21 additional new ones.
[67] Kinesiology may be used to confirm correct frequency by testing an indicator muscle after one second intervals of stimulation, each at a different frequencies. The frequency that facilitates the strongest muscle test is likely to be the most beneficial.

treatments. Electro-massage, a procedure in which microcurrents are run through the therapist's hands, requires higher intensity levels of 300 - 600 µA.

- *Frequency* - the number of waveform cycles per second, measured in Hertz, or cycles per second (CPS). This parameter is very important according to the Law of Resonance as mentioned earlier in Chapter 3. Each part of the body is most affected by a specific frequency or group of frequencies. Reinhold Voll and other German doctors did extensive research on the frequency resonance of specific tissue systems.

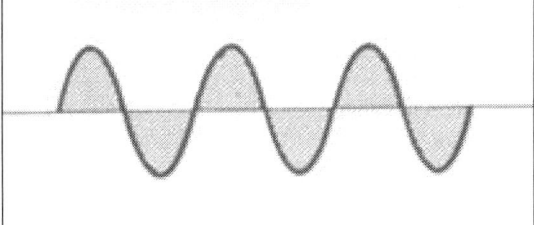

There are several sources of information about choice of electro-therapeutic frequencies, and of course contradictions exist between different sources. At least two basic frequency ranges are used therapeutically. One is the very low range of 0 – several hundred Hertz, which is most commonly used in most devices for pain management. Another is the medium kilohertz – megahertz[68] ranges that have been used in Rife generators and Lachovsky oscillator devices. These devices, which were developed in the earlier part of the 20th century, use these high frequencies for destruction of pathogens and restoration of homeostasis leading to healing, respectively. These devices are still not legally accepted into the licensed healing arts in the United States.

GENERAL CONSIDERATIONS FOR FREQUENCY SELECTION

The lower the frequency the more applicable for tissue healing acceleration and gentle treatment. The higher the frequency, the more applicable for relieving acute pain and inflammation, yet with less healing properties. These guidelines are not true in all cases, as some patients with sensitive and chronic pain may respond better to high frequencies of several hundred Hertz at times.

Two milliamp protocols that utilize kilohertz carrier frequencies to deliver lower frequencies deep into the tissues of the body are Classic interferential and Russian stimulation. Classic interferential uses 4000 Hz carrier frequencies to deliver "beat" frequencies of 10 – 100 Hz. Russian stimulation uses a carrier frequency of 2500 Hz to deliver a 50 Hz beat frequency. These complex protocols are generally preset by manufacturers and therefore require minimal user set-up.

---

[68] Kilohertz – thousands of Hertz, megahertz – millions of Hertz

- *Polarity* - the all-important Law of Polarity has been discussed in Chapter 3. In my opinion, it is lack of understanding of the application of proper polarity that is the most common reason for poor clinical results in electro-therapy and electro-acupuncture. A quality stimulator device allows the user to choose negative, positive, and biphasic treatments. In truth there is no difference between negative and positive selections on a stimulator except for reversal of electrode orientation. In other words, at any given time current is being delivered, there will always be one negative pole and one positive pole, or else current cannot flow. It is in reference to a particular electrode that polarity is designated. One electrode is often referred to as the *active* electrode, with the other as the *passive* or *dispersal* electrode. Active is usually negative polarity, as that is more stimulating due to being electron donating. Electrode lead cord tips are sometimes color-coded by manufacturers for ease of polarity recognition. Each lead cord bifurcates into two wires, each with a small metal pin that plugs into the pad electrode. For example, on the lead cords provided with the Acutron Mentor device, if polarized treatment is selected the black tipped pin is negative and the red tipped pin is positive.

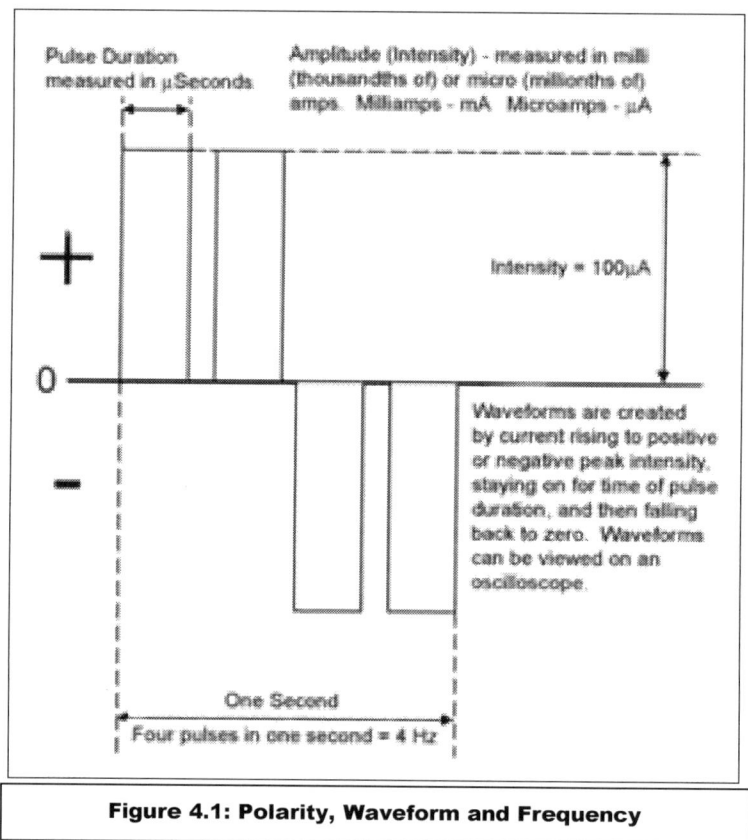

Figure 4.1: Polarity, Waveform and Frequency

The Acutron Mentor unit probe system has one probe called the trigger probe because it has a trigger switch that starts or pauses delivery of treatment currents. The other probe is called the counter probe. Each probe has an LED indicator that glows when that electrode is of the polarity selected by the user. If negative polarity is selected for a probe treatment, the trigger probe, which is the reference point, will be negative, and the counter probe positive. The LED indicator on the trigger probe will glow, confirming that that one is the negative or active probe.

Biphasic refers to an alternation of electrode polarity, thereby making the electrodes equal in clinical effect. When biphasic is chosen, the glowing of the LEDs alternate every few seconds and it is not necessary to be concerned about current polarity. Although this can simplify treatment a bit, biphasic treatments will not be as effective as polarized treatments for many meridian treatments and those involving the extremities. Many stimulator devices only offer biphasic treatments, and this factor significantly limits their versatility and effectiveness. See Chapter 8 for instructions for applying polarized and biphasic treatments.

- *Waveform* - the shape or configuration of current as it oscillates. A waveform is produced as current increases and decreases in intensity. Waveforms can be visualized on an instrument called an oscilloscope in patterns like these:

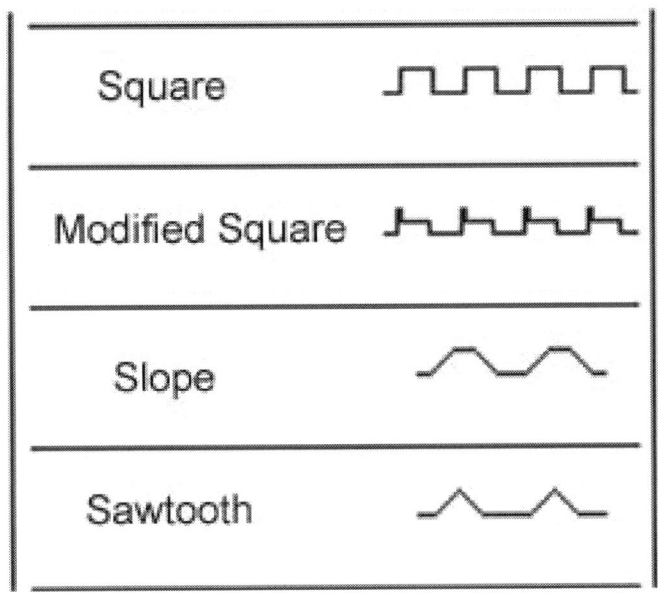

Figure 4.2: Microcurrent Waveforms

- *Modulation* - the process of patterning a treatment current to prevent accommodation or to create a special effect. Setting the correct modulation option in an electro-therapy treatment can often make the difference between success and failure. This principle is explained in Chapter 2.

- *Timer* - the function that delivers treatment currents for a specified period, then shuts treatment off. Microcurrent probe treatments are generally activated by pressing a small trigger switch on one of the probes. This activates a relay that starts treatment for a period of a few seconds up to several minutes. Treatment periods are alternated with conductivity measurements of the skin surface, also called "searching". These measurements help the practitioner to choose treatment points and evaluate changes in the points or meridians after treatment.

- *Sequence Treatments* - a form of modulation that helps to prevent accommodation and extend effectiveness of treatment. Advanced microprocessor controlled devices can offer preset treatments that have two or more parts, each for a specified time. The first part is usually more intense for relieving acute pain and tissue constriction, while the second part is gentler to support restoration of homeostasis and healing.

Treatment Presets

The parameters involved in an electro-therapy set up include the above-mentioned parameters of intensity, frequency, waveform, modulation, timing and polarity, as well as pulse duration and other variables. It can be quite intimidating and time consuming to program each of these parameters individually. Modern microprocessor technology has simplified this process by using presets. A preset is a group of pre-selected electronic parameters that have been found to be effective through long experience for a particular type of clinical condition, and which can be programmed together with the push of one button.

For example, the Acutron Mentor device has four menus of treatment presets: Probes, Microamp Pads, Milliamp Pads and Interferential. Each menu contains 4 – 6 presets, each of which contains parameters that target a particular clinical need. To illustrate an example of preset protocols, the four presets in PROBES menu are summarized below.

ACUTRON MENTOR PROBE PRESET PROTOCOLS

PRESET NUMBER	PRESET NAME	METHOD	SYMPTOMS	POLARITY
Probe #1	Local Treatment, Circling the Dragon	Local treatment of sets of acu-points that "sandwich" target tissues between the probes	Localized myofascial and joint pain, some headaches, arthritis and facial rejuvenation	*Biphasic* (alternating) (Not necessary to be concerned about + and - orientation of probes.) LED indicators will glow in alternation every few seconds
Probe #2	Dermatome / Distal Trigger Probe (-)	Pairs of local and distal acu-points treated together	Extremity disorders such as carpal tunnel syndrome and sciatica where polarized treatments are required. Used for meridian balancing.	*Fixed polarity* Trigger probe negative (LED continually glowing)
Probe #3	Acute	Local treatment of sets of acu-points that "sandwich" target tissues between the probes	Release of trigger points and areas of acute, inflammatory pain	*Biphasic* Most aggressive. Waveforms, frequencies, intensity and modulations programmed to have strong influence on stimulated tissues
Probe #4	Gentle / Chronic	Local treatment of sets of acu-points that "sandwich" target tissues between the probes	Treatment of infants and chronic pain patients that have poor tolerance for electrical stimulation	*Biphasic*

Table 4.3: Acutron Mentor Probe Preset Protocols

The other menus on the Acutron Mentor have similar choices.[69] Again, each preset described above has a specific combination of intensity, frequency, polarity, modulation, waveform and timing to optimize treatment results for the conditions for which it is indicated

---

[69] See Acutron Mentor Instruction and Training Manual for more details on presets.

CHAPTER 5

PRINCIPLES OF PAIN MANAGEMENT EAST AND WEST

Many lengthy volumes have been written about the theory and physiology of pain from a Western scientific perspective. Pain, by its very nature, is an urgent message from our bodies demanding immediate response. It is estimated by one prominent educator that Americans spend over *one hundred billion* dollars a year on various phases of pain control and management. This staggering figure includes the cost of medication, treatment by health professionals, hospital stays, and time lost at work due to back pain, headaches and other pain maladies. Since you are reading this book, it is likely that much of your income is derived from people seeking relief from the urgent message of pain, and you are motivated to find more effective ways to help these patients.

With all this money and expertise being directed toward the problem of pain, there is little clear scientific understanding of exactly what pain is. To quote from the landmark book *The Challenge of Pain* by Melzack and Wall:

> "Pain is such a common experience that we rarely pause to define it in ordinary conversation. Yet no one who has worked on the problem of pain has ever been able to give it a definition that is satisfactory to all of his colleagues. Pain has obvious sensory qualities, bit it also has emotional and motivational elements. It is usually caused by intense, noxious stimulation, yet it sometimes occurs spontaneously without apparent cause. It normally signals physical injury, but it sometimes fails to occur even when extensive areas of the body have been seriously injured; at other times it persists after all the injured tissues have healed and becomes a crippling problem that may require urgent, radical treatment."[70]

It is common knowledge among pain professionals that many patients who show significant physical findings in x-rays and MRIs live relatively pain free. These findings include protruding and herniated disks, massive scar tissue impinging on nerves, bone on bone in joint due to

---

[70] Melzack and Wall, The Challenge of Pain, 1983, from preface

worn away cartilage and bursae and other similar conditions. Yet, so many others who have no such physical findings complain of severe chronic pain. Pain is a complex phenomenon that involves much more than just injury or damage to nerves.

Western medicine and traditional Asian healing systems evolved independently for thousands of years, and therefore offer strikingly different explanations for many body functions, including pain. These different understandings of the causes of pain have led to development of treatment interventions based on those understandings. In this chapter, we will briefly examine the theories of the origin and control of pain in Eastern and Western medicines.

Western Pain Electro-physiology

In Western medicine and research, pain is regarded as a neurochemical phenomenon. Extensive research has been done to explain exactly how pain impulses travel from the injury site through the central nervous system, and how pain is modified.

Pain impulses start as stimulation of sensory nerve fibers, that exists in skin, muscle, internal organs, bone and most other body tissues. Interestingly, most of the brain, the largest part of the nervous system, contains no pain receptors.[71] Pain nerve fibers overlay each other in branching clusters. When any part of the sensory nerve network is damaged or sharply stimulated, then it sends multiple electrically coded signals through various afferent[72] nerve pathways to the spinal cord, traveling at different frequencies and speeds. These signals enter the spinal cord through a region called the dorsal horn, containing a network of dense fibers called the substantia gelatinosa. Here the signals change frequency and speed and move up the antero-lateral tracts of the spinal cord toward the lower part of the brain. Some of the pain signals follow the tract that leads to the part of the lower brain called the thalamus, along the spinothalamic tract. Most of the signals go directly to an area called the reticular formation, where most pain processes of the brain take place. This acts as a switchboard from which pain signals are routed to other parts of the brain. One area receiving pain impulses is the limbic system, a site of much conditioning and emotional response. The little girl who cries after banging her finger in the car door is probably experiencing a stimulation of the limbic system. The same is true for a chronic pain patient who is depressed and suicidal about his pain. Some pain signals are routed to the cerebral cortex, which cannot feel pain directly, but can think and reason about it.

Pain messages do not just travel one way. The brain also sends signals back down the spinal cord that modify pain in various ways. Narcotic-like peptide substances called endorphins and enkephalins that naturally inhibit pain have been discovered in the central nervous system. These are particularly dominant in the spinal cord and midbrain, specifically the regions known as the corpus striatum, amygdala, periaqueductal gray area and anterior hypothalamus[73]. Many researchers have found that electrically stimulating the periaqueductal gray area can produce significant analgesic effects. Opiates such as morphine apparently mimic the effects of these substances by stimulating the receptors sensitive to endorphins and enkephalins. A substance can only affect the body if receptor sites already exist for it. The effects of injected morphine seem to be based on a descending pain control effect from the midbrain.[74]

Endorphin, enkephalins and dynorphins are classified as endogenous opiates, substances which have similar molecular structure to plant opiates such as morphine. In addition to

---

[71] This is why anesthesia is not needed for brain surgery, except to numb the scalp.
[72] See Glossary
[73] Zhong-yi Liu, M.D, Acupuncture For Chronic Pain AJA Volume 8, #4, 1980
[74] Ibid.,, Ref 1, p. 171

endogenous opiates, there are neurotransmitter substances that modify pain such as serotonin, noradrenalin, dopamine, acetylcholine and gamma aminobutyric acid (GABA). There is experimental evidence that pain can be reduced, and opiate drugs made more effective, by increasing neurotransmission via promotion of these substances.[75] This holds interesting parallels to the TCM principle that pain can be relieved by increasing flow of Qi through areas in which it is stagnant.

Much research has been done to determine how electro-acupuncture (EA) analgesia relates to endogenous neurochemicals. It has been confirmed that release of these substances is frequency-specific[76]. Low frequency stimulation of 2 Hz is mediated by enkephalins via brain receptors, while high frequency (100 Hz) is mediated by dynorphins via spinal cord receptors. Dense-Disperse is a form of electrical stimulation modulation that alternates between these two frequencies every 4 – 5 seconds, and has been found to promote longer lasting and more efficient analgesia by activating dual pathways of pain control.

Neurochemicals are not the only descending pain modulation system from the brain. It is now recognized that attitudes, beliefs and previous experiences modify the perception of pain. Stoic attitudes about pain, or a collapsing "crybaby" response, are each determined by deeply held attitudes in consciousness that derive from past experience. There are probably other electrical signals sent from the higher brain down through the spinal cord that can control pain by regulating input of noxious impulses from sensory nerves. Through a combination of release of neurochemicals, descending electrical nerve signals and the force of belief and attitude, the brain can strongly influence and modify the perception of pain. Many chronic pain centers offer meditation and biofeedback programs that help pain patients modify their pain sensations through mediation of higher centers of consciousness.

Western Pain Treatments

In North America and Europe, most pain complaints are initially treated by medical doctors, osteopaths or chiropractors. M.D.'s prescribe pain medication, refer to physical therapists or psychotherapists, or in severe cases perform or refer patients for surgery. Chiropractors and some osteopaths manipulate the spine and other joints to take noxious pressure off the nervous system.

In response to the need for alternative treatments for the growing amount of chronic pain patients, many hospitals and other institutions have founded pain clinics. Anesthesiologists have often been asked to work in these clinics. These doctors have had to learn new methods beyond operating room anesthesia such as trigger point injections and pharmaceutical nerve blocks. Many of the more innovative pain clinics also offer consciousness based pain management such as bio-feedback training, meditation, counseling, visualization and yoga, as well as utilizing the services of acupuncturists and chiropractors. Physical and occupational therapists usually direct most of their treatments to rehabilitation, work hardening, exercise and other methods to help patients regain strength and function in the injured part of their bodies, and are generally less focused on pain treatment in itself.

Most of these interventions deal primarily with symptomatic relief of pain. The main exceptions are some of the alternative pain clinic treatments and physical therapies and chiropractic treatments that help patients strengthen and balance their body mechanics and adjust perceptions and attitudes.

---

[75] Hing-Gwan Kho and Eric Robertson, The Mechanisms of Acupuncture Analgesia, AJA, Vol. 25, #4, 1997
[76] Chen Xiao-Hong et al Optimal Conditions for Eliciting Maximal Electroacupuncture Analgesia with Dense and Disperse Mode Stimulation,_, AJA Vol. 22, #!, 1994

The tremendous surge of interest in acupuncture and other so-called alternative therapies is evidence that the Western model of pain management is incomplete. Western medicine is at its best for emergency, life-saving interventions, but has less to offer in the diagnosis, prevention and treatment of many types of chronic and complex disorders. This also applies to pain management. There is no better system than modern Western medicine to help an accident sufferer with severe physical trauma, but skilled acupuncture and/or bodywork treatments is often superior for treatment of chronic pain and mysterious, hard to diagnose maladies.

This discussion of the Western view of pain physiology is brief and by no means complete. This is an abundance of published literature available on the subject. This summary is offered to show the basic mindset of Western medicine, which is a search for physical and bio-chemical explanations and treatments for pain and disease. The rigorous methodology of Western research into pain has offered many valuable explanations how our bodies transmit and modify pain sensations that are left unexplained by traditional healing systems. Now let's look at the view of Chinese medicine on this subject.

Traditional Chinese Medicine Pain Theory and Practice

TCM[77] diagnosis is based on an inductive approach, assessing a myriad of signs and symptoms to arrive at the recognition of a pattern of disharmony. Treatment is therefore directed toward addressing the overall pattern as a means to address specific symptoms. Such pattern treatment is often combined with symptomatic treatments using acupuncture and other methods of stimulation of the meridians. While Western research regards pain primarily as the perception of noxious stimulation to the nervous system that can be modified by neurochemistry or surgery, TCM views pain as a sensation that arises from a multidimensional pattern of dysfunction.

One of the great gifts of Chinese medicine is the recognition of these patterns of disharmony. When pain is addressed through treatment of a correctly identified pattern, results are likely to be far better and longer lasting than when pain is treated as an entity in itself, as is commonly done with Western pain treatments. The bogeyman of "side effects" that plague drug-based modern medicine are in large part due to using techniques to silence the messengers of pain and disease symptoms without addressing the underlying pattern.

A good example of the more comprehensive nature of TCM diagnosis is the diagnosis and treatment of back pain. Western doctors will generally use orthopedic tests and MRI or x-rays to look for mechanical abnormalities such as bone spurs, herniated disks, scoliosis or stenosis. They may also check internal organs for severe disorders such as kidney or gallstones. Treatment will generally consist of physical therapy, surgery or drugs. Chiropractors of course use manipulation of the spine to treat back pain. In the practice of TCM, there are over 30 possible etiologies of back pain including Stagnant Qi and/or Blood, Liver Fire, Kidney Yin deficiency, Kidney Yang deficiency, Phlegm affecting the Lower Warmer, as well as traumatic injury. Treatment will involve a combination of acupuncture and/or herbal formulas specific to the diagnosis, as well as Oriental physical therapies such as shiatsu, tuina and manipulation. A course of such pattern-specific treatment is more likely than most Western approaches to clear up the underlying condition by bringing the whole body into improved homeostasis.

---

[77]TCM stands for Traditional Chinese Medicine. TCM has been somewhat sanitized by the Chinese government to avoid ambiguities that seem "unscientific", and so is not necessarily fully expressive of the depth of this art. In this text, we will use the abbreviation TCM to refer to true holistic pattern-based treatment, beyond the limitations of the politically correct official version.

Complete training in TCM diagnosis is beyond the scope of this book. For further reference, a list of excellent texts can be found in the bibliography. In this chapter, we will offer an overview of the aspects of TCM that are relevant to pain management.

Etiology of Pain According to TCM

The most fundamental understanding of pain in TCM is that it is the experience that arises when some aspect of our body/mind complex is in a holding pattern, and not moving and circulating freely and harmoniously. The specific substances in our bodies that can be so constrained are primarily Qi and Blood. The spiritual essences described by Chinese medical classics, Shen[78], Hun[79], and Po[80] may also give rise to pain when not functioning in harmony with the body. This is in accordance with the new understanding in the West of "psychosomatic" etiologies of pain and disease.

Chinese medicine and philosophy are based on the view that human beings represent the marriage of Heaven (Cosmos) and Earth. Heaven and Earth represent the two poles of existence that encompass our being – the most high and subtle vibration and most gross, dense and grounded energies. We are meant to function as open channels or intermediaries between Heaven and Earth. When we are thus open, harmony, good health, prosperity and happiness are our predominating experiences.

When we use our will and thought to act and think in ways that are out of harmony with Universal Law (Tao) pain arises. These choices away from the Tao lead to blockages and constrictions in the vital substances of our body/mind, which are experienced as pain. Even pain from traumatic injuries may be looked at as a result of living out of harmony with Tao, which may attract disharmonious events such as accidents and attacks due to being in the wrong place at the wrong time. The implication is that acupuncturists and other practitioners of the healing arts are foremost teachers to help patients learn to live in harmony with Tao, and secondly relievers of symptoms.

According to Chinese medicine, there are exogenous, endogenous and miscellaneous "Evils" (influences that can cause pain and dysfunction). The following sums up these influences:

Exogenous Environmental Evils

The exogenous (or externally created) evils, as described in classics of Chinese Medicine are: *Wind, Cold, Dampness, and Heat / Summer Heat.*

Rather than just dutifully memorize this list as I did in acupuncture school, it is worthwhile to reflect on its meaning. During flu season, it is easy to see the effects of Wind and Cold, as so many people manifest symptoms of runny nose, body aches, fevers and chills and malaise. In addition, here in Phoenix, Arizona, it is very easy to see the effects of pathogenic Heat, especially among those brave souls who attempt to hike in the summer! Yet, it is also obvious that, exposed to the same climatic influences some people get sick and most don't. Wind is only an Evil to those individuals who lack sufficient bodily homeostasis and defensive Qi[81]. So

---

[78] Shen, which dwells in the Heart, integrates all aspects of consciousness and is master of the central nervous system.

[79] Hun, which dwells in the Liver, is somewhat analogous to the Western concept of Soul, and harmonizes mental and emotional balance.

[80] Po, which dwells in the Lungs, gives rise to primal sensations, including pain.

[81] Defensive Qi is called Wei Qi in Chinese. It is a coarse (lower vibratory) level of Qi that is abundant on the surface of the body in a healthy person, and protects against climatic extremes. Strict vegetarians often lack abundant Wei Qi, as it is often the coarse vibration of meat that is most helpful in replenishing it.

none of the climatic influences is really "evil." Again, it is our lack of harmony with Tao that allows the "evil" to be a problem for us.

Endogenous Evils

Endogenous (or internally created) evils are extremes of emotions that bring the person out of harmony.

EXTREMES OF EMOTIONS IN CHINESE MEDICINE

Normal, Healthy Emotion	Associated Organ/ Element	Spirit Essence	Emotion Out of Harmony
Joy	Heart / Fire	Shen (Spirit)	Manic, too much mental / outer focus which disperses energy
Introspection	Spleen / Earth	Yi (Thought)	Overly detached from life, lack of spontaneity, heavy
Grief	Lungs / Metal	Po (Corporeal soul)	Obsessed with loss, can't let go, "wasting away"
Fear	Kidneys / Water	Zhi (Will)	Frozen, phobic, chronic tension and holding in body, intense fear, fright
Anger	Liver / Wood	Hun (Ethereal Soul)	Chronic raging, violence to self and others, depression

Figure 5.1: Extremes of Emotions in Chinese Medicine

Again, it is clear that the entire range of human emotions is normal and healthy in appropriate circumstances. "To all things there is a season". It is only repeated extremes of emotion that become pain and disease causing factors. So why do we indulge in such extremes? From some careful "introspection" it appears that all the "out of harmony" emotional patterns are adaptations to an ongoing feeling of disconnectedness with the Tao, the Universe, inner truth. The antidote to all these patterns is deep love and awareness of unity consciousness, the ultimate harmonizer of all separate aspects of self. To be an effective healer, it is necessary to ask ourself why and how our patient has come out of harmony with inner love and harmony in his life, and how he can return to it.

One of the amazing gifts of acupuncture is that stimulation of appropriate points and balance of the meridian system can actually assist a person in finding inner balance and harmony with the Tao, therefore emotional and spiritual healing. In the West, we usually consider all treatment of emotional and spiritual issues to be strictly in the province of psychotherapists, counselors and psychiatrists, or part of religious or spiritual practice. We would usually not think of sending a person to a physical therapist to treat depression. Yet the physical intervention of stimulating acu-points can help remove some of the blockages to the free flow of Qi and Blood, as well as supporting the Spiritual Essences in being full and balanced. Such interventions help the patient to feel a new alignment of energy in her body, in effect teaching her how to manage her energy in a more abundant and healthy way.

This is similar to biofeedback, which trains people to regulate their brain waves to stay in "alpha"[82] frequency. Once a person feels what it is like to be aware of balanced energy in his body, proper breathing, relief of pain and ease of mobility, it can be easier for him to adjust to staying in this state. The microcurrent electro-acupuncture techniques explained in the following chapters are very useful toward this end, especially the meridian balancing and kinetic interferential procedures.

---

[82] Alpha is the brainwave ranges of 8 – 14 Hz that is associated with alertness and well being.

Miscellaneous Evils

The classics of Chinese medicine mention a few other pathogenic influences besides those from weather and emotional excess. They are: *improper diet, sexual excesses, pestilence (infectious disease), parasites, lifestyle not in harmony with Tao*

In modern times, we can certainly identify many new Evils that adversely affect our health and potentially lead to pain and disease. These would include: *radiation, electromagnetic pollution, air and water pollution, increased stress from fast paced life, breakdown of traditional family and society structures, repeated negative and violent images from media, denatured foods, pesticides, herbicides, food additives, hormones given to livestock and chickens, exposure to viruses from all over the world through increased travel and trade, thinning of ozone layer of atmosphere exposing us to new pathogenic influences, drug and alcohol use*

The Liver and Pain Management

While dysfunction of any vital Organ can lead to pain due to deficiency or stagnation of Qi and/or Blood, the Liver is the Organ most intimately connected with pain. Western medicine recognizes the physical liver as a factory and processing center for metabolic substances and by-products, while TCM views the Liver in a more expansive way. In addition to its metabolic functions, the Liver has the following functions:

- *Storing Blood* – The Liver regulates the volume of circulating Blood, thereby influencing the functions of all Organs and tissues as well as menstruation. Therefore, dysmenorrhea and many types of myofascial pain are related to Liver dysfunction.

- *Controlling tendons* – The Liver supplies Yin and Blood to the tendons, keeping them flexible and strong. Tendinitis, a common cause of pain from overuse and athletic injuries, occurs most commonly in people with Liver imbalances.

- *Influencing the eyes* - The Liver directly communicates with the eyes through internal meridian pathways. When the Liver is not functioning optimally in regulating Qi and Blood, this predisposes the eyes to diseases such as poor vision, conjunctivitis, cataracts and macular degeneration.

- *Regulating the smooth flow of Qi* - As mentioned above, when we are in balance with Heaven and Earth, we freely circulate and blend energies in our bodies. The Liver is the function in our bodies that is most responsible for this free circulation of energy. When the Liver is healthy in this way, we feel energized, relaxed, confident and empowered. When it is not smoothly regulating the Qi, some combination of anger, depression, rage, nervous tension and physical pain result. This is why the Hun, or the spiritual Soul, is said to reside in the Liver. Back and neck pain and chronic headaches and migraines are common in people with constrained Liver Qi. Understanding this connection of the spiritual Soul and energy stagnation helps us to see the common relationship between spiritual disconnectedness and chronic pain.

  The proper functioning of the Liver, based on it's function of qi flow regulation, is of prime importance in acupuncture pain management. The acu-point combination the "Four Gates", consisting of bilateral stimulation of LI 4 and Liv 3, is a harmonizing treatment that relieves many kinds of pain and tension through the Liver. The Four-Step protocol described in Section III starts with measuring and balancing the Organ/meridian system, which often addresses the root Liver imbalances. This is of great value in administering effective and long lasting therapy.

Chinese Medical Diagnosis

Fig. 5.2 Diagnostic Patterns and Treatment Protocols

Pattern	Examples of Painful Conditions	Pulse & Tongue Indications	Treatment
Stagnation of Qi	Traumatic joint and muscle pain, dysmenorrhea with bloating, purplish blood and distended breasts, Raynaud's phenomenon	P: Wiry T: normal or purplish	Acupuncture Electro-acupuncture Qi moving herbs
Stagnation of Blood	Stabbing low back pain after traumatic sprain, myocardial infarction (M.I.), angina pectoris	P: Choppy or irregular T: purplish with possible red spots	Western medical intervention for M.I. Blood letting[83] Blood moving herbs
Accumulation of Cold	Abdominal pain made better with warm drinks and applications Painful groin / testicles with cold feelings	P: Deep, tight or slow T: pale or white coat	Moxibustion Hot compresses Warming herbs
Accumulation of Heat	Painful diarrhea with fever, rheumatoid arthritis in inflammatory stage	P: Rapid T: red material with possible yellow coat	Acupuncture Microcurrent therapies Cold applications Cooling herbs
Accumulation of Phlegm	Headache with feelings of heaviness and possible vertigo, cystitis with greasy discharge, distended abdomen with heavy feeling	P: Slippery T: greasy white or yellow coat (white greasy coat on pale tongue for cold phlegm and yellow greasy coat on red tongue for damp-heat)	Acupuncture Dampness clearing herbs Dietary changes
Deficiency of Qi	Mild intermittent cramping and bloating pain due to PMS with low energy and/or anemia, dull, "spacey" headaches	P: Weak and thready T: pale or lusterless with little or no coat	Tonifying acupuncture Microcurrent meridian balancing Moxibustion Tonifying herbs
Accumulation of Phlegm and Heat	See above for phlegm and heat	P: Slippery and rapid T: red with greasy yellow coat (combining Phlegm and Heat patterns)	See above for Phlegm and Heat

---

[83] Bloodletting is the practice of bleeding a few drops of blood out of distended arteries or veins on affected meridians to relieve the intense pain of blood stagnation.

In order to arrive at an accurate diagnosis for a painful complaint, it is necessary to understand the patterns that involve painful sensations. The Eight Guiding Principles of diagnosis are a way to quickly put the complaint into a perspective that leads to a suitable treatment approach. The Guiding Principles are:

HOT	**COLD**
EXCESS	**DEFICIENT**
EXTERNAL	**INTERNAL**
YANG	**YIN**

Is the pain of a hot or cold nature? Is it relieved by ice or better relieved by hot compresses? Is it Excess, which is felt as more intense, acute pain due to stagnation of Qi and Blood or stagnation due to Cold, or is it Deficient, which is felt as duller, milder pain associated with weakness and retarded circulation? Is the pain of of the skin or myofascial tissues (External) or of the deeper organ and tissue (Internal) level? These principles provide a framework to understand the overall nature and location of the complaint. TCM recognizes six main diagnostic patterns that produce painful symptoms. Two essential diagnostic tools in TCM are pulse and tongue observation. Each pattern produces a distinctive effect on these indicators. Again, for complete information about these tools the reader is directed to other acupuncture texts.

It should be clear from the chart on the next page that TCM diagnosis cannot be arrived at from a symptomatic description only. In each case other data is needed, such as cold sensations, better by hot drinks, distended breasts or abdomen, as well as pulse and tongue evaluation (see below).

Microcurrent electro-acupuncture is at its best for relieving painful conditions due to stagnation of Qi, and may be all that is required for such conditions. This is the most common presentation in a pain management practice, including most myofascial and many joint-related pain syndromes. Microcurrent treatment may also be used as part of a complete treatment plan in all the other above categories except for stagnation of Blood, for which its benefits appear to be less pronounced. Yet even in this case, such treatment may help to prevent Blood stagnation.

There are two main styles of acupuncture pain management are in use in the West today. One deals with identifying and treating the overall patterns of disharmony according to the principles of traditional Chinese medicine, along with some symptomatic treatment. (A few schools of acupuncture, notably the so-called Five Element schools,[84] discourage their students from offering any direct symptomatic treatment.) The other is cookbook, symptomatic acupuncture based on formulas of acu-points for treating each presenting problem with minimal understanding or treatment of the overall pattern of disharmony. I do not condemn the second approach, but simply state that it is highly limited, and will not yield positive results nearly as much as the first. I do not condemn symptomatic treatment because it does relieve pain in many cases, and is particularly valuable for first aid and patient self-treatment with acupressure

---

[84] Five Element, or Five Phase acupuncture is a system that is totally holistic, and based on Five Elements of Fire, Earth, Metal, Water and Wood, and elaborate Elemental correspondences of Organs, colors, sounds, directions, foods, emotions, and much more. These are used to determine key aspects of the transformation of energy in the body that are "calling for help". Practitioners of this system are generally more inclined toward treatment of emotional and mental complaints than are most other acupuncturists, and rarely treat pain and injury directly from a symptomatic perspective.

and moxa rolls.[85] Symptomatic treatment can be remarkably effective with microcurrent electro-acupuncture. I have heard from many practitioners who have reported surprisingly powerful results in pain control to me using simple microcurrent treatments through localized applications, prior to studying any of the instructions or techniques.

It will take a more comprehensive approach than symptomatic treatment, however, to adequately deal with the needs of many of the modern patients who walk through our doors. It is common to have patients presenting complex and multi-layered disorders, combining aspects of chronic injuries and pain with Organ weakness, consequences of poor diet, environmental toxins and/or low-grade viral infections, and stress-related emotional and mental imbalances. Even if symptomatic treatment gives these patients some pain relief, it is likely to be short-lived and unsatisfactory.

Root and Branch

The terms Root and Branch go back to complex ancient Chinese astrology systems, many of which are still used by modern acupuncturists to select "open" treatment acu-points based on specific dates and clients' astrological signs. A much simpler understanding of Root and Branch can be used as a triage[86] tool for determining the correct priority and sequence of treatment for a patient.

In this simplified view, the Root represents the deeper TCM pattern of disharmony, or a specific causative factor from a Western perspective such as low-grade infection, toxicity, genetic predisposition or unhealthy lifestyle habits. The Branch represents the actual symptomatic complaint. For example, a patient comes to you with a complaint of migraines aggravated by emotional stress. The actual pain she is complaining about is in her head. Your diagnosis reveals a wiry pulse, normal tongue, and electronic meridian testing[87] and abdominal diagnosis show a Liver imbalance. According to these diagnostic signs, in this case the Root is constrained Liver Qi[88], and the Branch is vascular pressure in the head causing severe pain. So, do you treat the Root, the Branch, or both?

This is an important question. In each profession dealing with pain management, treatment decisions concerning Root and Branch come up frequently. In the above case example, should an acupuncturist try to first sedate or disperse Qi and Yang in the head with local treatment, or stimulate Liver Qi circulation throughout the body? Or should she support the Yin to cool the Liver? Should a chiropractor adjust to give as much fast relief of neck pain as possible, or work on overall soft tissue balance and teach the patients exercises and stress relieving methods to get to the cause? Should a M.D. treating severe arm pain first inject anesthetics to produce a nerve block, or use more extensive testing to determine the underlying cause and prescribe conservative physical therapy before drug therapy?

Understanding when to treat the Root and when to treat the Branch is a prime art of the acupuncturist and other pain management professionals. A few simple guidelines can be offered here. These are general guidelines only and not rules for all situations:

---

[85] Acupressure is the act of using manual pressure on acu-points to relieve pain and other problems. Moxa is a dried wool of the *Artemesia Vulgaris* mugwort plant that is burned over or on acu-points to add heat and energy to selected acu-points and body areas.
[86] Triage is the practice of determining the clinical priorities of treatment, either in an emergency room setting or for an individual patient's treatment plan.
[87] This is explained in Section IV
[88] Constrained Liver Qi is a TCM diagnostic pattern that is common among people with so called "stress-related" complaints. According to TCM, the Liver is responsible for the free flowing circulation of Qi throughout the body, and when it is impaired in this function, many types of physical pain, digestive problems and emotional instability result.

Treat the Branch first when:

- A patient comes to you with intense acute pain that is significantly limiting movement, and is causing severe muscle tension and cramping.
- The pain or injury is acute and of recent origin in an otherwise healthy person, such as with many athletes or workers compensation patients.
- The patient is highly skeptical of acupuncture, and needs some rapid reassurance that it "works" so he or she will continue treatment.
- In other emergency first aid situations.

Treat the Root first when:

- You have tried skilled symptomatic Branch treatment and the pain is not relieved.
- The patient presents with chronic pain that has defied many types of treatments.
- The patient has significant Deficiency of Qi and/or Blood.
- The patient's pain is clearly tied to mental and emotional imbalances.
- The patient is hypersensitive, and may react with aggravations to direct symptomatic treatment. This is often true in cases with reflex sympathetic dystrophy, fibromyalgia, and various types of neuropathic pain.
- The patient presents with pain associated with violence and abuse with which there are significant traumatic emotional overlays.
- The patient is presenting with "rebellious Qi" or *nobose* (same concept in Japanese). This is a condition presenting troublesome symptoms of the head and upper body such as headaches, hypertension, chronic shoulder tension, dizziness and sense organ disturbances due to rising Yang Qi. The Yang is inappropriately rising due to weak and deficient root energies in the lower abdomen, also called the Tantien in Chinese or Hara in Japanese. The Yang that should be freely circulating throughout the body is moving too much in an upward direction, like a helium balloon without ballast, and causing problems because it is not sufficiently anchored by the Yin Qi of the Tantien.

Treat the Root and Branch together when:

- It is appropriate to treat the Root, as mentioned above, and it is also possible and a priority to relieve pain and bring about structural balance of the body. This is appropriate in a wide range of modern patients, and is excellently addressed by the Four-Step Protocol described in Section III.
- You only have a limited amount of time or visits to resolve the patient's complaints due to geographical or financial constraints, and she needs both Root and Branch treatment.
- Treating inflammatory diseases such as rheumatoid arthritis or inflammatory bladder infections. Support the Yin and cool Fire (Root), and it may also be appropriate to perform local microcurrent treatment on the affected joints or body regions to move the stagnant Qi and reduce inflammation.

Root and Branch Treatments

The table on the next page provides some guidelines to understand which treatments address the Root and which more address the Branch. Please understand that most of the treatments in each list could potentially be used for Root or Branch treatment. This is why what we practice is called the "healing arts". These lists are provided to help you understand the practical applications of this principle.

PRINCIPLES OF ROOT AND BRANCH TREATMENTS

BRANCH TREATMENTS	ROOT TREATMENTS
- Local dispersion of ah shi acu-points with needles or microcurrent probes	- Extraordinary vessel acupuncture or microcurrent treatment[91]
- Treatment of the tendinomuscular meridian system[89]	- Most treatments addressing the internal Organs
- Most treatments to reduce symptoms around the head, neck, shoulders and extremities	- Strengthening and balancing the lower abdomen to root and ground Qi
- Auricular therapy symptomatic points, Korean hand points, foot reflexology	- Meridian balancing work
- Herbal formulas and singles that clear the surface, purge fire, drain fluids or other symptomatic relief	- Auricular therapy Master point formulas
	- Auricular medicine[92]
- Local electric stimulation: interferential currents, Russian stimulation, TENS, high volt galvanic	- Constitutional acupuncture and herbal medicine
- Most milliamp (high intensity) electro-therapies	- Treatment to tonify and harmonize Qi, Blood, Shen and Essence[93]
- Trigger point physical therapy treatments (may address the Root as well)	- Dietary therapy, cleaning up lifestyle excesses
- Drug injection treatments - nerve blocks, trigger points	- Myofascial release work, Rolfing, shiatsu, core energetics (these treatments can be more directed toward either Root or Branch depending on the intent and skill of the practitioner)
- Osseous manipulation (this can address Root as well in many cases)	
- Work hardening physical therapies	- Homeopathy and other vibrational medicines
- Most aspects of rehabilitation work	- Most kinds of emotional and spiritual healing
- Most types of surgery	- Treatments to strengthen the immune system
- Antibiotics, steroids, anti-inflammatory, NSAIDS[90], cocaine derivatives, opiates (these drugs can in some cases treat the Root, but are rarely used that way)	- Meditation, prayer, breath work, bio-feedback
	- Qigong, tai chi exercises
- Most psychotropic drugs	

Figure 5.3: Principles of Root and Branch Treatments

For specific suggestions on choosing acu-points for Root and Branch treatments, see Section III and the Treatment Formulary.

---

[89] Tendino-muscular meridians are a network of superficial channels that circulate Yang Qi through the muscles and tendons. These channels exchange Qi with the principle meridians, and can become Excess when the principle meridians are Deficient, and vice versa.
[90] Non-steroidal anti-inflammatory drugs such as aspirin, ibuprofen, etc.
[91] Extraordinary vessels are a system of deep energy regulatory channels that drains Excess or replaces Deficiency from the principal meridians. They can be treated to correct structural and Organic imbalances from a Root level.
[92] Auricular therapy is the practice of stimulating ear points for mostly symptomatic relief. Auricular medicine is using the ear in conjunction with the pulse to choose energetic remedies and regulate the body/mind
[93] Essence is pure and distilled Yin substance that is involved with genetics, sexuality and reproduction

Four-Step Pain Mastery Protocol

The Four-Step pain mastery protocol described in Section III is a valuable and practical system that systematically combines Root and Branch treatments within single treatment sessions. This system is straightforward and highly accessible, even to those who have not yet mastered the intricacies of traditional Chinese diagnostics. It allows truly holistic patient treatment, yet also maintains a strong focus on giving the relief and rapid resolution our patients come to us for. Diagnosis in this system is simpler than in TCM, in which understanding of a more detailed and accurate pattern must be arrived at to allow for selection of complex herbal formulas.

Section II

Microcurrent Electro-Acupuncture Treatment Techniques

INTRODUCTION

"The journey of a thousand miles starts with the first step."

Some of my students have expressed feeling overwhelmed by how much new information there is to assimilate in the practice of microcurrent electro-acupuncture. My usual response is that it is necessary to walk before one is ready to run. In this case, walking refers to learning the basic techniques of microcurrent therapy first, and then running with it by expanding to more precise or complex meridian based methods later.

In this Section, Chapter 6 will discuss why most practitioners do not have more consistent and positive clinical successes, and how your patients can enjoy far superior results. Chapter 7, the lengthiest, details a comprehensive range of hands-on microcurrent therapies using probe electrodes including whole-body meridian therapies. Chapter 8 deals with one of the most powerful pain-relieving methods for the extremities -- polarized probe treatment of the Great Loops of the meridian system. Chapter 9 covers electro-stimulation through pad electrode techniques, including interferential, Russian stimulation and kinetic methods.

The techniques presented here have been synthesized from many sources in several countries. Some of the microcurrent techniques have been compiled and taught by several microcurrent device developers, including myself, Dr. Thomas Wing[94], Daniel Kirsch[95] and others. The interferential and milliamp treatment techniques in Chapter 9 are based on electro-therapeutic techniques commonly practiced in the chiropractic and physical therapy professions plus some of my own innovations. Many of the techniques described do not require specific acupuncture knowledge, and are largely based on anatomical selection of stimulation sites.

Microcurrent Therapeutics

Like many healing disciplines, microcurrent therapy is an art form as well as a set of techniques. In order to enjoy superior results, a versatile and flexible approach is needed. This involves learning a range of pad and probe techniques and applying them in conjunction with other indicated treatments such as acupuncture, physical therapies, manipulation, allopathic medicine and bodywork. The practitioner should frequently monitor the response of the patient, adjusting the approach as needed to achieve positive results.

Such a flexible and experimental approach will allow you to enjoy positive results within a single clinical session more of the time. I have humorously called the experience of administering a treatment technique to a patient, and then having to wait until the next session to see if it was effective or not "acupuncture hell"! I prefer a clinical approach in which I give brief applications of treatment, frequently re-testing the patient to see its effects. If the first approach tried does not provide noticeable positive change, I adjust and try another set of treatment points, different current polarity or frequency, or new preset treatment protocol. I often administer these techniques while the patient is mobilizing his affected bodily area, or

---

[94] Wing developed the MENS line of stimulators and has written many articles about microcurrents
[95] Kirsch is the developer of the Alpha-Stim line of stimulators

positioning it in a way that challenges his movement limits. After a few minutes of such experimentation, I usually discover which approach works for that patient. This does not imply that the patient always has major relief of their complaint right away, although they usually do. Improvement can be measured through many signs, including reduced pain, increased range of motion or improved readings of energetic diagnostic indicators.

Probe treatments are used to treat specific acupuncture points or trigger points, or small anatomical areas such as finger joints, the temporo-mandibular (jaw) joint, sinuses or sense organs. Most probe treatments involve placing a set of two probes on complementary acupoints. Pad treatments are used for more generalized flooding treatment of soft tissue and joint regions, while four-pad interferential treatments are most applicable for treating the large joints of the low back, hips, shoulders and knees. It is usually more effective to combine probe and pad treatments in the same visit. When probe stimulation is used to disperse blocked acupoints and balance the meridian system, the body generally responds more readily to direct local stimulation and/or manipulation of the symptomatic region. Even within a pad treatment session, a two-step sequence treatment can add to the effectiveness.[96]

It has been challenging to set up meaningful research studies on the subject of microcurrent therapeutics. Some past studies into the efficacy of microcurrent for pain management have not clearly demonstrated microcurrent to be more effective than TENS units or non-treated controls. In examining these studies, I have noticed that in very few of them were microcurrent therapy applied to the subjects in the actual ways that are required for good results. For example, one study I read at a poster exhibition at the American Physical Therapy Association (APTA) yearly convention involved applying microcurrent stimulation through pads directly bracketing an area of low back pain. The paper compared the results to the same treatment performed with a milliamp TENS unit. The study revealed no advantage of microcurrent stimulation. This is because simply bracketing an area of low back pain with microcurrent pads is rarely the most effective method! In order to set up meaningful studies, treatment must be applied in the manner that has been found clinically effective and based on an individual constitutional and physical assessment.

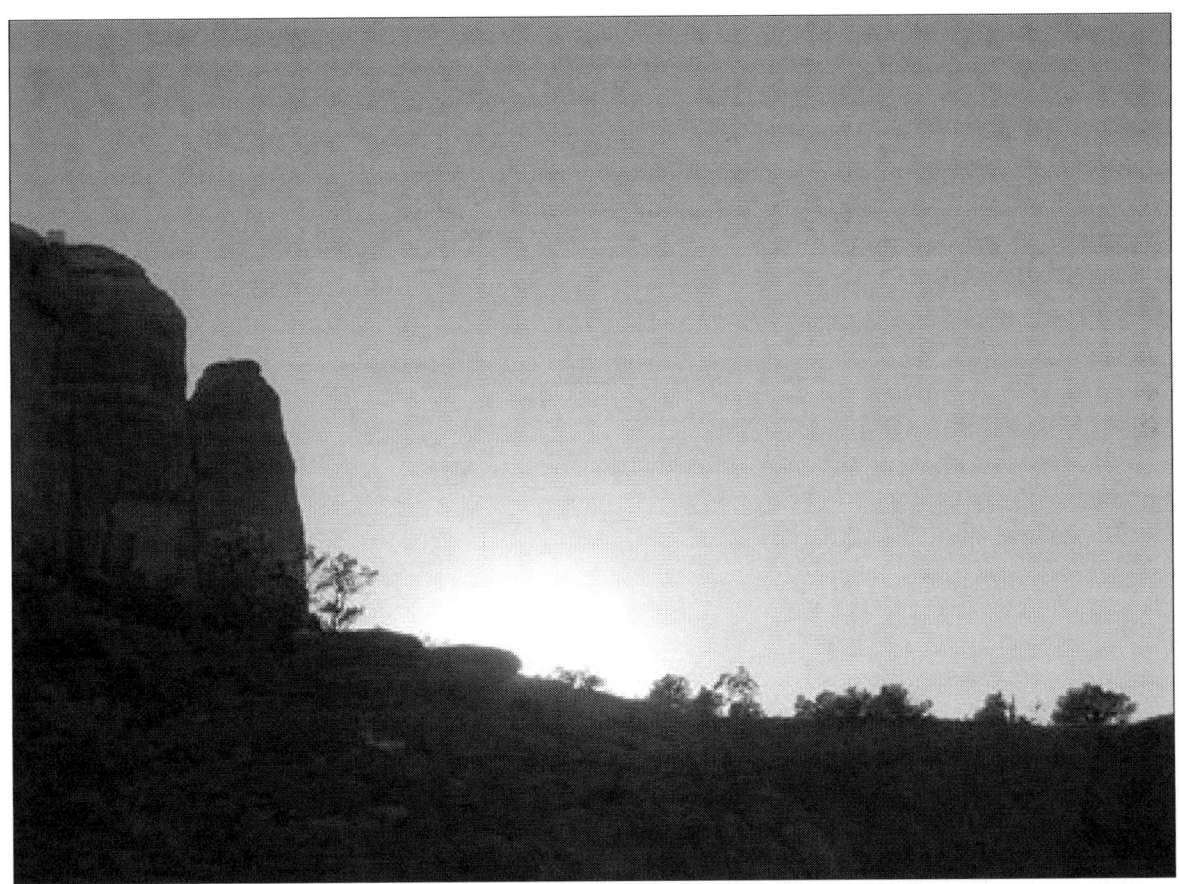

Chapter 6

SHORTCOMINGS OF MODERN ELECTROTHERAPY ... AND SOLUTIONS

Now that you have read this far, you understand some of the basic principles of energy medicine and electrical theory. In this chapter, we will examine the ways electro-therapy is taught and practiced in the United States. You will learn why most practitioners do not have more consistent and positive clinical successes, and how your patients can enjoy far superior results. Chapter 7 will detail the techniques of microcurrent electro-acupuncture that will allow you to put these principles into action.

Before going into the specific shortcomings, it is helpful to briefly reflect on how electro-therapy has historically developed. The earliest recorded use of electricity for pain relief was recorded by Scribonius Largus in ancient Rome. His narrative explains how Roman doctors fished the Mediterranean for torpedo fish, creatures that have electrical organs that can deliver a nasty 220-volt shock when in danger. These fish were put into buckets of water, and suffering gout victims placed their feet in the bucket to agitate the torpedo fish, and voila, instant electro-therapy! Apparently, this technique was credited with the relief of a lot of pain, although this was far from a non-invasive approach.

Jumping ahead hundreds of years, Ben Franklin also left writings about healing his neighbor's shoulder pain with shocks from a crude electrical battery he constructed[97]. We have all heard about Franklin's experiments with electricity – remember the famous kite and key story?

In The Body Electric, Robert Becker goes through a fascinating account of the history of research into the electrical nature of life and healing over the last centuries.[98] I highly recommend this book to all practitioners of microcurrent electro-acupuncture.

In the United States of the 1800's, the Industrial Revolution was booming, and this quest into new technologies also brought about the creation of scores of electro-therapy devices. Many of these were fanciful and without any reputable scientific basis, while some were, no doubt, effective for some conditions[99]. There are many health problems that do respond favorably to local stimulation

---

[97] Kahn, Joseph, Principles and Practice of Electrotherapy, p 1
[98] The Body Electric, Ch 1 - 4
[99] Nelson & Currier, Clinical Electrotherapy, Ch10

to clear energetic obstruction, a common principle of Chinese acupuncture, and many of these devices worked on this basis. The devices of the 19th and early 20th century tended to create intense and sometimes burning stimulation, as modern electronics was not yet available to deliver precise or subtle stimulation. It appears that most or all of these devices applied electrical energy directly to painful or dysfunctional parts of the body, or bathed the whole body in electrostatic energy. Of course, these were also the days when anyone could order morphine or cocaine through the Sears and Roebucks catalogue!

In 1910 the infamous Flexner Report[100] delivered to Congress discredited many of the so-called alternative therapies in favor of allopathic medicine, and this eventually led to the creation of laws against the practice of homeopathy and prejudice against electro-therapies. There is evidence that the Rockefeller family, who had huge financial stakes in the pharmaceutical companies, championed this report. It was mainly chiropractors and naturopaths who kept the use of electro-therapy alive between the 1920's and 1960's. In the 1960's, chronic back pain research by Norman Shealy and others led to the creation of implantable spinal column stimulators. The obvious drawbacks of surgically implanted devices then led to the creation of Transcutaneous Electric Nerve Stimulator (TENS) units that used surface patch electrodes.

Since the 1960's several improvements over the TENS units were developed. These include interferential, high volt galvanic, Russian stimulation, and microcurrent stimulators. While each of these devices offer an improvement in some aspect of treatment, the style of treatment generally taught for utilizing them in health care schools and texts has not changed significantly since the freewheeling 1800's. An examination of the training manuals or training courses offered with most of these devices mostly reveals directions for local stimulation of the painful zone. While this may appear logical, it is actually rarely the most effective way to apply therapeutic stimulation to the body.

A major event in the 1970's was the opening of increased communication between the U.S. and China during the Nixon presidency. Part of the information exchange involved the importation of acupuncture to the U.S., and its increasing acceptance here. Now, at the start of the 21st century, the practice of acupuncture and Chinese herbal medicine has become a well-established and growing profession in the U.S. One of the greatest gifts acupuncture has brought to our health care system is the understanding of whole-body treatment, and the use of distal acu-points for pain relief and energy balancing.

This book is about the marriage of the invaluable principles of acupuncture with modern electro-therapy, a topic that has not been adequately addressed until this time. By using modern microprocessor technology to deliver specific therapeutic currents in a whole-body treatment fashion, our clinical successes with challenging chronic pain and certain disease conditions can greatly improve. It is most specifically the combination of gentle microcurrents with an energetic meridian-based approach that is responsible for so many of the surprisingly effective and rapid results we are frequently seeing and hearing about from colleagues and students. Now let's examine the specific shortcomings of modern electro-therapy practice and the solutions necessary to attain effective and rapid results.

Shortcoming #1: Overemphasis on Local Stimulation

Most electro-therapy manuals and treatment formularies largely recommend placing electrodes over the local area of pain or injury. In my experience, this yields clearly positive results 25 – 50% of the time at best. There are several reasons. First, pain is often perceived in areas of referral, that is, not

---

[100] for more information, see website http://www.healthy.net/naturopathicjournal/vol4no1/rbpratn.htm

in the actual area of injury.[101] Secondly, the area of pain is often inflamed, which is associated with excess energy and concentration of electrons. Adding further stimulation to that area may be equivalent to pouring gasoline on a fire – not a good way to put it out. Appropriate distal acu-points in a sense are escape valves for this excess energy, and stimulating them is a far more reliable way to reduce the excess at the injury or pain site. It is true that release of ah-shi[102] or myofascial trigger points in the local area can also provide good relief, and so it is often a combination of local and distal treatment that yields the most balanced and effective results.[103]

The solution to the overemphasis on local stimulation is more utilization of dermatome[104] treatments and distal acu-points and body zones for a balanced treatment approach.

Shortcoming #2: Use of "Overkill" Stimulation Currents That Inhibit Healing and Carry-over of Relief

The innate electrical activity of the human body has been measured in the pico, nano and microcurrent levels. Picoamps are graduated in trillionths of an amp, nanoamps in billionths of an amp, and microamps in millionths of an amp. Therefore, even applying microcurrents to the skin surface is an introduction of currents generally far in excess of our innate biological electrical activity. Yet because the resistive and capacitive qualities of bodily tissue greatly reduce and modify the actual current that penetrates to the target tissues it is rare that these tissues actually receive the level of stimulation set on a device[105]. Apparently one of the ways therapeutic currents benefit the body is by stimulating somewhat above the normal level, thus creating an intervention that can move "stuck" Qi and tonify, or add energy to areas lacking sufficient energetic charge to heal themselves. Although microamps are rarely felt by patients, in fact they are much stronger than most of our innate currents. Research has shown that microcurrents in the 10 – several hundred μA levels can accelerate healing of wounds and fractures.[106]

With this understanding that microcurrent stimulation is already stronger than our innate currents, it is easy to see why the milliamp currents[107] used in most modern stimulators are often way too much current for our bodies. Milliamps are measured in the thousandths of an amp range, 1000 times more intense than microamps. By the time our sensory nerves can clearly feel treatment currents, they are already at levels that can significantly disrupt our subtle bioelectrical systems, thus *slowing the healing process*[108]. The common practice of running milliamp currents directly through acupuncture needles has several dangers as well. The first is electrolysis of the metal of the needles, which is the process of breaking down a substance with electrical currents. Potentially toxic metal ions can migrate from the needle into the tissues, an undesirable effect. This type of electro-acupuncture can also literally burn the tissues the needles are in contact with, and there is a danger of needle breakage when the muscles it is inserted into are twitching.

---

[101] Tortura and Anagnastokos, Principles of Anatomy and Physiology pp 361-362
[102] Ah Shi points are acu-points that spontaneously appear in painful and inflamed parts of the body. Acupuncture dispersal methods on these points is an important part of pain control through the tendino-muscular meridian system. Treating ah-shi points alone, however, is generally not a complete treatment.
[103] For a good book on acupuncture treatment of trigger points, see A New American Acupuncture by Mark Seem
[104] Dermatomes are regions of superficial tissues of the body that are each innervated by a specific spinal nerve. Dermatomes run down the arms and legs and circle the torso.
[105] Clinical Electrotherapy, Ch 2
[106] for example, see Carley and Wainapel: Electrotherapy for Acceleration of Wound Healing: Low Intensity Direct Current Archives of Physical Medicine and Rehabilitation, Vol. 66, July 1985. Many other abstracts on electrical healing acceleration can be found at website www.eastwestmed.com
[107] Milliamps are currents graduated in the thousandths of an amp range, and can be clearly felt by the sensory nerves as tingling, prickling or throbbing sensations. Most electro-therapeutic devices in current use only deliver milliamp stimulation.
[108] See study Cheng, et Al: The Effects of Electric Current on ATP Generation, Protein Synthesis, and Membrane Transport in Rat Skin Clinical Orthopaedics and Related Research, #171, Nov/Dec. 1982

Because the body responds so well to gentle microcurrents, we can conclude that it is rarely necessary or desirable to use milliamp stimulation on your patients. I would suggest that you start to use microcurrent stimulation as your first and primary treatment, and only use milliamp if necessary after that if the patient's pain is not relieved. You will be surprised to find how rarely milliamp currents are needed!

There are some exceptions, however. When a patient is presenting acute pain, inflammation, muscle spasm and edema these symptoms can greatly reduce blood and lymph circulation to the affected area. Because of this impaired circulation, it is hard for the body to eliminate waste products from the area, which is essential for reduction of inflammation and healing.[109] In cases like this, it may be appropriate to use milliamp stimulation to, in effect, force the body to relax its tension and to stimulate local muscles to pump out excess fluids. This can help restore proper circulation, which can carry off the toxic waste products, thereby promoting healing.

I start almost all electro-therapy sessions with microcurrent stimulation through local and distal areas, and only use milliamp currents when this is not successful in reducing some acute pain cases.[110] In my experience with pain patients, milliamp stimulation is necessary less than 20% of the time.

The solution to the overuse of overkill currents is simply greater use of microcurrents as a first approach to pain, only using milliamps when necessary in some acute conditions.

Shortcoming #3: Simple Treatment Current Patterns That Cause Adaptation

When a repetitive stimulation of any kind is applied to the body, it stops being effective very quickly as the body accommodates, or adapts, to the stimulation.[111] Most electro-stimulators deliver repetitive stimulation. Applying therapeutic currents that have constantly varying frequency, intensity, and timing have greater clinical value. These will tend to create longer lasting pain control and other healing effects. Ask the manufacturer of a device you are considering buying what current modulations are available from it.

The solution to the shortcoming of adaptation is use of modulated and multi-step protocols.

Shortcoming #4: Incorrect Choice of Electrode Polarities Leading to Inappropriate Treatment of Extremities and Radiculopathies

The Law of Polarity is an all-important, all-pervading reality of our physical and energetic existence. It is totally applicable to electro-therapy. The healthy human body has an electrically positive orientation on the head and central spinal area, and a negative orientation at the extremities.[112] By following this pattern with electrode placements, we are working *with* the body, and it is much easier to bring about pain relief, healing and homeostasis. Unfortunately, most electro-therapeutic devices, including some microcurrent devices, offer most treatments only in biphasic, or alternating polarity, and this often is not what is needed. Biphasic currents are generally more successful for treatment of the neck and trunk of the body, but inconsistently effective for problems of the extremities and radicular[113] pain. In the realm of meridian balancing work, only properly polarized current will be effective.

---

[109] Clinical Electrotherapy, Ch 3

[111] Clinical Electrotherapy, Ch 3
[112] The Body Electric, Ch 4
[113] Pain or numbness that radiates, usually down the arms or legs.

In my seminars, I often use a very dramatic illustration of this principle. I use kinesiology, or muscle testing, to determine the overall energetic response of the body, first testing the baseline strength of the indicator muscle before applying any stimulation. I then place a positive probe on a proximal acu-point and a negative probe on a distal point, and test the muscle. I then reverse the polarity on the same points, and test the muscle again. In 100% of the cases, the muscle will be strong with one polarity placement, and "blow out" or go weak in the opposite position. This procedure can be repeated many times and the same effect will continue to happen.

In my experience, it is the misunderstanding of the Law of Polarity as it applies to electro-therapy that is the single most important factor in poor clinical results and aggravations of pain.

The solution is the use of properly polarized treatment currents for treatment of extremities, radiculopathies and meridian balancing.

Shortcoming #5: Passive Electro-stimulation

Our experience has shown that, during certain stages of treatment, electrical stimulation is much more effective if applied while the patient is in motion. This makes a lot of sense if you think about it. There are two main stages of pain and injury treatment – the acute phase and the rehabilitation phase. During the acute phase, it is not desirable or sometimes even possible for the patient to move or exercise – the first objective is relief of pain and inflammation so that suffering is reduced and healing can proceed. Once the acute pain has reduced, however, the most important objective besides continued pain relief is restoration of normal, healthy movement and function. Much of physical therapy consists of exercises and movements to re-educate the body for that end. By gradually increasing the pain-free range of motion and strengthening weakened muscles and tendons, the patient can gradually regain as much normal posture and movement as possible. Yet this process can often be painful and difficult as guarded and sore areas are exercised.

When microcurrent stimulation is applied during exercise, it makes the whole process easier. The patient feels less discomfort during movement, and the muscles and tendons often become more flexible and capable of re-education with less stress. There is also a strengthening effect on some weak muscles, which assists in rehabilitation. I have seen wheelchair bound patients find it easier to practice standing up and sitting down when microcurrent interferential pads were placed on their lower back during their exercise.

There is still no proven scientific explanation for this phenomenon (like most commonly accepted medical procedures), but here are some likely reasons:

- Studies have shown that microcurrent stimulation increases ATP[114] concentrations in the cells, and this can promote muscle softening.

- The meridian blockage clearing properties of microcurrent increases Qi flow in the area, freeing up available energy and promoting ease of movement.

- Proprioception is the feedback system between peripheral muscles, tendons and sensory nerves and the central nervous system that adjusts muscle tone to allow smooth movement.[115] It is likely that microcurrent stimulation during movement in some way augments proprioception, accelerating the re-education process of injured muscles and joints.

---

[114] ATP- Adenosine triphosphate, the energy currency of the cell.
[115] Principles of Anatomy and Physiology, pp 361-363

- Because microcurrent stimulation often immediately reduces pain during exercise, patients can increase their range of motion with less resistance. This expanded movement helps the neuromuscular systems of the body to adapt to fuller and easier movement patterns.

There is one caution about this practice. Because it is easier for patients to extend their range of motion during stimulation, they may attempt so much increased movement that they create post-exercise soreness after underused muscles and tendons are activated. I have particularly seen this with rheumatoid arthritis patients. To avoid such pain rebound, ask the patient to extend their range of motion in gradual increments over a series of treatments using this technique. Massage, hot packs, analgesic plasters and hot baths may help alleviate soreness after therapy.

Whatever the reasons, it is clear that "microcurrents with motion" is a far superior rehabilitative therapy than passive electro-stimulation, during which there is no movement.

The solution to the limitation of passive electrotherapy is kinetic treatments – microcurrents in motion.

SUMMARY OF SHORTCOMINGS AND SOLUTIONS

Shortcoming	Problems with Traditional or Milliamp Therapy	Benefits of Alternative or Microcurrent Therapy	Solution
Overemphasis on local stimulation (electrodes on site of pain/injury)	Not consistently effective. Area usually inflamed (excess energy / electron concentration)	Distal points are "escape valves" Whole-body treatment superior for long-lasting results	Use microcurrent dermatome treatments, distal acu-points and body zones
"Overkill" stimulation inhibits healing and carry-over relief	Milliamps disrupt body's bioelectrical systems, slowing healing. Milliamps can cause needle electrolysis →broken needles	Microcurrents are more harmonious with body's innate bio-electricity	Use microcurrents as first mode of treatment Use milliamps in acute pain, inflammation and muscle spasm
Simple treatment current patterns cause adaptation	Most electro-therapy devices deliver repetitive stimulation	Variable frequency, intensity, timing create longer lasting pain control	Use modulated, multi-step protocols
Incorrect polarities → inappropriate treatment for radiculopathies and extremities	Most electro-therapy devices deliver biphasic (alternating) polarity; may aggravate pain Improper polarity placements may aggravate pain	Polarized treatments (validated with muscle testing) work with body's polarity to relieve pain and promote energetic balance	Use polarized treatments along dermatomes and meridian pathways, and to link body zones (Positive Probe Proximal)
Passive electro-stimulation	Passive therapy does not promote restoration of normal healthy movement and function	Microcurrent relieves pain during movement; increases muscle/tendon flexibility; strengthens muscle for rehab	Use kinetic treatment - "Microcurrents in Motion"

Figure 6.1 - Summary of Shortcomings and Solutions

Summary

The principles presented in this chapter are fairly simple and easy to apply, yet it is remarkable how little they are understood and practiced. This lack of understanding is responsible for much of the mediocre reputation electric stimulation has had in the health care community, and is partially responsible for cutbacks in reimbursement for these procedures we have seen in recent years. It is highly recommended for you to internalize these important principles. It is the combination of electro-therapies with knowledge of meridian energetics that yields the most positive results, far beyond that commonly experienced by practitioners using standard electro-therapy methods. An understanding and application of this information will certainly take a practitioner from "stone age" electro-therapy to highly effective holistic treatment with rapid, tangible results.

Chapter 7

MICROCURRENT TREATMENT: PROBE TECHNIQUES

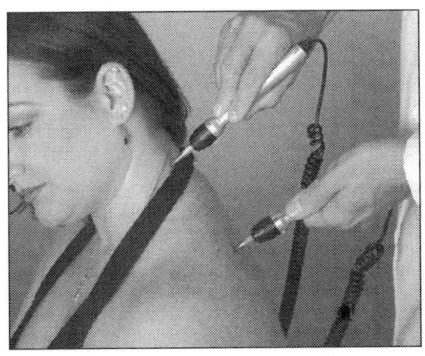
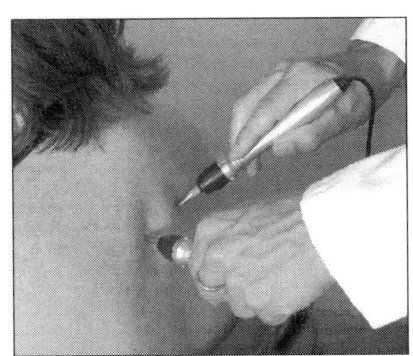
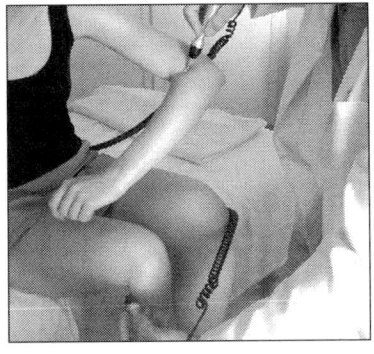

Figure 7.1 Probe Techniques

User Interface

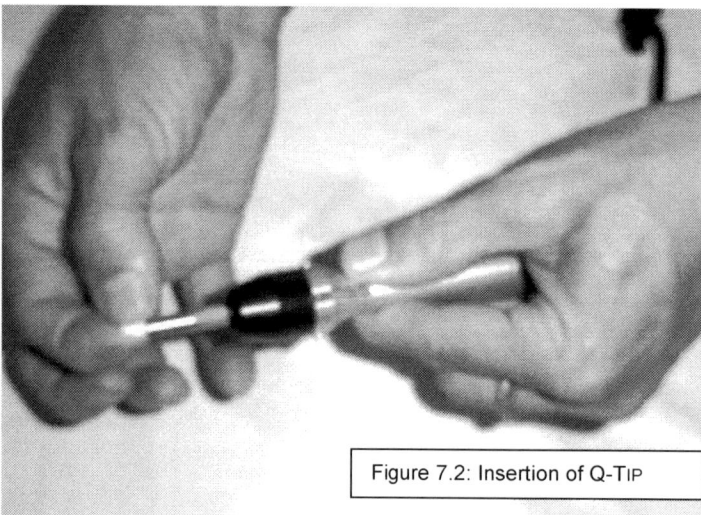

Figure 7.2: Insertion of Q-Tip

Most probe electrodes use wetted cotton swabs to transfer treatment current to the patient. Some use metal tips that must be regularly cleansed. I highly recommend the use of the Q-Tip brand[116] of cotton swabs.

Insertion technique for cotton swabs varies according to probe design. For MENS units, cut the swab in half and place each half into the hollow probe tip. For the Acutron Mentor, break or cut off the handle or stem of the swab so only the cotton bulb area at each end is retained. Screw this into the hexagonal metal probe tip in a clockwise manner so the inner threads will grab the cotton and hold it in place.

The cotton tips must be kept wet throughout use to assure good conductivity[117]. I recommend cutting or breaking off a generous supply of swap tips and keeping them handy in a small bowl next to a small container of water next to your device. Replace the cotton tips when crushed or soiled.

There are other probe tips available, depending on device manufacturer. These may include specialized probe attachments or tips for auricular treatment, meridian testing and intra-oral stimulation[118].

Search and Treat Modes

Probe techniques involve more than just delivering stimulation. The most effective methods involve a rapid, dynamic alternation between measuring and treating. Quality microcurrent stimulators offer two probe modes - search mode and treat mode. During search mode, the device acts as an ohmmeter, a device to measure changes in electrical resistance[119]. In this mode, which is factory set and requires no user adjustment of parameters, the user moves the probes lightly over the skin surface to search for the areas of maximum electrical conductivity. This information gives valuable guidance in selecting points for treatment. Search mode also gives guidance about how long to treat each set of points. Search mode measurements of acu-points can be interpreted in general or highly specific ways, depending on the intent of the practitioner and the part of the body being measured.

---

[116] A product of Cheeseboro Ponds Corp. These cotton swabs have cardboard rather than plastic handles. Most other brands do not have as much cotton on the tips.
[117] Tap water generally works well for this purpose, as it has plenty of dissolved minerals that transfer electricity. If your water comes from a well or is particularly pure, add a few pinches of sea salt to it to improve conductivity
[118] The Acutron Mentor device offers all of these probe attachments. Other manufacturers offer these or others.
[119] Resistance is the inverse of conductivity. The meters on microcurrent devices rise to higher levels as the resistance decreases and conductivity increases, therefore higher readings indicate areas in which the treatment current will encounter less resistance in penetration into the body.

The general measurements, such as those taken during "chasing the dragon" treatments for local muscle and joint pain, are not so useful for meridian diagnostics, but can offer guidance as to how long to treat. Changes in skin resistance over master acu-points distal to the elbows and knees can be interpreted much more accurately to evaluate the meridian system and arrive at an energetic diagnosis. Details on electronic meridian testing (EMT) can be found in Chapter 17.

When your device is turned on, and a probe treatment selected, the unit is automatically in search mode. The probe tips can be applied to the skin surface to start searching immediately. During this time the ohmmeter will display the % of conductivity, with 100 indicating complete conductivity and 0 no conductivity. Touching the metal probe tips together should drive the meter up to 100, and separating them should read 0[120]. The human body acts as a partial conductor, so most readings on the body between the two probe tips will read some value between 0 and 100.

One of the probes is called the trigger probe and will have a small button or switch on it for starting delivery of treatment currents. When this trigger switch is pressed the unit switches from search mode to treat mode, which stays on for the length of time set on the timer control. During treat mode the patient receives treatment currents through the points the probes are placed on. While treatment is being delivered, the meter no longer reads out % of conductivity. Instead, it reads out the % of commanded current actually delivered. For example, if the device is set to deliver 75µA, the meter will read out 100% during treatment periods as long as the full 75 µA is being delivered. If the resistance of the skin exceeds the voltage capacity of the stimulator, this display will read below 100%[121].

How to Search With A Microcurrent Device

These instructions are for searching in conjunction with "circling the dragon" method, in which pairs of local points are stimulated around an injured or painful area. The same method can be used to search for single point treatment as well, for body or auricular points, and for local and distal point combinations. For the instructions below we will be using the example of a painful rotator cuff of the shoulder. The method is similar for most other regions of the body.

These instructions are for units that have a conductivity meter with a 0 – 100 numerical range, and audible tones that rise and fall with the fluctuations of the meter. The higher the meter reading, and the higher the pitch of the sound, the greater the electrical conductivity. Remember, conductivity is inverse (opposite) to resistance, so the higher the skin conductivity, the lower the resistance to the flow of currrent. You are measuring the conductivity reading between the two electrodes, which will consist of two probes, or one trigger probe and a grounding hand mass.

It is recommended that you adjust the unit sound volume so that it is clearly audible, yet not annoyingly intrusive. Once you gain skill with searching, it will be possible to be guided by the sound alone, which is quicker and more intuitive than having to keep turning your head to look at the device meter.

---

[120] This is the case for the Acutron and MENS units. The search criteria for other devices may vary.
[121] These descriptions are true for the Acutron and MENS lines of devices, and may not be applicable to other brands of microcurrent stimulators.

1. Insert wetted Q-tips into the ends of the probes and turn on the unit. For Acutron unit, choose any probe preset from the probe menu, or the top Quick Key labeled "Circling the Dragon." For other microcurrent devices, set up probe treatment according to manufacturer's instructions.

2. Place one probe tip on the posterior portion of the painful region. Place the other probe tip on the anterior portion of the same region, so that the painful area is sandwiched between the two probe tips. Do not yet press the trigger probe switch. (To do so will activate treatment currents.) If you inadvertently activate treatment, pull the probes away from the skin until the treatment expires (usually 5 – 6 seconds), and begin again.

3. Hold the probe on the posterior portion of the painful area and search with the probe on the anterior portion by moving its tip very lightly on the anterior skin surface. Make sure the Q-tip is wet and *touch the skin as lightly as possible. Deep pressure will create artificially high readings.* Slowly glide the cotton probe tip around the anterior area and listen to the sound. When the sound reaches its highest pitch, that is the point of greatest conductivity. Once you have located the most conductive point on the anterior aspect, now hold that probe steady and search with the posterior probe in the same way. When this is completed, you will have located the most conductive anterior and posterior points of the region.

4. You have now completed searching and are ready to treat

The meter feedback can do much more than just locate optimal treatment points. It can also show you how long to treat each set of points, using the following procedure:

1. Follow above steps for searching. Note the numerical meter reading after you find the most conductive points. Example: Meter reading after searching on shoulder is 35 on the 0 – 100 scale. This is your baseline reading prior to treatment. Press the switch on the trigger probe and release to apply treatment through the points. You may use a firmer or massaging motion with the probe tips during treatment to enhance results.

2. After the timer expires (usually 5 – 6 seconds), release most of the pressure on the points and note the new meter reading. It will often be higher than the baseline, as therapeutic microcurrents will usually decrease electrical resistance of the skin.[122] If the meter reading stays the same after treatment, it is probably an indication that other treatment points will be more beneficial. Occasionally the reading will be lower if the treated area was highly inflamed (Excess).

3. If the meter reading did not change after the first treatment period, move to different points that may be more responsive. If the reading did go higher after step 1, press the trigger again to initiate another treatment period on the same two points. When the treatment time expires, note the meter reading again. Is it higher again? If so, press the trigger a third time. To continue our example, the new reading is 45, that is 10 points higher than the baseline reading.

4. Continue this procedure until the meter does not read higher after a treatment period. To complete the example, it now has climbed to 68 and won't go any higher, although you administer another 6- second treatment period. Once the meter reading reaches its plateau in this way, it generally means that this set of points has accommodated to

---

[122] This is due to increase of microcirculation of blood and increased nerve and cellular ionic activity stimulated by the applied current.

the treatment current, and does not require any further stimulation. It is now appropriate to move onto another set of points.

It is important to point out that the actual numerical readings on the meter are not as important for this technique as the degree of change. A change from 20 up to 45 is just as significant as a change from 60 up to 85. As mentioned above, the exact numerical values read out by the meter during search mode are only significant when measuring the Command, or Five Element, points distal to the elbows or knees[123].

THE BODY AS COMPUTER

At this point it is useful to draw a comparison between the acupuncture meridian system and a computer keyboard. When a key of a computer keyboard is pressed, it sends an electrical signal to the processor. This signal causes a response in the software operating system that brings about a function, such as a letter appearing on the screen, or a numerical value entered into a formula. To achieve this function, it is only necessary for you to press the key on the keyboard momentarily. Holding it down for a long time will not add to the function, and in fact will usually cause unwanted effects. In a similar way, once you have driven the conductivity reading as high as possible while treating a set of points, the body's internal processing systems are properly activated to achieve a function, such as opening flow of Qi or adjusting neuro-hormonal balance. In most cases with microcurrent electro-acupuncture, continuing to stimulate the points will not add to the desirable effect. As usual, there are exceptions to this principle, such as some cases of acute inflammation.

A Brief Discussion Of Myofascial Trigger Points

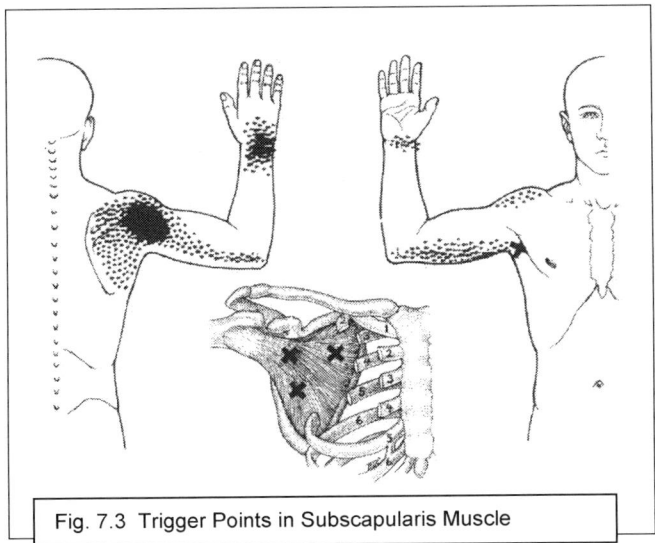

Fig. 7.3 Trigger Points in Subscapularis Muscle

A major part of acupuncture pain management is the local treatment of painful and constricted tissues. This is the more superficial level of treatment, while meridian balancing and distal point stimulation work on a deeper, systemic level. Yet both levels are important.

An important part of acupuncture is needling of ah shi points, which are local points of tenderness and soreness. These are not precisely mapped out, and must be located by palpation. These points block Qi and Blood at their sites. Ah shi points are traditionally treated with dispersing needle

---

[123] See Ch 17 for details on Electronic Meridian Testing

techniques, direct moxibustion, cupping[124] or gua-sha.[125] Ah-shi points can be quickly reduced with microcurrent probe stimulation, or a combination of manual pressure and manipulation with simultaneous microcurrent stimulation (electro-massage)[126].

Japanese acupuncture describes similar areas called kori. These are also defined as areas of myofascial stiffness and constriction that block local physiological functioning. Kori impedes blood and lymphatic circulation and nerve conduction in the areas in which it appears, and in addition to local pain and stiffness, kori can lead to many types of organic and systemic dysfunction and disease.

The works of Janet Travell, M.D. and David Simons[127] are very valuable for charting common trigger points in muscles throughout the body. Travell defines trigger points as foci of hyperirritability in a tissue that are painful when compressed. They may either be locally painful only, or radiate pain toward other body areas. There are several types of trigger points: myofascial, cutaneous, fascial, ligamentous and periosteal. According to Travell and Simons, most people have latent trigger points in muscles. When a person is stretching and exercising regularly and is free of traumatic injury, the trigger points have no effect. Through trauma, inactivity and lack of stretching, however, the trigger points can be activated. Like classical Chinese medicine, Travell recognizes the ability of exposure to wind and cold (and air conditioning, which was not mentioned in the Nei Jing) to also activate trigger points. Some viral illnesses can activate them as well.

If a person in the early stage of trigger point activation obtains treatment or self-treats through proper stretching and exercise, the trigger point is likely to go back into latency. Unfortunately, many people do not do this, and instead guard the affected area by chronically limiting its movement. Thus the trigger point becomes more established, causing more protracted problems. This, and viral activation, are major factors in the painful and stiff areas that proliferate in persons with fibromyalgia, lupus, and chronic fatigue syndrome.

An excellent book detailing the relationship between Travell and Simon's work with trigger points and acupuncture is <u>A New American Acupuncture</u>[128] by Mark Seem. Dr. Seem has spent much of his career integrating hands-on palpatory methods with traditional acupuncture systems.

Microcurrent therapies, in conjunction with needle or non-needle acupuncture, stretching and hands-on bodywork, is a powerful and effective method to reduce the limiting effects of trigger points and restore full motion. Trigger points generally have different electrical characteristics than surrounding tissues, as can be confirmed with Galvanic Skin Response (GSR) measurements. In effect, they are acting as insulators, which block flow, and capacitors, which store charge. Pulsed microcurrent stimulation can open the local electrical circuitry, thereby reducing or eliminating both these phenomenon.

---

[124] The practice of placing suction cups over acu-points to reduce local pain or pull out atmospheric evils such as wind and cold.
[125] The practice of rubbing a hard and smooth object repeatedly over an affected area to increase local blood circulation and in some cases causing minute capillary bleeding.
[126] See Chapter 13 for a description of electro-massage
[127] Travell, Janet and Simons, David, <u>Myofascial Pain and Dysfunction, The Trigger Point Manual</u> Williams and Wilkins
[128] <u>A New American Acupuncture – Acupuncture Osteopathy</u> by Mark Seem, Blue Poppy Press

Probe Techniques

MICROCURRENT PROBE TECHNIQUE SUMMARY

Probe Technique	Qi Effect	Symptom / Problem
Circling the Dragon	Disperse blockage	Local myofascial pain, swelling and constriction, back, neck and extremity joint treatments, arthritis, some headaches
Dermatome and Distal	Balance meridians and body regions	Meridian treatment, radiculopathy, distal joint treatment, headaches
Acute	Disperse Yin accumulation	Release myofascial masses and trigger points
Gentle / Chronic	Tonify, gently disperse	Treat very sensitive patients and babies
Specific Muscle Techniques (Origin / insertion and cross muscle)	Disperse, adjust tone and communication between muscles and CNS[129]	Whiplash, muscles overuse, piriformis syndrome treatment for sciatica
Nerve Root Stimulation (Hua To points)	Stimulate yang	Neck and back pain, nervous system stimulation through dermatomes and myotomes
Microcurrent Mu-Shu technique	Balance yin and yang of viscera	Visceral balancing, chakra stimulation
Micro-macro technique	Promote free flow of Qi and blood in channels, collaterals and Organs	Acute pain control, brain and endocrine balance, addiction control

Figure 7.4: Microcurrent Probe Techniques

Each technique works by adusting the body's bio-electricity in a different way, as presented here. Complete instructions for each technique follows.

Circling the Dragon

Purpose: To disperse blocked Qi and Blood through local stimulation. In this case the word "Dragon" refers to the painful or injured area. Use this technique to reduce pain and improve range of motion. This is a dynamic technique, rapidly alternating between searching and brief treatment periods that pass current directly through painful and injured areas[130]. Circling the Dragon is directed toward points of pain, ah-shi points, trigger points, nerve roots and other acu-points of local effect.

Most commonly used to treat:

- Neck pain
- Shoulder pain
- Knee pain
- Arthritis of finger and toe joints

---

[130] This technique is largely detailed by the explanation above of searching and knowing how long to treat.

- Sinus congestion and pain
- Tennis elbow and carpal tunnel syndrome, when used in conjunction with Dermatome and Distal
- Some types of headaches

Time required: 2 – 3 minutes per body area treated

Set-up: Acutron Mentor: Probe Preset #1, or top Quick Key (biphasic polarity)[131]

Other devices: Intensity: 50 – 100 μA (75 μA for most persons, less if very sensitive)

Frequency: 10 Hz or other specific frequency

Waveform: Square

Polarity: Biphasic

Timer: 5 – 6 seconds per press of trigger

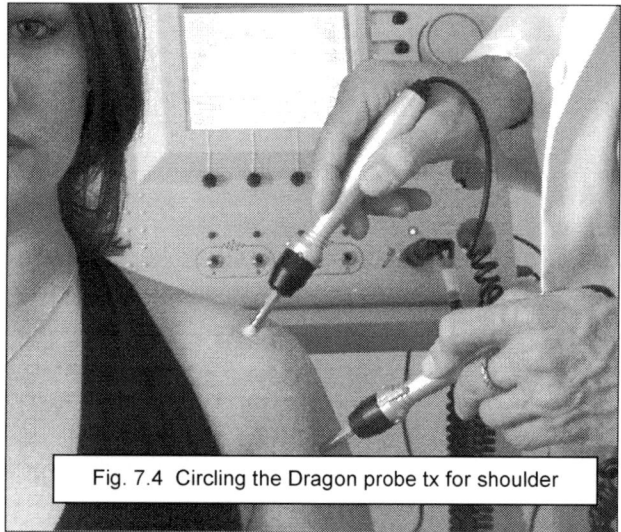

Fig. 7.4 Circling the Dragon probe tx for shoulder

Steps:

1. Choose pairs of points to treat together. Visualize an imaginary energy beam between the probe tips, and place them so the "beam" intersects the painful or injured area from several different directions. For example, to treat generalized shoulder pain, you could select the following sets of points:

- From anterior shoulder to posterior shoulder (acu-points Jianneling to S.I. 10)
- From base of neck to deltoid muscle (C6 nerve root to L.I. 15)
- From armpit to top of shoulder (Ht 1 – L.I. 16)

These points are for example only. The exact points to be treated will be based on the actual area of pain and the results of searching. With Circling the Dragon technique, it is more favorable to treat the points with the highest meter readings in each region than exact anatomical locations of known acu-points.

2. Treat each set of points until the meter reading in search mode reaches its highest plateau, as described above, then move onto the next set of points.

3. To assess your results, check the pain-free range of motion of the area to be treated prior to probe treatment. Frequently recheck throughout the session. This will allow you to confirm which sets of points are effective and which are not.

---

[131] the polarity of the probes will switch back and forth every few seconds. This in effect makes both probes equal and eliminates the need to deal with polarity discrimination

4. Results can often be enhanced by placing the affected area in a stretch position that challenges the limits of pain-free motion while applying probe treatment. By doing this you will often be able to see the ROM increase as microcurrents are applied. For example, if a patient cannot fully abduct the shoulder, ask him to abduct as far as possible without significant pain or restriction. Place one probe near acromial extremity and the other down the arm on a distal acu-point or tender area. If points are well chosen, patient may be able to raise arm further during stimulation period.
5. Circling the Dragon technique can be freely combined with other probe and pad techniques such as Dermatome and Distal or interferential therapies.

Dermatome and Distal

Purpose: To treat extremity pain and injuries, radiculopathy, most headaches and sciatica. This is the most appropriate technique for treatment of local and distal acu-points.

Most commonly used to treat:

- Tennis elbow
- Carpal tunnel syndrome and other wrist sprains and strains
- Brachial plexus "pinched nerve" syndrome
- Knee, ankle and heel injuries and pain
- Peripheral neuropathy
- Most headaches (one probe on head and other on distal acu-points on extremities)
- Acu-point treatment through the Great Loops of the meridian systems and electronic meridian balancing
- Micro-systems such as auricular and Korean hand points

Time required: 2 – 3 minutes per body area treated, or as short as 30 seconds for local and distal acu-point combinations, longer for meridian balancing sessions

Set-up: Acutron Mentor: Probe Preset #2

    Other devices: Intensity: 50 – 100 µA (75 µA for most persons, less if very sensitive)

    Frequency: 10 Hz or other specific frequency

    Waveform: Square

    Polarity: Negative (make sure you correctly identify negative probe)

    Timer: 5 – 6 seconds per press of trigger

Basic principles: It is vital for you to know which probes are negative and positive to perform this technique. Unlike circling the Dragon, accurate placement of your positive and negative probes is vital. In most cases it is appropriate to place the positive (+) probe proximally and the negative probe (-) distally. The "3 P's" principle is: Positive Probe Proximal.

Polarized Probe Techniques

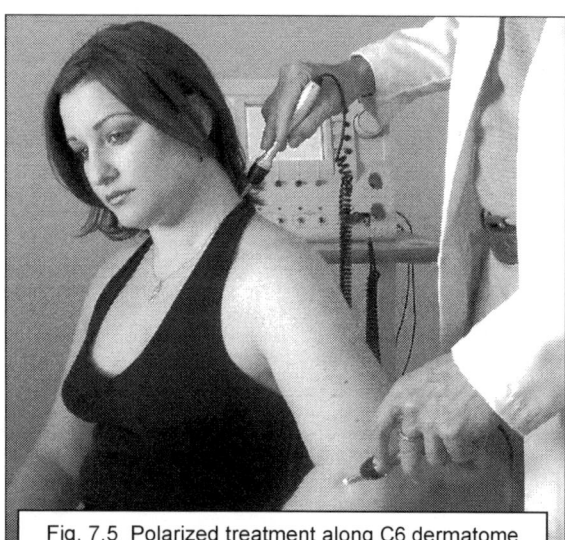

Fig. 7.5 Polarized treatment along C6 dermatome

For all of the following techniques, insert clean Q-tips into probe tips. (Remember to keep the tips wet throughout procedure.)

1. Dermatome Treatment:

Place positive probe on or around the spinal nerve root of the affected dermatome. Start negative probe close to positive, and then in Search mode move it distally down the pathway of the dermatome, looking for points of high conductivity on the surrounding skin. As you find each one, treat up to maximum plateau of conductivity. Keep moving probe distally, searching and treating high conductance points in this way, including main points of pain or paresthesia.

An alternate method of dermatome probe treatment is to place the positive probe on the nerve root in the same way, and the negative on the most distal area of the dermatome, on the hand or foot. Move the probes together in increments of several inches each time, again searching for sets of high conductivity points and treating them. Eventually the two probes will meet in the midway area.

2. Radiculopathy[132] Treatment:

The method is the same as 1. Above

For example, when treating sciatica due to L-5 lesion, place the positive probe over the affected L5 nerve root. Use the negative probe to search for high conductance points along the pathway of pain or paresthesia, and treat them to plateau reading. You can treat a number of points in this way, ranging from more proximal points in the buttocks and thighs to distal points at the furthest radiation of pain, as far as the foot. A similar approach may be used for "pinched nerve" syndromes of the arms, including carpal tunnel syndrome.

---

[132] Radiculo = radiating, pathy = pathology or illness of. Radiculopathy is radiating pain or numbness.

Polarized Probe Treatment – Option 1 and Option 2

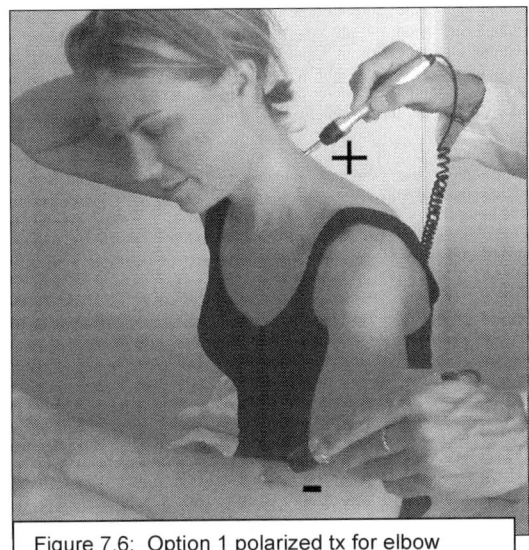

Figure 7.6: Option 1 polarized tx for elbow

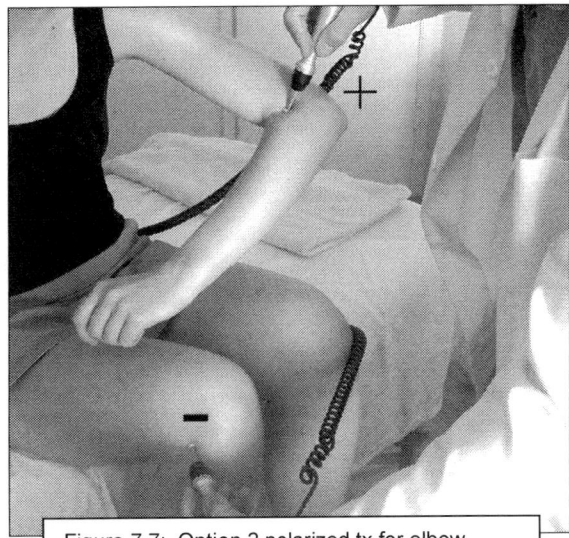

Figure 7.7: Option 2 polarized tx for elbow

3. Acu-point Pairs for Balancing:

   The use of polarity agents on related acupuncture Master points is a very powerful method for balancing body energetics to relieve pain and promote healing. Polarity agents include polarized microcurrent probe electrodes, magnets, and even some aspects of hands on healing. The common factor of these methods is treating pairs of complementary acu-points that have a regional or global balancing effect. In the case of microcurrent probe therapies, the **positive** pole of the stimulator, or the anode, **reduces the charge** at the point it is touching. This in effect **sedates** the point. The **negative** pole, or the cathode, **increases the charge** at the point it is touching, which **tonifies** it. By sedating and tonifying pairs of related Master points, rapid and profound balancing is accomplished. Chapter 11 details effective ways to balance the meridian system.

PROXIMAL TO WHAT?

Proximal means "close to", or "in proximity to". There are two anatomical areas that can be considered proximal – **close to the body center or close to the local site of pain.**

The first refers to a region that is close to the <u>center of the body</u>, specifically the spinal column and head. From this perspective, you can treat sciatica by placing a positive probe on an anatomically proximal region, such as the L5 nerve root, and the negative probe distally down the leg on a tender point within the pain radiation area, or treat a temporal headache by placing the + electrode on the side of the head and the – electrode on acu-point TW 5 on the wrist.

The other type of proximal probe location is proximal to the <u>site of pain</u>. From this perspective, you can treat carpal tunnel syndrome by placing the positive probe on the painful wrist area and the negative probe on an acu-point on the opposite ankle, according to the principle of the Great Loops (see Chapter Eight). In this case both electrodes are about the same distance from the midline of the body, yet one is clearly closer to the area of complaint.

Therefore, the principle of **Positive Probe Proximal** can apply to either of those probe placements. I suggest that you try a brief treatment using each of these placements, noting which provides the most pain control. In my seminars I call these two methods of treatment Option 1 and Option 2. See the photos on the previous page for examples of each.

As with most principles of energetic medicine, there are exceptions to this one as well. It is my experience in testing hundreds of patients that well over 90% do better with positive probe proximal and negative probe distal. Yet there are some that require the reverse. So how can you tell?

There are three main ways to confirm which polarity placement is appropriate.

One is through clinical results- if the patient's symptoms are clearly decreased, and range of motion improves, the polarity placement was correct. If their pain worsens, you have likely used incorrect polarity. The second way to determine correct polarity is through **kinesiology**, or muscle testing. Instructions for this method are detailed in Section IV. The final way is through the conductivity meter of your microcurrent device. The polarity placement was probably beneficial if the meter rises 15 or more points after a single 6-second polarized treatment period. In many cases it will go "off the chart", that is, rise from the initial reading to 100%. This is due to the fact that correct polarity placements on extremity acu-points will tend to move large amounts of Qi. This increased Qi circulation immediately increases electrical circulation through the Law of Resonance.

More subtle signs that confirm correct energetic treatment:

- Her breathing deepens
- Her facial color is a more healthy, ruddy glow
- She tells you she feels better in some way
- She releases a sigh
- The Chi, Cun and Guan pulse positions on the radial artery of the wrists equalize.

4. Tendino-Muscular Meridian Treatment:

   A strategy that comes from the classics of acupuncture addresses the tendino-muscular meridians (TMM), which are the channels most directly affected by microcurrent stimulation. These channels roughly follow the pathways of the principal meridians on a more superficial level, and mostly circulate Yang energy to facilitate physical movement and defenses from environmental Evils. When the TMM are in an excess condition, as is the case with most acute pain and injury, the rule is to disperse the local ah-shi points and tonify the underlying principle meridian.

   This can be approximated by placing the positive probe on various local points of pain and the negative probe on the tonification point of the principal meridian most closely coursing through the painful area. For example, the Large Intestine meridian is most associated with lateral shoulder pain. To treat according to this method, place the positive probe on the painful zone around LI 15, and the negative probe on LI 11 on the lateral elbow, the tonification point of this channel. For low back pain on the Urinary Bladder channel, place the positive probe on various painful back points, and the negative on the lateral nail bed of the little toe, UB 67. This is only one possible way to choose the distal point for this method. Source points, Xi-Cleft points, or other points of special effect can be used to good effect as well.

Some other uses of polarized probe treatments:

- Pain control through the Great Loops of the meridian system (Chapter 8)
- Extraordinary channel balancing (Chapter 11)
- POLAR MERIDIAN PAIR BALANCING (CHAPTER 11)

Acute Probe Treatment

Purpose: Utilizes more intense and dispersive electro-therapeutic parameters to release myofascial nodules and reduce trigger points and areas of acute inflammation. The parameters used for this style of treatment may be considered to be more "aggressive" in that they will more powerfully relax and reduce areas where actual trophic changes have taken place. This is a form of sedation. This is in contrast to the gentler "circling the dragon" treatment parameters which primarily move energy blockages, similar to acupuncture. These acute settings are not applicable to all patients, only those that can tolerate a more intense stimulation. When uncertain about this, try a brief 6-second application of acute settings and note results.

Most commonly used to treat:

- Muscular knots that do not release with other gentler probe treatments, especially around shoulders, back and hamstrings
- Myofascial trigger points
- Inflamed nerve roots
- Inflamed joints, as with rheumatoid arthritis
- Distal point treatment of acute low back pain

Time required: 2 – 3 minutes per body area treated

Set-up: Acutron Mentor: Probe Preset #3

Other devices: Intensity: 150 - 300 µA

Frequency: 80 – 130 Hz, sometimes several hundred Hz can be applicable

Waveform: Modified Square[133]

Polarity: Biphasic

Timer: 5 – 6 seconds per press of trigger

Note- these settings are generally too strong for very weak or hypersensitive patients. For such patients, you can use the same techniques as described below, but use Circling the Dragon or Gentle/Chronic settings of microcurrent device.

Steps:

1. Insert clean Q-tips into probe tips. (Remember to keep the tips wet throughout procedure.)

2. Pinch the nodule or trigger point between the probe tips and treat for 6 seconds. Check for possible aggravations of pain. If no aggravation, continue for another 15-20 seconds. Then pinch the area perpendicularly to the first placement and treat in the same way. Another way to describe the placements is east and west, then north and south. In most cases this approach will relax the affected tissues.

3. If a localized approach is not successful, and the knot or trigger point is still tense and active, a polarized local – distal treatment will probably be effective. In this case use the Dermatome and Distal settings listed above. Place the positive probe directly over the affected tissue, and the negative probe on an applicable distal point. For example, if treating the trapezius–levator scapulae area of the shoulders and a resistant point does not release with other treatments, first try applying acute probe setting as mentioned above. If area does not release, set polarity to negative, and try placing positive probe on resistant nodule and negative probe on acu-point GB 41 on same side. This will often release the resistant area.

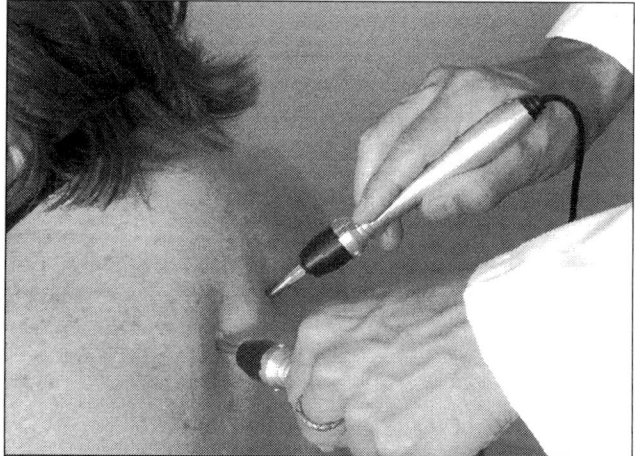

Fig. 7.8 Pinching trigger point with Acute probe technique

---

[133] Modified square waveform is a microcurrent square wave with a brief milliamp spike at the start of the wave. It is available only in the Acutron Mentor and Electro-Acuscope at the time of writing. If not available, use regular square wave.

> **ABOUT HYPERSENSITIVE PATIENTS**
>
> Research with microcurrents has suggested that acceleration of healing is promoted through increasing migration of charged ions through cell membranes, which increase production of ATP.[134] Such physiological effects are promoted by increasing electrical charge at the cell membrane within a specified threshold. As long as patients have a normally functioning nervous system and good circulation of Qi within the meridian system, the excess energy from the microcurrent stimulation is dispersed as needed throughout the body. Patients become hypersensitive when their body slackens its ability to circulate and disperse energy in this way. This can be due to general Deficiency, lymphatic or tissue toxicity, or lack of proper Liver function.
>
> People with this condition often experience painful aggravations of their complaint when continuous electrical stimulation is applied because their bodies cannot disperse the charge. It then builds up and creates local Excess. The settings listed below help prevent such aggravations by utilizing very gentle and low settings, and allowing pause periods (Burst mode) to make it easier for the body to prevent excess buildup of electrical charge.
>
> When aggravations are experienced, it is usually due to one of the following factors:
>
> - current and/or frequency too high
> - Improper polarity of current – patient may require a specific polarized approach, such as + local and – distal instead of local biphasic currents.
> - Improper placement strategy – may require different acu-points or shifting focus from local treatment to overall meridian balancing
>
> When confronted with hypersensitive patients that require pain control, it is especially important that the practitioner use the precise treatment required. When using improper treatment parameters as mentioned above, it is likely that the patient's pain may be aggravated. A very useful tool for confirming precise parameters needed is muscle testing, or kinesiology. Once a positive and negative indicator muscle response is clearly demonstrated, it is possible to try very short treatment periods utilizing the parameters or presets you think are best. The indicator muscle will weaken if the treatment is not beneficial, and other treatments may then be tried until the appropriate one is confirmed. Longer therapeutic treatment can then be administered. Complete instruction for "O Ring" kinesiology can be found in Chapter 16.

Gentle/Chronic Probe Treatment

Purpose: Apply microcurrent treatment for patients who are hypersensitive, weak, or negatively reactive to energy stimulation, or for treatment of babies.

Most commonly used to treat:

- Pediatric complaints such as earache, colic or other health disorders in infants and babies
- Pain control for hypersensitive patients with RSD, causalgia, and some other forms of neuropathy

---

[134] See www.eastwestmed.com website for research citations

- TMJ intra-oral treatment

Time required: 2 – 3 minutes per body area treated. Start with very brief stimulation periods of 6 – 12 seconds and check patient's reaction before proceeding.

Set-up: Acutron Mentor: Probe Preset #4

    Other devices: Intensity: 25 µA

    Frequency: 0.3 – 0.6 Hz

    Waveform: Sloped

    Modulation: Burst (alternating on and off periods)

    Polarity: Biphasic

Timer: 5 – 6 seconds per press of trigger

Methods: See Treatment Formulary at end of book for treatment for specific conditions utilizing this approach, such as TMJ treatment, earache in children, reflex sympathetic dystrophy (RSD), and more.

Specific Muscle Treatments

Purpose: To adjust tone and promote healing in injured or dysfunctional muscles. This technique is called specific muscle treatment because it is used to treat one muscle at a time, in contrast to other probe techniques that treat groups of muscles and fascia in a bodily region.

Most commonly used to treat:

- Whiplash
- Facial problems such as Bell's palsy and facial pain
- Cosmetic facial rejuvenation treatments
- Athletic overuse injuries of shoulder girdle, hamstrings, groin and other areas
- Treatment of patients who have had central nervous system damage, such as from massive head injury, stroke or cerebral palsy, for the purpose of helping to relax high-tone muscles

Time required: 1 – 4 minutes per muscle treated

Set-up: Acutron Mentor: Probe Preset #1 and set frequency as mentioned below

    Other devices:

    Intensity: 50 - 75 µA

    Frequency: Set according to muscle length (see below)

    Waveform: Square or Slope (Slope for more sensitive patients)

    Polarity: Biphasic

    Timer: 5 – 6 seconds per press of trigger

Setting Frequency: By the Law of Resonance, each tissue system of the body is most resonant with a specific frequency or set of frequencies. This is also true for this technique. Each muscle has a correspondence to an internal organ and a resonant frequency. This is the basis for the systems of Applied Kinesiology[135] and Touch for Health[136]. One anecdotal system for choosing frequency for specific muscle treatment is the Baker Formula. Measure or estimate the length of the muscle in inches, then set the frequency of your microcurrent device to 1/10th of that number. Here are some examples:

- Treat masseter muscle of cheek- It is about 3" long, so set frequency to 0.3 Hz
- Treat vastus medialis muscle of hamstrings. It is about 14" long, so set frequency to 1.4 Hz

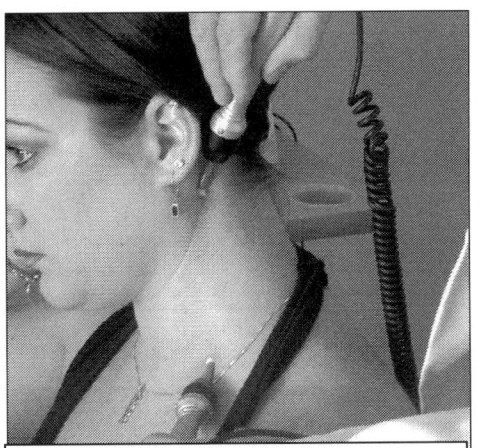

Fig. 7.9 O/I Tx of Sterno-Cleido-Mastoid M.

Steps:

There are two main techniques, Origin-Insertion and Cross Fibre:

1. *Origin-Insertion (O/I) technique:*

This is based on the principle of proprioception, which is the feedback system between the peripheral neuromuscular systems of the body and the central nervous system. Proprioception enables the muscles to grossly and subtly adjust their individual tone, or degree of tension, as well as coordinating interacting muscle systems to work together to facilitate smooth and graceful movement.

The relay centers in each muscle that transmit information on muscle tone to the CNS are nerve bundles called Golgi tendon organs (GTO). These bundles are found in the tendinous areas of the muscles, near the origins and insertions. Origins are the place where the muscle attaches to a relatively stable part of the skeleton, while insertions are the places where the other end of the muscle attaches to a bone that is moved by contractions of that muscle. As the muscle contracts and relaxes, this information is relayed via the GTO to the lower brain, which then sends back signals that adjust the muscle tone as needed.

The basis of O/I technique is using pressure and electrical stimulation over the origin and insertion of the affected muscle to goad tense muscles into relaxing, and flaccid and weak muscles into tightening. Dr. George Goodheart, who popularized the manual aspect of this technique, discovered that inward pressure toward the belly of the muscle, tends to increase tone, while outward pressure, away from the belly of the muscle tends to relax and decrease tone.

The addition of microcurrent stimulation to such manual pressure increases the results of this method. There are several ways to do this. Set up your device as mentioned above, preferably setting the Hz according to the Baker formula. Place the two probe tips of your device over the GTO and press inward or outward depending on the situation.

---

[135] More information on Applied Kinesiology can be found at www.kinesiology.net and other searchable web sites

[136] Information on the Touch for Health kinesiology system is available at: http://home.inforamp.net/~centre/kinesio.htm

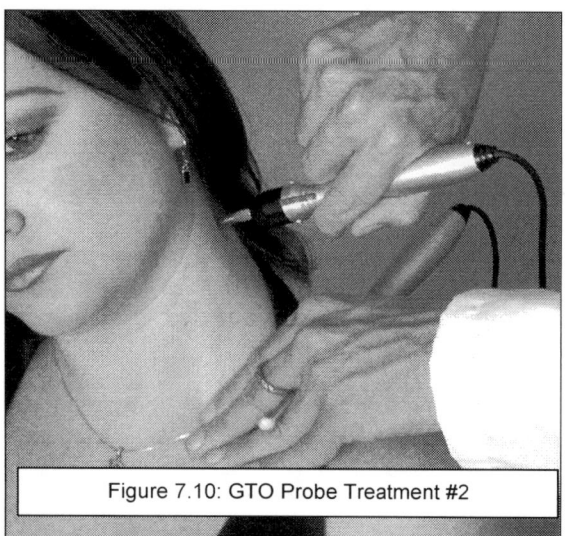

Figure 7.10: GTO Probe Treatment #2

Another method is to hold one probe tip on the origin of the muscle and the metal tip of the other probe between the third and fourth finger of your other hand to make an electrical connection with your hand. Use that hand's thumb to manually press over the GTO area. Your hand holding the first probe should remain insulated from the probe tip so no electrical connection is made.

Goodheart found that it takes a strong degree of manual pressure to adequately adjust the GTO system, so this favors the second system described in the preceding paragraph.

It is possible to use this method to adjust sets of muscles by increasing the tone of one that is weak (press inward) and decreasing the tone of one that is tense (press outward). This is valuable in some cases of whiplash or post-stroke syndrome. For example, in cases of whiplash of the neck.the sterno-cleido-mastoid muscle may be weakened and require strengthening of tone, while the levator scapulae may be too tense and require reduction of tone. See below:

2. *Cross-Fibre Technique:*

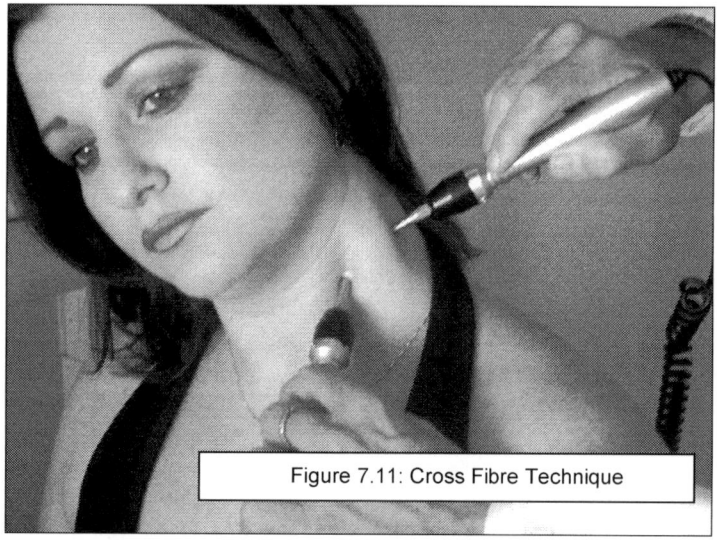

Figure 7.11: Cross Fibre Technique

This related method uses the same electrical parameters as above. While the origin-insertion technique sends current and pressure along the length of the muscle, this is done across the muscle fibers. Place the probe tips across from each other near one end of muscle and treat for 6 – 12 seconds. Move both probes down the muscle in ½" segments and treat for same time at each location. Continue until all segments of the muscle are treated. Use same Hz as for O/I treatment.

A combination of origin-insertion and cross-fiber techniques may be freely used.

Nerve Root Stimulation

Purpose: Relax paraspinal muscles, dermatome pain relief, rib pain, treat viscera through autonomic nervous system

CHAPTER SEVEN – MICROCURRENT TREATMENT: PROBE TECHNIQUES   103

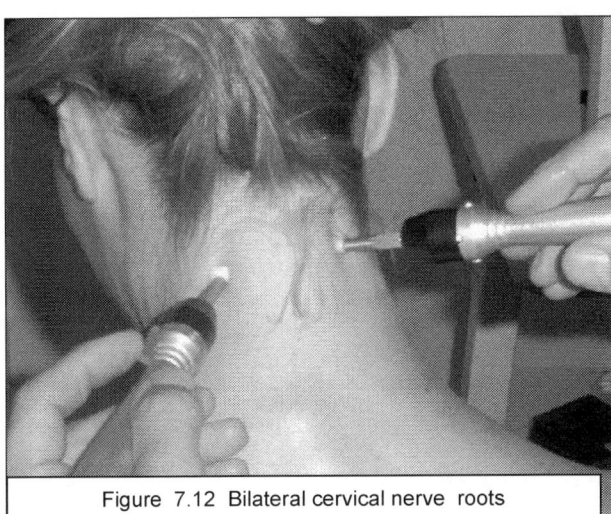

Figure 7.12 Bilateral cervical nerve roots

Most commonly used to treat:

- Extremity pain and dysfunction
- Peripheral neuropathy
- Tight and painful back and neck muscles
- As part of treatment of viscera and glands through the autonomic nervous system

Set-up: Acutron Mentor: Preset # 1 for treatment across spine, Probe Preset #2 for dermatome treatment. Default frequencies of 10 – 5 Hz is applicable for upper back nerve roots. Modifying Hz to 20 may be more resonant for low back nerve roots.[137]

Other devices: Intensity: 50 - 75 µA

Frequency: 5 Hz - upper back nerve roots, 20 Hz - low back nerve roots

Waveform: Square or Slope (Slope for more sensitive patients)

Polarity: Biphasic or Negative for dermatome tx

Nerve roots are the proximal portions of spinal nerves, each of which is associated with a specific vertebral segment. Spinal nerves connect to the spinal cord through an anterior root containing motor fibers and a posterior root containing sensory fibers. These unite to form the spinal nerve as it exits from the intervertebral foramen. Once the nerve root leaves the foramen, it divides into branches called rami. One that is called the ventral rami innervates the extremities and superficial muscles of the back, sides and front of the body. These ventral rami form nerve plexi in all spinal areas except the thoracic spine, which directly innervates its related body parts.

Spinal nerve roots are needled in Chinese acupuncture through acu-points called Hua-To points. These are located about one half to one inch from the spinal midline at each thoracic vertebral segment, and slightly wider at the lumbar spinal segments. Hua-To points are indicated for the treatment of pain and stiffness of the back, and organic diseases that are associated with the functions of the Back-Shu points at that segment. This pattern is similar to the distribution of the autonomic nervous system as described by Western science.

This is a place where contemporary anatomy and physiology correlates with TCM. We now know that each spinal nerve forms a preganglionic neuron that connect to antonomic ganglia, where they synapse with postganglionic neurons. Postganglionic neurons lie entirely outside of the central nervous system, and terminate in visceral effectors that innervate muscles, glands and organs. There are two branches of the autonomic nervous system, the sympathetic and parasympathetic. Each has its own separate effectors acting

---

[137] This information on Hz is derived from the work of Paul Nogier, M.D., who mapped ear and body areas for most resonant therapeutic frequencies.

on the target tissues. Most organs have both kind of effectors, and are considered to be dual innervated. One of the two systems initiates activity in the target organ, while the other inhibits activity. The stimulating aspect can be either sympathetic or parasympathetic. For example, parasympathetic activity stimulates digestive action, and sympathetic inhibits it, as is necessary when a person is confronted with emergency fight-or-flight situations. Yet the sympathetic system stimulates heart activity, while parasympathetic decreases it. In general, the parasympathetic division is concerned with rest and conservation of body energy, while the sympathetic system is more concerned with expending energy to deal with stress and life demands.

Stimulation of the Hua-To point associated with each segment of the autonomic system has a direct effect on the organs, glands and muscles innervated by that spinal nerve, as is indicated in traditional acupuncture texts. Therefore, nerve root stimulation can have local as well as far reaching systemic effects. There are two main techniques associated with nerve root stimulation:

1. *Bilateral nerve root stimulation:* This is the simplest approach. Use biphasic polarity, and set parameters according to above specifications. Place probes bilaterally on right and left nerve roots of affected area. When applied to the cervical spine as shown above, this method is very useful for all kinds of neck pain and dysfunction, and many types of headaches.

    Bilateral stimulation can be applied to the thoracic, lumbar and sacral spine as well. It has been successfully employed by many chiropractors as a quick and easy lead-in to spinal manipulation. They have found that patients have less stiffness and resistance, and the adjustments often last longer, when preceded by microcurrent nerve root stimulation. It is especially valuable when treating the neck and sacral regions, with probes placed bilaterally over each affected segment of the affected region. In the treatment of lumbar disk protusions and herniations, stimulation of the nerve roots at the affected level can support other kinds of interventions, and in some cases, help the local muscles to adjust their tone to better support the spine.

Great care must be exercised when applying nerve root stimulation to the thoracic region due to the innervation of the heart. Although application of microcurrents are unlikely to have any effect on the heart pacemaker, it is wise to not pass any current across the spine or through the chest of any patient with any level of cardiac disease, or with those using an electronic pacemaker or defibrillator. In many cases, electrical stimulation of any kind around the chest is contraindicated for such patients. When the patient is stable enough to receive microcurrent therapy to the thoracic region, the next technique, dermatome nerve root stimulation, is more applicable.

The following chart may offer helpful guidance[138]:

SYMPATHETIC AND PARASYMPATHETIC SYSTEM EFFECTS

FUNCTION	SYMPATHETIC EFFECTS	PARASYMPATHETIC EFFECTS
Eye	Dilates pupil	Constricts pupil
Sweat glands	Stimulates secretion	No effect
Adrenal glands	Stimulates secretions	No effect
Lungs	Dilation	Constriction (as seen in asthma)
Heart	Increases contraction strength, dilate vessels,	Decrease contraction, constrict vessels
Liver	Promotes glycogenolysis, decreases bile secretion	Promotes glycogenesis, increases bile secretion
Stomach	Decreases digestive action	Increases digestive action
Intestines	Decreases digestive action	Increases digestive action
Kidneys	Constricts vessels, decreases urine volume	No effect
Pancreas	Inhibits secretions	Increases secretions
Spleen	Discharge of stored blood into circulation	No effect
Urinary bladder	Relaxes muscular wall, increases tone in sphincter	Contracts wall, relaxes internal sphincter
Uterus	Inhibits contraction if not pregnant, promotes contraction if pregnant	Little effect
Sex organs	Promotes ejaculation in male, reverse uterine peristalsis in female	Vasodilation and erection in both sexes; promotes female secretion

Figure 7.13: Sympathetic and Parasympathetic Effects

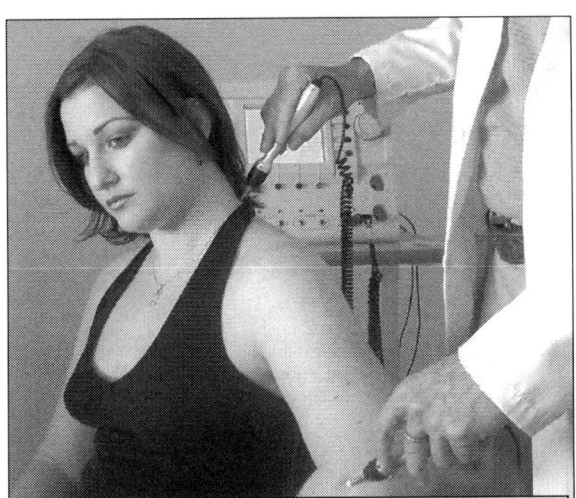

Figure 7.14: Polarized dermatome probe treatment along C 6 dermatome for treatment of radicular pain

Dermatome nerve root stimulation: This is an extenstion of the Dermatome and Distal technique detailed above. For this style of treatment, set up your microcurrent stimulator with negative polarity, that is, the trigger probe negative and the counter probe positive. Place the positive probe on the nerve root of the affected dermatome, and place the negative probe on a distal point, either within the dermatome, or on an acupoint that relates to the function being treated.

---

[138] by Tortora and Anagnostakos Principles of Anatomy and Physiology, Third Edition, Harper and Row

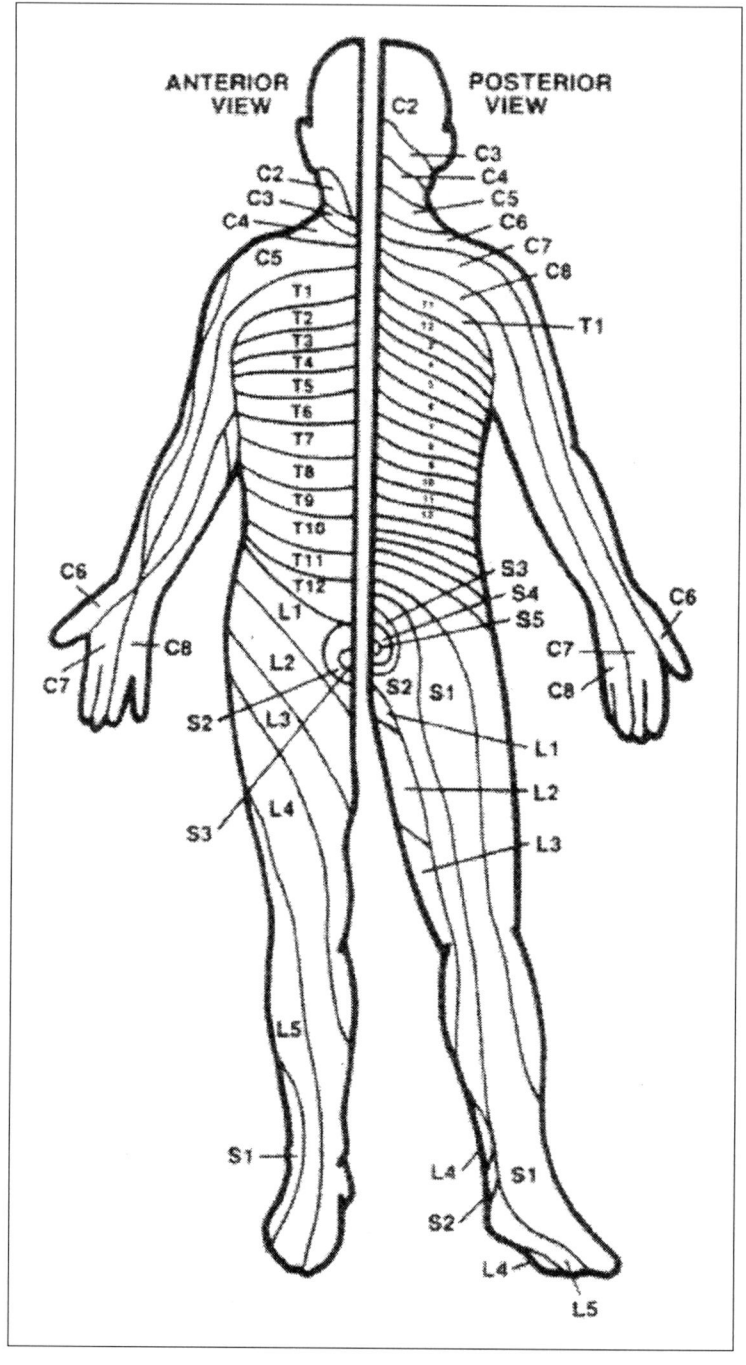

Figure 7.15: Dermatome Chart
Courtesy of Uni-Patch Co., Wabasha, WI

Some clinical examples follow:

- *Brachial plexus constriction causing pain and numbness along C6 dermatome of right arm-* Place positive probe on C6 nerve root on right side, negative probe on several painful locations along arm within C 6 dermatome. Use searching function of device to locate and treat most conductive (hot) points along pathway. Some practitioners have found it effective to place one probe at the spinal nerve root and the other at the farthest radiation of pain, and then move them closer together several inches at a time, searching and treating at each set of points, until the probe have met midway on the arm.

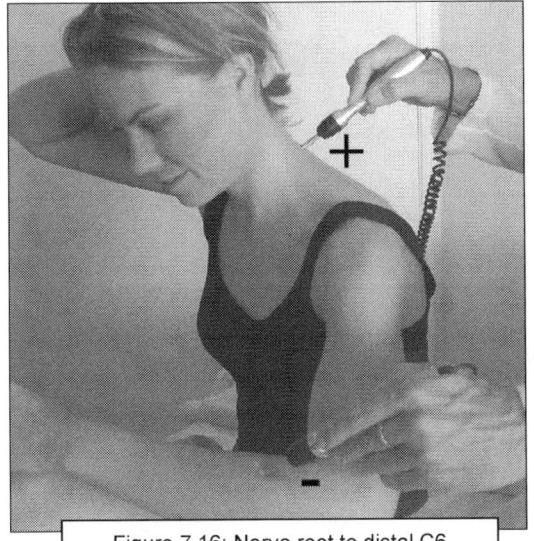

Figure 7.16: Nerve root to distal C6 dermatome

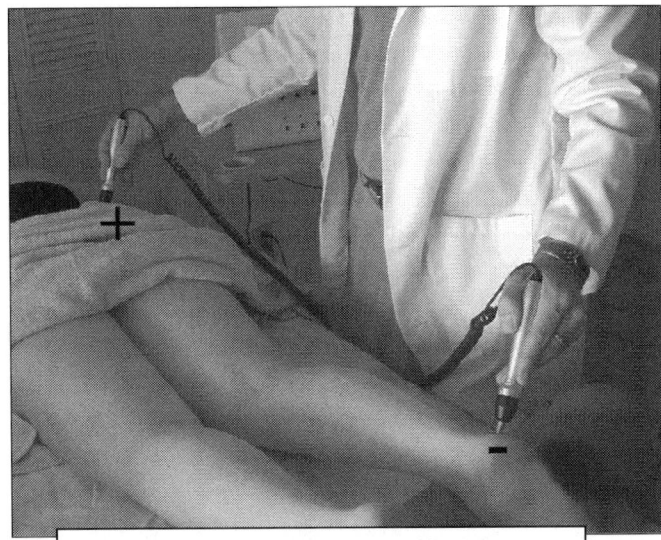

Figure 7.17: Dermatome treatment of sciatica

- *Sciatic pain running down Urinary Bladder meridian of back of leg to calf-* Use same method as described for brachial plexus. Either hold positive probe on nerve root and move negative probe distally in several increments, or start the probes far apart and move them together until they meet in the center of the affected pathway on the back of the thigh.

- *Stiffness of paraspinal muscles of thoracic spine-* Place positive probe on tight muscle area, and negative probe on acu-point UB 2 above inner canthus of eye socket, on same side, and/or UB 58-59. These points have empirical effects on relaxing the paraspinals.

- *Digestive weakness, with slow digestion, gas, possible diarrhea or constipation-* To treat through autonomic system, place positive probe on Hua-To points at levels of T11 and T12 vertebrae. Use both sides in turn. Place negative probe on distal acu-points that enhance digestive function, such as St 36, LI 10, Sp 4, or P 6, also bilaterally. The negative probe may also be placed on appropriate abdominal points such as Liv 13,

Ren 6 or Ren 12. Polarity may need to be reversed in some cases depending on condition. Test to check when not sure.

This treatment can be enhanced by stimulating UB 10 on the nape of the neck, the Master point of the parasympathetic nervous system (according to French acupuncture teachings). Digestion is often weakened by deficient parasympathetic tonus, or excess sympathetic tonus, which can arise from chronic emotional stress. UB 10 can be needled during microcurrent nerve root treatment, or stimulated with the negative probe while the positive probe is held on the indicated Hua-To points. In any treatment in which parasympathetic tonus needs to be enhanced, you can stimulate UB 10. For any treatment in which sympathetic tonus needs to be enhanced, stimulate GB 20.

Polarized microcurrent stimulation may potentially be used for any visceral or glandular disorder by placing the positive probe on the associated Hua-To point, and the negative probe on distal acu-points that are traditionally used to treat that function. This is an area where TCM can be blended with Western physiology. For that reason, some experimentation may be necessary to find the most useful point combinations. In some cases, the patient may require reversed electrical polarity of the probes as well, with negative on nerve root and positive on the distal point. Therefore kinesiology or other indicator system can be very helpful in confirming these choices.

Here is another example that combines nerve root stimulation with glandular treatment through the Extraordinary Vessels:

- Thyroid disorders- Place positive probe on cervical nerve roots at level of C3 – C5, and negative probe on Pc 6, Pc 8, Sp 4, or Ren 22. This treatment regulates the thyroid through the Yin Wei Extraordinary Vessel. This is a treatment that particularly requires accurate polarity, so it is best to briefly muscle test before administering treatment. Polarity may need to be reversed depending on whether the patient has a hypo or hyperthyroid condition.

Microcurrent Mu-Shu method

Purpose: Regulate internal Organs, balance Yin and Yang of Organs[139]

Most commonly used to treat:

- Disorders of the viscera
- May be valuable for some kinds of back pain

Time required: 20 – 45 seconds per set of Mu-Shu points treated

Set-up: Acutron Mentor: Probe Preset #2

    Other devices: Intensity: 75 μA
Frequency: 10 Hz
Waveform: Square or Slope (Slope for more sensitive patients)
Polarity: Negative
Timer: 5 – 6 seconds per press of trigger

---

[139] In this book, the word organ with a small "o" refers to the physical internal organs recognized by Western medicine, while Organ with a capital "O" refers to the more expansive energetic orb of influence described by traditional Chinese medicine. These terms overlap in many ways, yet have some significant differences.

Method: Place positive probe on Front-Mu point, also know as Alarm point, corresponding to the Organ to be treated. Place negative probe on associated Back-Shu point.[140] Treat right Mu to right Shu, then same on left side. Treat each set of points for 15 – 30 seconds.

I have used kinesiology to test the recommended polarities many times. So far, this test has always shown the recommended polarities to be indicated. I suggest that you experiment with this for yourself, so you don't just take my word for it!

There are two major systems of Front-Mu points. The first is that which is taught through TCM. Manaka taught the other.

From a look at this chart, you can see that the Mu points on the chest are the same in both systems, while those on the abdomen are mostly different. Manaka came up with his points through rigorous research. He found that the Chinese abdominal Mu points were correct when a person was standing or walking, while his were correct when a person was lying supine. This is a good guideline to follow. Use Manaka's points when the patient is lying on a treatment table, and use the Chinese points if he is sitting up or standing.

FIGURE 7.18: TCM AND MANAKA MU POINT COMPARISON

ORGAN	TCM Mu Point	Manaka Mu Point
Lungs	Lu1	Lu 1
Pericardium	Ren17	Ren17
Heart	Ren14/Ren15	Ren14/Ren15
Stomach	Ren12	Ren12
Gall Bladder	GB24	GB 24, ASIS area
Spleen	Liv13	Liv13, axillary line
Liver	Liv14	Soft tissue just below angle of right costal region
Kidney	GB25	K 16
Triple Warner	Ren5	St 25
Small Intestine	Ren4	Slightly medial to St 26
Large Intestine	St25	Slightly lateral to St 27
Urinary Bladder	Ren3	Ren 2/Ren 3, K 11

---

[140] Also know as Associated points in some acupuncture traditions

Fig. 7.19: Back Shu Points

Organ	Back Shu Point	Spinal Level	Symptoms / Problems
Bones, vertebra	UB11	T1	Stiffness of neck and spine, flu, arthritis
Wind gate	UB12	T2	Cold, flu, fever, neck & back stiffness, asthma, nose problems
Lungs	UB13	T3	Cough, asthma, empty heat conditions of lungs
Pericardium	UB14	T4	Cough, chest fullness, angina, depression
Heart	UB15	T5	Cough, irritability, epilepsy, insomnia
Blood	UB17	T7	Disorders of heart, lungs, diaphragm, skin & blood disease
Liver	UB18	T9	Liver and eye diseases, irritability, intercostal pain
Gall Bladder	UB19	T10	Jaundice, bitter taste, pleurisy, tuberculosis, headache
Spleen	UB20	T11	Weak digestion, diarrhea, bloating, vomiting, edema, anorexia
Stomach	UB21	T12	All digestive problems, bloating, nausea, back pain
Triple Warmer	UB22	L1	Indigestion, bloating, edema, pain, stiffness of low back
Kidneys	UB23	L2	Bladder and sexual disorders, **fatigue**, back pain, deafness, edema, blurred vision, thirst, tinnitus
Qi Gate	UB24	L3	Low back pain, hemorrhoids, connects to Ren6
Large Intestine	UB25	L4	Abdominal distension and pain, diarrhea and constipation
Source Gate	UB26	L5	Low back and abdominal pain, connects to Ren4
Small Intestine	UB27	S1	Sacral pain, female discharge, hemorrhoids, enuresis, enteritis
Urinary Bladder	UB28	S2	Cystitis, enuresis, diarrhea, constipation, low back pain

Mu Points are often called Alarm points in English translation. This is because they can get very sore and distended upon palpation. Because they are infused with the Qi of the Organs after which they are named, these points directly register related organic disorders. The same is true for Back-Shu Points, sometimes called Associated points. Both Mu and Shu points can be palpated as diagnostic tools.

Although both types of points reflect the condition of the physical organs, Mu points register more of the Yin, or physically substantial and nutritive aspect of the Organs, while Back-Shu points register more of the Yang, or energetic, aspect. This makes sense because Mu points are generally located right over the physical organs, while the Shu points are mostly located over the regulatory autonomic ganglia. The nervous system is more Yang in relation to the Organs themselves. I believe it is for these reasons that the kinesiology tests have shown correct electro-therapy polarity of the Mu-Shu technique to be positive on the Mu points and negative on the Shu points. Negative polarity, being more stimulating[141] than the positive pole, is more Yang.

---

[141] The negative pole is electron donating. Electrons are negatively charged.

By placing negative microcurrent polarity over the Shu point and the positive polarity over the corresponding Mu point, an electrical circuit is infused through both the physical organ and its energetic control systems. This polarity pattern sets up a powerful balancing effect on the organ.

Microcurrent Mu-Shu technique is offered as a new and very useful interface between TCM and modern microcurrent technology. It has many valuable applications to internal medicine, pediatrics and meridian balancing. It can be used as an alternative to moxibustion for Step Two of the Four-Step protocol described in Chapter 12. The following table shows the Mu-Shu point combinations:

FIGURE 7.20: MU-SHU TREATMENTS

ORGAN TO BE TREATED	MU POINT: + PROBE	SHU POINT - PROBE	COMMENTS
Lung	Lu 1	UB 13	Use caution with cardiac/elderly patients with this combination
Pericardium	Ren 17	UB 14	Do not pass current through heart – substitute Kidney Mu-Shu
Heart	Ren 14	UB 15	Do not pass current through heart – substitute Kidney Mu-Shu
Liver	Liv 14	UB 18	Use Manaka Liver 14- in soft tissue below R costal angle
Gall Bladder	GB 24	UB 19	
Spleen	Liv 13	UB 20	In this case the TCM Spleen Mu works better
Stomach	Ren 12	UB 21	
Triple Warmer	St 25/Ren 5	UB 22	Either Manaka or TCM Mu point will work, test to select
Kidney	Ki 16	UB 23	Manaka Mu point better here
Large Intestine	St 25/27	UB 25	Either Manaka or TCM Mu point will work, test to select
Small Intestine	St 26/Ren 4	UB 27	Either Manaka or TCM Mu point will work, test to select
Urinary Bladder	Ren 3/Ki 12	UB 28	

There is an important caution/contraindication to observe when performing microcurrent Mu-Shu method. When passing microcurrents through the Mu-Shu combinations of the Pericardium and Heart, electrical currents will pass directly through the region of the heart organ. While this is unlikely to have any negative effect on healthy people, it is an unacceptable risk for patients with cardiac disease or with pacemakers in place. To be on the safe side, it is best to avoid utilizing electrical Mu-Shu method through these points. When the patient's evaluation calls for treatment of the Heart or Pericardium functions, you can substitute treatment of the Kidney or other lower back functions. The Kidney is intimately related to Pericardium through the Ministerial Life Gate Fire, and to the Heart through the Shaoyin Great Loop circuit. For example, if your diagnosis calls for treatment of the Spleen and Pericardium, you could choose the Mu-Shu combinations of the Spleen and Kidney.

Micro-Macro Technique

Purpose: Control acute pain and regulate disorders of body through connection of local area and corresponding micro-system point(s) of ear or hand.

Most commonly used to treat:

- Acute myofascial or musculoskeletal pain
- Balancing of head/brain and rest of body
- Potentially any organic disorder

Time required: 12 – 30 seconds per set of points to be treated

Set-up: Acutron Mentor: Probe Preset #2, modify frequency to ear region treated, or universal ear frequency of 2.5 Hz. Reduce current intensity to 25 – 50 µA for sensitive persons. Place special auricular probe tip on trigger probe.

Other devices: Intensity: 25 - 75 µA

Frequency: See following chart, or set to 2.5 Hz

Waveform: Square for pain, Sloped for other disorders

Polarity: Negative

Timer: 5 – 6 seconds per press of trigger

Steps:

1. Set up microcurrent unit with probes polarized. If available, place a 2 – 3mm auricular probe tip on the trigger probe, which should be negative. In most cases, it is appropriate to place the negative probe on the micro-system point, and the positive on the macro body point. The micro-system point is acting as the distal point in this system, which usually requires the negative polarity. In some cases, the polarity may need to be reversed.

2. Place wetted Q-tip of counter probe (positive) on symptomatic part of the body such as painful elbow, shoulder or back, or on acu-point that directly registers the Qi of that part, such as St 36 for the Stomach. For ease, you can usually have the patient hold the counter probe. In pain cases, just tell her to touch it to where her body hurts the most.

3. Dip auricular probe tip of trigger probe into water and shake off excess, and apply it to area of ear or hand point that directly corresponds to affected body region. For example, in cases of shoulder pain, patient holds counter probe on shoulder, while you place trigger tip on Shoulder point of ear.

4. Use searching feature of device to find exact micro-system point with highest conductivity reading. You can then search with counter probe on body area to locate most conductive point there as well.

5. You have now created an electrical circuit between the macro (body) and micro (ear) point. Treat in 5 – 6 second periods until the reading on the unit meter goes as high as possible. You can then move onto other applicable point combinations and repeat the procedure.

6. It can be valuable to have the patient move or exercise the affected body region while performing this technique. Movement draws more Qi and Blood to the area for correction of stasis, and helps re-educate the neuro-muscular system through proprioception.

The same instructions may be used in connecting a Korean hand point or any other micro-system with the corresponding body region.

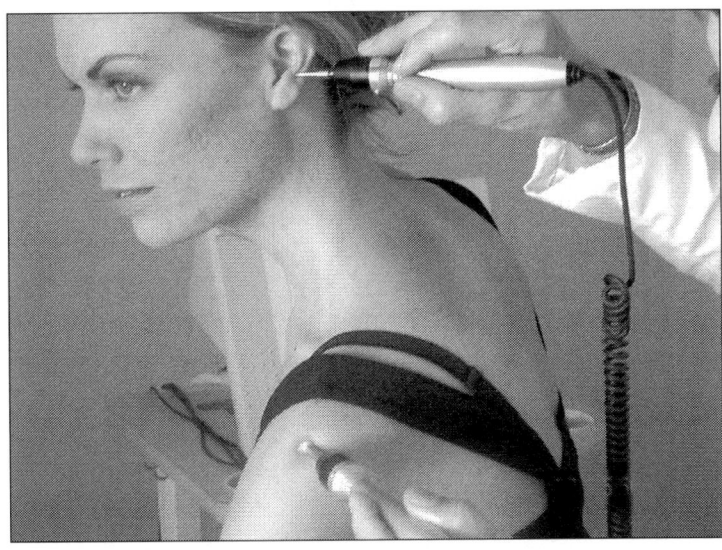

Figure 7.21: Auricular micro-macro technique connecting actual shoulder and ear-shoulder point

Chapter 8

TREATMENT OF GREAT LOOPS

General principles

The tremendous success of acupuncture for pain control is based on whole-body treatment through the meridian system. This is the vital difference between microcurrent electro-acupuncture and localized electro-therapies as commonly practiced.

One of the simplest and most common methods taught in introductory acupuncture courses is to combine the needling of local and distal points. In many cases, the distal points utilized are on the meridian that passes through the affected areas. Powerful distal acu-points treatments have been described in excellent books such as Master Tong's Acupuncture[142] and Twelve and Twelve In Acupuncture.[143] Most of the points described in these books are not traditional acu-points on the fourteen main meridians, and require additional study and memorization in order to use them.

While it is of great value to learn and apply these new points, it is equally beneficial to understand for ourselves the energetic principles by which we can select effective distal points. This involves learning and internalizing the energetic relationships between meridians of the upper and lower extremities. I refer the reader to the excellent work of Dr. Richard Tan. His Balance Method of acupuncture is a clearly explained system for utilizing these relationships in acupuncture practice. Due to the electrical nature of the meridian systems, I have found that microcurrent is an excellent tool for utilizing such methods.

In the more reductionistic ways of Western society, acupuncture courses usually refer to meridians as individual entities, such as the Lung channel or the Spleen channel. This is not how meridians are usually understood in the classics of acupuncture. A "Great Loop", on the other hand, is a complete meridian, consisting of one branch beginning or ending on the upper extremities, and the other branch beginning or ending on the lower extremities. For example, the Lung and Spleen channels are part of one Great Loop called Taiyin. The proper, full name for the Lung channel is the "Lung channel of Arm Taiyin", and the full name for the Spleen channel is the "Spleen channel of Foot Taiyin". Each Great Loop is composed of two Yang meridians or two Yin meridians.

The Nei Jing, or Yellow Emperor's Classic of Internal Medicine states: (in paraphrased form):

> "For diseases of the upper body, treat the lower, for diseases of the lower body, treat the upper, for diseases of the front, treat the back, for diseases of the back, treat the front, for diseases of the right, treat the left, for diseases of the left, treat the right."

Great Loops treatment works according to this understanding. Utilizing these principles in selecting acu-points gives added power to treatments. The understanding of the Great Loops is

---

[142] Translated by Miriam Lee, pub. Blue Poppy Press
[143] This and companion volume Twenty Four More is written and pub. by Richard Tan, O.M.D and Steven Rush

very important for pain management and is a powerful key to successfully healing painful conditions on one part by treating points on the opposite part of the Loop.

The clinical approach of the Great Loops brings together three powerful principles of pain management into one, easy to perform technique. The three principles are:

1. **Treating opposite quadrants** of the body through related meridians on the upper and lower extremities Again, taking advantage of the advice "for disease of the upper treat the lower, for diseases of the right treat the left (and vice versa)."

2. **The Law of Polarity** as applied to the relationship between electrical currents and the natural polarities of the human body

3. The receptivity of the body to correctly applied **subtle energy stimulation** (microcurrents)

The Great Loops can be understood as layers of energy (Qi). Thus the "top" layer, Taiyang (Urinary Bladder and Small Intestine channels) represents the most superficial energies of the principal meridian system, and the "deepest" layer, Shaoyin (Heart and Kidney channels), represents the most vital bases of life. Therefore, the Taiyang layer is most affected when one is exposed to external environmental conditions or pathogens and gets a simple cold or flu, with body aches, sneezing, runny nose, fever and chills, etc. When the body's defenses (Wei Qi) are unable to expel the pathogenic influence, it may penetrate to deeper energy layer, causing diseases that are progressively more serious and chronic pain conditions. The stages of disease according to energy layer are described in the Chinese classic the <u>Shang Han Lung</u>[144]. When a disease penetrates to the deepest Shaoyin layer there is clearly a life and death situation present (heart and kidney disease).

There is also an energy layer even more superficial than Taiyang – this is the network of Tendino-Muscular meridians (TMM), which is not considered to part of the principal meridian system. This layer is most affected by simple trauma to the body, and is where the body's defensive Qi initially reacts to external invasion or trauma. *The TM meridians, which have electro-magnetic qualities, are what is probably the most directly affected by microcurrent stimulation.* It is likely that the TM system exists primarily in the fascial system of the body, as some Japanese researchers espouse. I believe that, although electrical stimulation and electro-diagnostics mainly deal with this most superficial energy layer, the deeper principal and Extraordinary meridians are affected as well through the Law of Resonance. This has been clearly confirmed in my clinical experience and experimentation.

---

[144] by Zhang Zhong-jing, circa 220 C.E.

ENERGETIC LAYERS OF THE BODY
Tendino-Muscular Meridians
Taiyang, or Greater Yang (UB + SI)
Yangming, or Sunshine Yang (St + LI)
Shaoyang, or Lesser Yang (GB + TW)
Taiyin, or Greater Yin (Sp + Lu)
Jueyin, or Absolute Yin (Lv + Pc)
Shaoyin, or Lesser Yin (K + Ht)
Shaoyin, or Lesser Yin (K + Ht)
Bone

Figure 8.1: Energetic Layers

Great Loops treatment is most useful for extremity conditions such as, but not limited to:

- Tennis elbow
- Shoulder injury and restricted ROM
- Carpal tunnel syndrome and other wrist injuries
- Hip pain
- Knee pain and sprain
- Ankle pain and sprain
- Peripheral neuropathy

In this chapter, I use the term Great Loops more loosely to refer to the method of creating an electrical circuit between a local painful area on the extremities and a distal point on the opposite aspect of the body. You will learn how to use actual Great Loops meridian pairs as listed above, such as treating the leg Gall Bladder channel for problems along the Triple Warmer channel of the arm. In other cases, a different meridian relationship between local and distal point(s) will be required, and this is explained as well.

Treatment Principles

There are two important principles to understand before you can perform microcurrent Great Loops therapy. They are proper polarity placement and the anatomical relationship of joints.

Polarity Placement

> **THE THREE P'S**
>
> The principle of polarity treatment in this application is the *Three-P's*, or *Positive Probe Proximal*. The term proximal can be understood in two ways. The first and most common anatomical definition of proximal is a region *closer to the head or spine*, while distal means farther from the head or spine. This more common anatomical definition is applicable to dermatome treatment. In this case, the positive probe is applied to a spinal nerve root (Hua-To point), and the negative probe is applied to a distal area within the dermatome related to that spinal nerve. For example, placing the positive probe on the C6 nerve root and the negative probe down the arm on the radial area of the wrist for pain and numbness caused by some "pinched nerve" syndromes. The second definition of proximal uses a different perspective. In this perspective, proximal is <u>on or near a painful body part</u>, while distal means going to an opposite anatomical body part as follows (the sides of the body in this chart can be reversed):
>
> | PAINFUL BODY AREA | DISTAL OPPOSITE AREA |
> |---|---|
> | Right shoulder | Left hip |
> | Right elbow | Left knee |
> | Right wrist | Left ankle |

Anatomical Relationship of Joints

The wrists and ankles are the most distal main joints, while the elbows and knees are the next up the extremities, while the shoulders and hips are the major joints closest to the trunk of the body. Get it? So in this definition of **P**ositive **P**robe **P**roximal, place the + probe on the painful body area, and the – probe on a tender point on the opposite joint according to above chart.

Correspondences

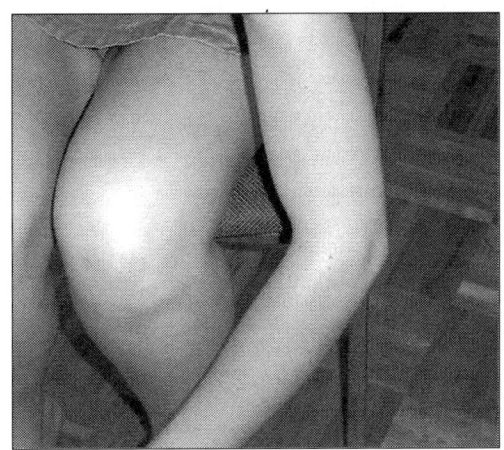
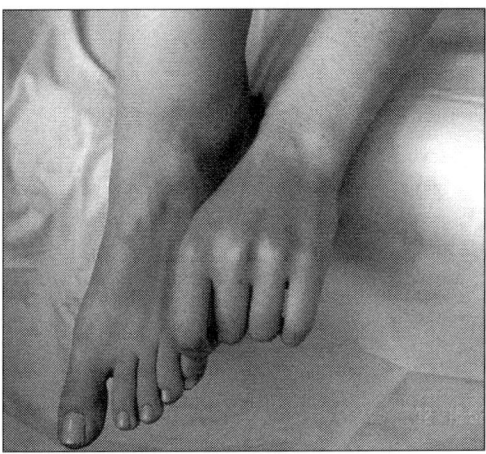

Figure 8.2: Anatomical Symmetry of the Major Joints of the Extremity

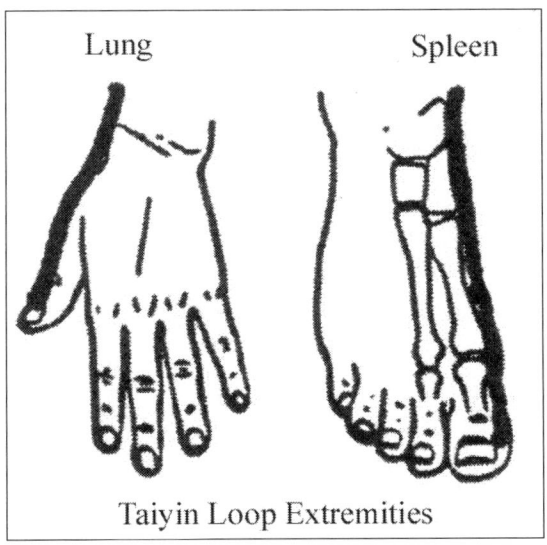
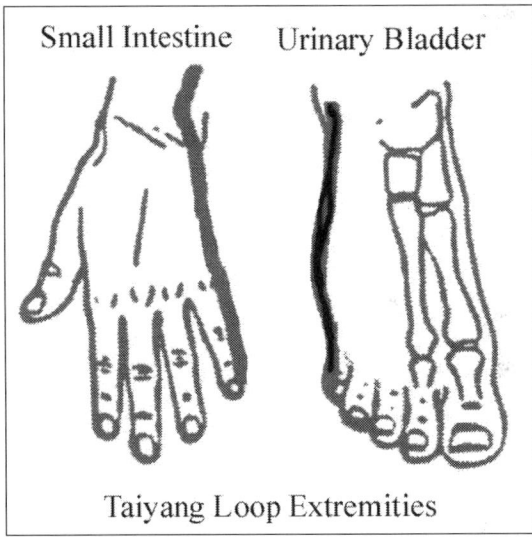

Figure 8.2a: Meridian Symmetry – Taiyin and Taiyang Great Loops

Besides understanding meridian relationships, hands-on palpation is also essential for locating key distal points, as they tend to be tender and sore. The most effective distal points will not always be on or around the opposite joint, they can be above or below them, on the inner or outer aspects of the limb. Skill in Great Loops treatment is based on synthesizing your knowledge of the meridian relationships with palpation skills, and some trial and error, until a circuit is found that powerfully alleviates the complaint.

Step-by-step Great Loops treatment

Great Loops treatment is simple:

1. Choose the painful area to treat. Ask the patient to let you know how painful it is when she moves through its range of motion, or while you press on it, so you can compare before and after treatment status.

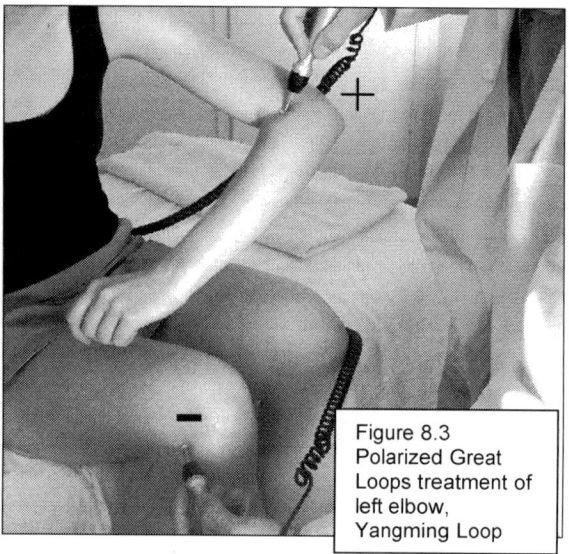

Figure 8.3 Polarized Great Loops treatment of left elbow, Yangming Loop

2. Go to the opposite anatomical area and carefully palpate for tender points. Start on the meridian pathway that is related to the painful area through the Great Loops, i.e., if painful area is on the Lung channel (hand-Taiyin), then first palpate the Spleen channel (foot-Taiyin) on the opposite side of the body. See Meridian Relationship chart on next page for details on selecting distal points.

3. If you find a tender zone on that meridian, use that for treatment. If you do not find one there, palpate other areas on, above and below the opposite joint until you find a highly reactive point. Once you select the most indicated distal point, place the negative probe on it, and the positive probe on the most tender focus of the painful area you are treating.

4. Press probe trigger switch to initiate treatment for a 6 – 8 second test treatment.

5. Ask the patient to rate their pain again after moving the affected area or having pressure applied. If there is significant pain reduction, you have chosen good points.

6. If test treatment has given good relief, treat in the same way for an additional 30-45 seconds to reinforce the effect. Try doing this while the patient puts the injured part in several positions that were previously difficult or painful.

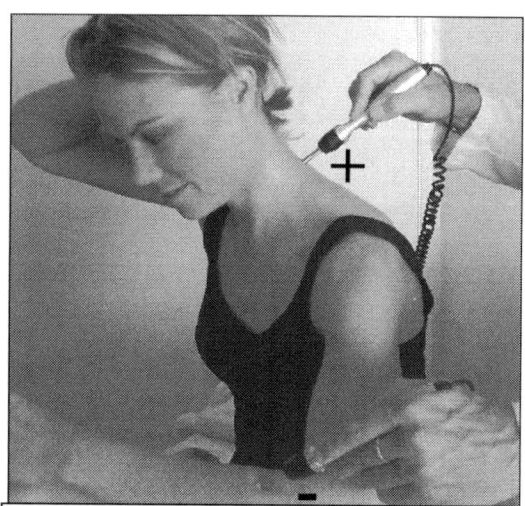

Figure 8.4: Polarized treatment of elbow from nerve root to local area

7. If the first points you use do not alleviate the pain, try other distal points, drawing on your knowledge of the meridian relationships listed below. If you have tried several opposite quadrant points and there is no significant relief, try a dermatome treatment. This is polarized treatment with both probes placed on the same quadrant of the body (see picture to the left).

8. Finish treatment by rechecking the pain level and range of motion of the painful area.

9. Great Loops technique can be freely combined with other techniques such as Circling the Dragon, electro-massage, acupuncture, manipulation and physical therapies. I generally recommend using Great Loops treatment or other

whole-body balancing as a first step in a session, and then follow with other appropriate treatment.

Meridian Relationships

Below are some examples of energetic relationships between the upper and lower body. You can draw on any of these. Feel free to palpate, experiment and use your knowledge and intuition. The points listed below are usually used by crossing the midline of the body from the local to the distal point[145]:

MERIDIAN RELATIONSHIP EXAMPLES

Relationship	Acu-points
Upper and lower aspect of same meridian	GB 21+ and GB 41- for tight trapezius
	UB10+ and UB 40- for vertebral problems and stiff neck or dizziness
Great Loops	LI 15+ and St 31- for lateral shoulder pain

YIN-YANG RELATIONSHIPS

Relationship	Acu-points
Taiyang - Shaoyin	Low back local UB points + and Ki 3- for low back pain
Shaoyang - Jueyin	GB 30+ and Per 6/7- for hip pain in elderly
Yangming - Taiyin	LI 11+ and Sp 9 or Sp 9a[146] for tennis elbow, mainly in women

POLAR MERIDIAN RELATIONSHIPS

Relationship	Acu-points
Urinary Bladder - Lung	UB 61+ and Lu 9 for heel pain
Small Intestine - Liver	SI 11+ and Lv11/12- for scapular pain (if Liver points tender)
Gall Bladder - Heart	GB 29/30+ and Ht 7- for hip pain in elderly
Triple Warmer - Spleen	TW 10+ and Sp9- for olecranon elbow pain
Large Intestine - Kidney	Kid 10+ and LI 11- for medial meniscus strain of knee
Stomach - Pericardium	Pc 6+ and St 36- for digestive problems (polarity may be reversed)

"TAI-TAI" MERIDIAN GROUPINGS

Relationship	Acu-points
Taiyang - Taiyin	Local area+ and Chung Tze/Chung Hsien on palmar aspect of hand for pain in the upper back (bladder or small intesting channel.) These points are approximately on the Lung channel of the hand
Shaoyang - Shaoyin	Use of distal Heart channel point, notably Ht 4, to relieve trapezius pain of neck (GB channel)
Yangming - Jueyin	The famous "Four Gates" acu-point combination uses LI 4 (Yangming) and Liv 3 (Jueyin) to powerfully calm the nervous system

---

[145] O Ring kinesiology is valuable for confirming whether crossing the midline is most beneficial, and for choosing most effective distal points. Alternatively, treat the side on which the distal point is most tender to palpation.

As you can see, there are many meridian connections through which to utilize this treatment principle. The bottom line is to understand the anatomical relation of the joints as mentioned above, and carefully palpate to find the most tender and reactive distal point. It will likely reflect one of the above meridian relationships. Understanding these relationships will certainly further the accuracy and overall diagnostic integrity of your treatments. Understanding that the patient's injury is in the realm of the "Large Intestine - Kidney" polar meridian pair, for example, points to a Root treatment that can be used to generally balance the meridian system before going after direct pain control. This is the heart of the Step One treatment explained in Chapter 11.

Combining microcurrent and needle stimulation

Acupuncture needle treatment may be combined with microcurrent Great Loops treatments to good advantage. To do this, place the needles in the most indicated opposite quadrant points, and gently stimulate to obtain Te Qi. Set up your microcurrent device for polarized probe treatment. Place the positive (+) counterprobe on the local painful area (or ask the patient to do so), and then touch the needles with the metal probe tip of the negative (–) trigger probe. Press the trigger button and stimulate the needles for up to 30 seconds. It is valuable to experiment with this to find out whether the addition of needles to this method increases the effectiveness. In my experience, the combination of needles and microcurrent is mainly indicated for long term, recalcitrant pain conditions, in which long needle retention periods give deeper results. Many less serious conditions respond very well to the non-needle technique alone. This is particularly true in the case of pediatric treatments.

Summary

How many times have you tried your best to help a patient with knee or elbow pain with local therapies, and not had clearly effective results? If your answer is a positive number, then the technique of the Great Loops is likely to significantly improve your results. As stated above, the power of this technique as taught here is based on the combination of appropriate distal point selection, the receptivity of the body to microcurrents, and the Law of Polarity.

Case Study - Peripheral Neuropathy

Here is a case history from my practice using this approach: A heavy-set man in his forties came to me because his profession was electronic assembly bench work, and he was losing fine motor control over his hands. This was a form of peripheral neuropathy where other medical approaches had failed. He also presented with chronic low back pain. Energetic diagnosis revealed Kidney Yang deficiency and stagnant Qi and Dampness. I placed acupuncture needles in the following points- Hua-To (nerve root) points of C 5-7 on the back of the neck, LI 15, SI 9 + 10, LI 11, TW 4 and the Baxie points of the hands.[147] These were placed bilaterally, as the neuropathy affected both arms. I also needled K 3 on both sides. The next step was to set up the Acutron microcurrent device on preset Probe #2, which delivers polarized microcurrent stimulation at 75µA and 10/5 Hz. I chose sets of needles to stimulate, always placing the + counterprobe on proximal points and the − trigger probe on distal points. For example, + on the Hua-to points with − on the Baxie points. I also used other channels of the device to simultaneously deliver microcurrent interferential pad stimulation to the patient's lower back. The next step was to set up the Acutron microcurrent device on preset Probe #2, which delivers polarized microcurrent stimulation at 75µA and 10/5 Hz. I chose sets of needles to stimulate, always placing the + counterprobe on proximal points and the − trigger probe on distal points. For example, + on the Hua-to points with − on the Baxie points. I also used other channels of the device to simultaneously deliver microcurrent interferential pad stimulation to the patient's lower back. After several days, this man reported to me that he had already gained at least 70% more use of his hands. He came in for two more treatments, after which his complaint was resolved. I have never heard from him again, which appears to show that the resolution was long term. This case utilizes microcurrent probe stimulation directly through needles.

---

[147] Baxie are Extra points found between the knuckle MCP joints in the soft tissue, inserted proximally

Chapter 9

ELECTRO-THERAPEUTIC PAD TREATMENTS

The previous two chapters dealt with microcurrent probe techniques. Such treatments constitute only a very small aspect of modern electro-therapy practice. Most commonly used electro-therapeutic devices mainly apply current through pad or vacuum electrodes that administer a much broader and more generalized stimulation than probe treatments. Those of us who have used both techniques correctly have found that probe treatments on specific acu and trigger points usually provide faster and more impressive results than general pad stimulation. We have also found that a sequence of specific probe treatments followed by more generalized pad treatments, often with simultaneous mobilization, offers many pain patients the most comprehensive and lasting results.

The simple reason probe techniques are not more commonly used is that most practitioners of electro-therapies are physical or occupational therapists, chiropractors or other physicians who have little or no knowledge of the acupuncture meridian system. Because their training is primarily based in Western anatomy and physiology, they are mainly taught to apply biphasic, milliamperage stimulation to the local injured region. Of course this practice can achieve many positive results, including relief of acute traumatic pain, improvement of blood and lymph circulation and reduction of acute muscle spasm and edema. Yet the results of such treatments are quite limited and inconsistent, and aggravations of many sensitive patients' complaints are common. To get the most from this chapter, you are recommended to review Chapter 6, which details these and other shortcomings, of traditional electro-therapies.

Electro-Therapy Devices

There are several types of devices that deliver therapeutic stimulation through pad electrodes:

1. *Transcutaneous Electric Nerve Stimulator (TENS) unit* - This unit is a very simple, portable milliamp stimulator that is prescribed for patients with chronic pain. The stimulation unit clips onto the belt, and has one or two sets of leads that attach to pads. The pads are generally placed on or around the painful area, and the patient is instructed to turn the intensity up to tolerance for several hours per day.

2. *Low-volt stimulator* - A larger, clinical version of the TENS unit. It offers higher voltages as well as more adjustments to the output currents, such as polarity shifts, pulse duration and

variable frequencies. These were the main units used by chiropractors prior to the popularization of interferential units in the 1980's.

3. *High-volt pulsed galvanic stimulator (HVPG)* - Utilizes a very narrow duration pulse waveform, sometimes with a twin peak shape. Stimulation with HVPG is more comfortable than low-volt units that produce longer pulse duration. Quite a bit of research has been done with these units. Studies have confirmed their efficacy for accelerating wound healing.

4. *Electric muscle stimulator (EMS)* - Similar to low-volt devices, this is a stimulator designed to relax tense and constricted muscles and to improve blood circulation in patients with circulatory impairments. In some cases, this device is used to stimulate the muscles of the pelvic floor to treat incontinence. An EMS often has additional features such as alternating on and off times, ramping frequencies and intensities that gradually increase and decrease the contraction of muscles.

5. *Classic Interferential stimulator (IF)* - Developed by Hans Nemec in Germany in 1950, and still largely used today, these devices use the principle of interference to drive treatment currents deeper into the body. IF utilizes out-of-phase 4000 and 4100 Hz carrier frequencies, each through a separate set of pad or vacuum electrodes. The interference effect between these two frequencies creates effective therapeutic frequencies of 100 (the difference) and 8100 (the sum). The lower, 100 Hz rate is most therapeutically significant. The two sets of electrodes are placed so that the pathways of current between each intersect in the painful bodily area. This crossing area will be most affected by the deep pulsing of the beat frequency.

Interferential Waveforms[148]

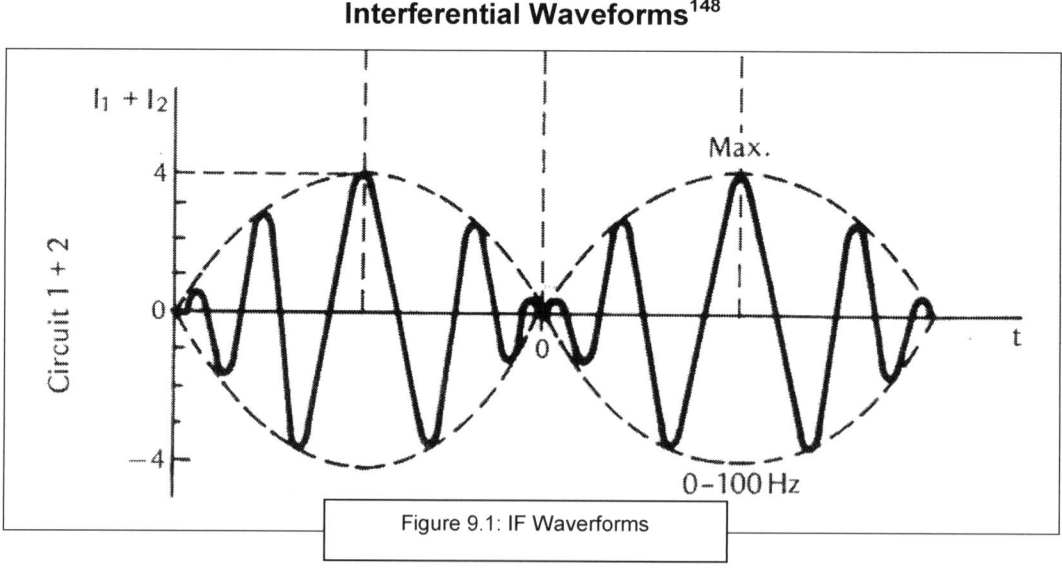

Figure 9.1: IF Waveforms

The advantages of IF treatment are the broader stimulation area due to four electrodes instead of two, and the reputedly deeper current penetration. Since the 1980's, IF units have become very popular among chiropractors and physical therapists. Although classic interferential units have shown themselves to be quite effective for temporary relief of many

---

[148] Interferential diagram courtesy of Appleton & Lange, from book <u>Clinical Electrotherapy</u> Nelson and Currier, editors, 1987

kinds of acute low back and other large joint pain, they are, in my opinion, greatly overused. The current pattern created by these units is very intense and highly dispersive of Qi. This can be beneficial when treating patients with strong physical constitutions for acute injuries. Yet it is often an "overkill" treatment for children, elderly, chronic and sensitive patients. Interferential stimulators have been used to produce electronic "nerve blocks". The ability of intense milliamp currents to block nerves are due to Wedensky inhibition, which is a sustained depolarization of nerve cell membranes leading to a continuous refractory state.

6. *Russian stimulation-* This is a more complex form of electric muscle stimulation developed for the Russian Olympic team to enhance muscular development. It utilizes a polyphasic sinusoidal waveform that produces an effective therapeutic stimulation of 50 Hz using a carrier frequency of 2500 Hz. Although one of the least versatile forms of electrical stimulation, Russian current has become widely used for muscle development, re-education and acute pain control.

7. *Microcurrent device-* Most microcurrent devices sold in the U.S. offer some form of probe and pad stimulation. In most cases two separate sets of pads can be administered in a frequency range of 0.1 – 1000 Hz. Some more advanced devices can produce out-of-phase frequencies through two sets of pads to produce what is called microcurrent interferential. Such currents offer many of the advantages of classic interferential, such as deeper and broader stimulation, yet without the overstimulation and excess dispersion associated with such devices. Microcurrent pad stimulation is excellent for kinetic electro-therapies, or "microcurrents with motion", and as a general flooding stimulation to complement meridian balancing with probe electrodes.

Therapeutic Effects Of Electrical Pad Stimulation

Electrical stimulation (ES) is used as therapy precisely because the human body is, by nature, exquisitely attuned to respond to endogenous and exogenous electric currents. As mentioned earlier in this book, most life processes are intimately associated with electrical activity, including the functions of the neuro-muscular systems, heart, brain, cellular respiration and repair, bone and so much more. Therefore, externally applied electrical currents may be used to influence any or all of these physiological functions.

A useful physiologic principle is the Arndt-Schultz Law of physiology. This states that high-intensity stimulation inhibits organic functioning while low-intensity stimulation increases organic functioning. This Law gives a good guideline for the choice of milli or microamp treatments. In view of the Arndt-Schultz ILaw, the physiological effects of ES may be divided into two categories- the gross and the subtle. The gross effects are those generally associated with high-intensity milliamp stimulation, while the subtle effects are brought about by microcurrents, or even subtler energies of healing touch, thought or color and light. Being in the middle of the spectrum, microcurrent stimulation offers balanced benefits.

Pad electrodes

The most important quality of a pad electrode is the ability to evenly disperse treatment current. If a pad fails to do this, "hot spots" will be created that can cause shocks and discomfort. The old style pad electrodes were made of black rubber impregnated with metal particles. The underside is coated with conductive gel and applied to the skin. These rubber electrodes are still of value due to their economy, as they can be used indefinitely as long as they are regularly cleansed. They are also valuable for stimulating hairy areas, as the gel can be coated on thickly for these treatment regions. The most popular type of pads used today are self-stick, disposable ones. These are coated with a reusable polymer that adheres to the skin and evenly conducts electricity. These kind of pads can last from 3 to 15 applications. Skin preparation is the main factor that determines how many applications the pads will serve.

The most important factors in pad longevity:

- Cleanse skin with alcohol wipes, or soap, water and a washcloth prior to applying pads to remove dead skin cells, oils and cosmetics which can all clog the adhesive of the pad.

- After using pads, place them back on the plastic sheet on which they come packed and slip them back into their pouch so they won't dry up.

- After the first few uses, it will be necessary to rub a drop of water all over the sticky side of the pad before each use to re-activate the adhesive.

If a patient complains of uneven stimulation or shocks, immediately discard that set of pads. If such complaints persist, contact your pad or device vendor.

Pad electrodes come in many shapes and sizes. Larger pads range in size from 2" x 4" up to 6" x 6", and may be used for generalized lower back pain. Smaller pads are about 2" x 2" or smaller. Microcurrent electro-acupuncture generally utilizes smaller pads because they can be used with greater precision over specific acu-points and for four-pad interferential stimulation of joints and body regions.

ELECTRO-THERAPEUTIC PAD TECHNIQUES

Treatment techniques to produce the gross effects of ES are mostly based on local stimulation of the affected body area with the correct form of stimulation. Many worthy books have been written about these principles and methods that may be referred to for further resources[149]. The basic techniques described herein are divided into milliamp and microamp categories. For each technique described, a preset on the Acutron Mentor unit will be referenced. Although there is significant overlap, the milliamp techniques described below mainly target the gross effects listed above, while the microamp techniques mainly target the subtle effects.

1. Milliamp pad techniques

- *Local low-volt stimulation (mA Pad #1)* - Pads may be placed on the body to bracket affected area. Useful for local pain relief and muscle tension and spasm that does not respond to gentler measures. See next section on microamp pad techniques for photos of single pad placements

- *Local high-volt stimulation (mA Pad #2)* - Due to its narrow pulse duration, higher intensities than conventional stimulators may be used with greater comfort. High-volt treatment is often administered in a two-step process – first with continuous current to recruit the maximum amount of muscle fibers, second with a burst mode that turns the currents on and off every few seconds. High-volt stimulation is also used for wound healing acceleration. For this purpose, custom electrodes are saturated with sterile saline solution and packed directly into open pressure sores and other wounds, with the counter electrode placed on healthy skin at some distance from the wound. The negative polarity has been found to be more useful for draining and disinfecting pustulent wounds, while positive is better for promoting granulation of new tissue.

---

[149] See Bibliography

- *Russian Stimulation (mA Pad #3)* - This protocol was originally designed for the purpose of passive muscular development by the Russian Olympic team. The most common technique of use is with burst mode, in which bursts of current alternate with off periods lasting from 6 up to 50 seconds. Intensity is turned up to the point of strong muscle contractions, with pads placed over major motor points of the muscles to be stimulated. This back and forth action creates the maximum muscle cell activation. The two most common burst protocols are 10 seconds on and 50 seconds off, or 10 seconds on and 10 seconds off. Russian Stimulation has also been used in the United States for acute pain control related to athletic injuries.

- *Milliamp-Microamp Combination (mA Pad #4)* - One of the drawbacks of high-intensity stimulation is potential aggravation of pain caused by the drastic and sudden changes caused to the electro-physiology of the body. According to Chinese Medicine, the Liver is responsible for assuring the smooth flow of Qi throughout the meridian system. When the Liver is functioning well, the body can adapt to and tolerate sudden energy changes relatively well, including changes of temperature, sudden movements, and emotional surges. This also includes changes of electrical stimulation levels to parts of the body. Many chronic pain patients have impaired Liver function. These patients are not able to adapt to such energy changes quickly and easily. When this is the case, the experience of a high level of ES being suddenly shut off at the end of a treatment may cause a rebound pain effect anywhere from immediately to several hours after the treatment. Milliamp-Microamp combination therapy was designed to minimize this effect by giving the patient several minutes of sub-sensational microcurrent after the termination of a period of milliamp stimulation. This has been found to minimize the pain rebound effect, and be "kinder and gentler" to sensitive patients who require milliamp treatment.

- *Classic Interferential (I.F. #4)* - This is the original form of interferential treatment from Germany. It utilizes two sets of electrodes, each set to a different frequency. The two frequencies are out of phase with each other, which creates a constantly varying modulation. Classic IF (IFC) has been used to treat acute pain, peripheral neuritis, vascular insufficiencies and urinary incontinence. It is the most effective form of transcutaneous electrical stimulation for inducing anesthesia. Thus it is sometimes used for electrotherapeutic nerve blocks, which can profoundly suppress the sensation of pain in acute or intractable chronic pain conditions. Because it is so strong, IFC currents are contra-indicated for frail and sensitive patients. All interferential treatments involve the use of two separate output channels of a stimulator, using four electrodes. Each set of two electrodes outputs a different out-of-phase frequency. The pads are arranged so the pathway of current flow between each set of pads crosses, or "interferes" in the target tissue to be treated. Therefore the most common and basic technique is to create a crossing, or "X" pattern surrounding the painful area.

EXAMPLES USING CHANNEL A AND B PADS - LOW BACK PAIN

Channel A's pads could be at the upper right and lower left of the painful back zone and Channel B's pads at the upper left and lower right of the same zone. Shoulder pain: Channel A's pads could be placed on the anterior and posterior aspects of the shoulder, and Channel B's pads could run from the neck nerve roots to the lateral shoulder.

The primary objective of Classic Interferential is to identify the target tissue, and arrange the pads so this zone receives the maximum area of current intersection. In placing interferential pads, it is important to remember that the area of strongest stimulation is not always directly under the pads, but in the intersection area in between them. Pads should be placed with a three dimensional view in mind, so that the area of intersection of the two current pathways will be in the painful or injured area.

INTERFERENTIAL PAD PLACEMENTS - SHOULDER, LOW BACK AND KNEE

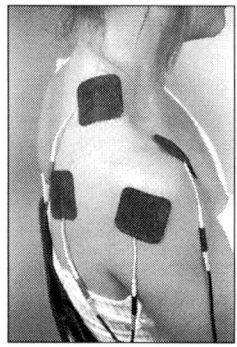 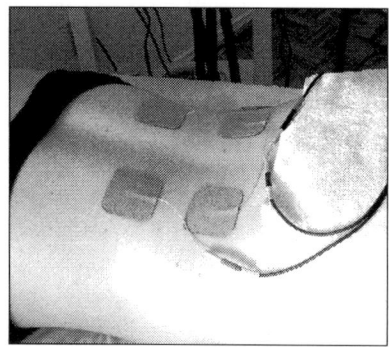 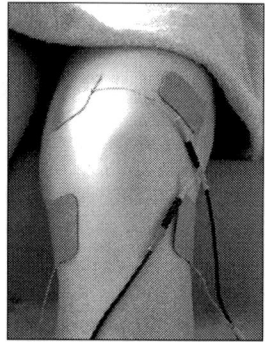

Figure 9.3: IFC - Shoulder, Low Back and Knee

This same principle of placement can be applied to other parts of the body. Remember, when treating elderly, frail or weakened patients, apply interferential currents with care, watching carefully to see if the treatment exacerbates the condition. As is the case with any intense and invasive treatment, classic interferential significantly disrupts the body's normal electro-physiology. I have heard about many patients treated with interferential that had initial pain reduction, but then experienced severe rebound of pain a few hours after the treatment. This can be prevented much of the time by following any classic interferential treatment with gentle, low frequency microcurrent stimulation. We call this the "cool down" period.

- *Interferential combination (I.F. #5)* - This is an Acutron Mentor innovation that uses the same principle as Milliamp-Microamp Combination above, yet through interferential style treatment. This combines the most useful aspects of IF and milliamp-microamp treatment. This has proved a very popular and valuable protocol among practitioners treating acute injury patients.

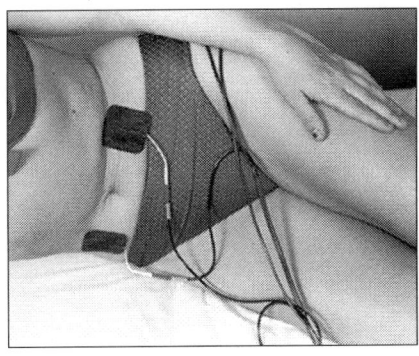 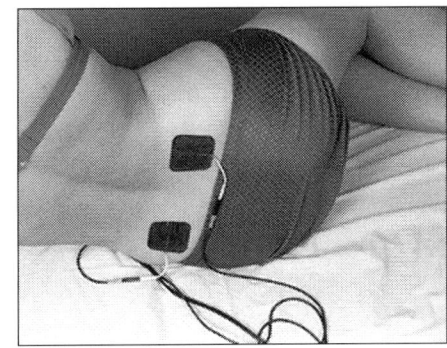

Figure 9.4: IFC – Anterior-Posterior IF pad placement for deep low back pain. Each set of pads crosses midline of body, i.e., from right front to left back and vice-versa.

2. Microamp pad techniques

The same pad placement arrangements as described above can also be used for microcurrent therapies, although the physiologic level of effect may be different. Some additional strategies utilizing polarized layouts can add important precision and effectiveness to extremity treatments. Because microamp pad treatments do not cause muscle contractions, possibilities are opened for kinetic electro-therapies, also called microcurrents with motion.

Basic microamp pad stimulation (µA Pads #1) - This is the simplest form, in which a single set of two pads, set to low frequency and biphasic polarity, is placed to bracket an area of pain or dysfunction. This can be applied anywhere on the body where there is not thick hair. Some valuable uses:

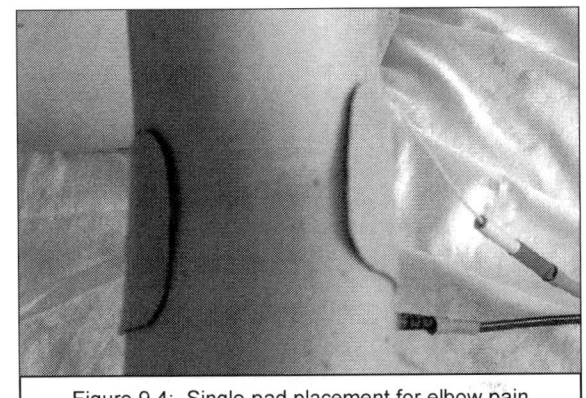

Figure 9.4: Single pad placement for elbow pain

- around small joints of the wrist, elbow, and ankle
- around finger and toe joints for arthritic conditions.
- facial pain and Bell's Palsy

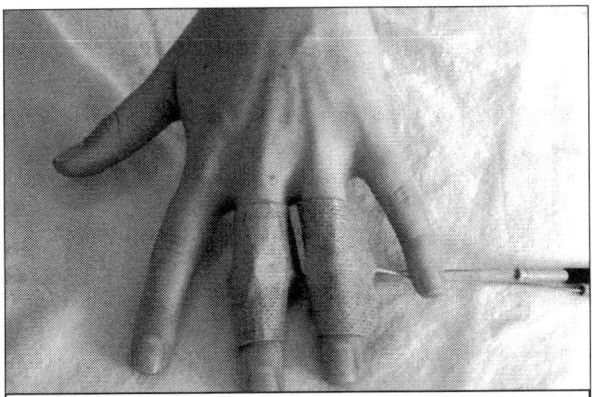

Figure 9.5: Single set of pads used for finger arthritis

surrounding skin lesions such as wounds, hematomas, lipomas, scars and bruises. (Make sure there is no malignancy before applying any electrical stimulation, as it may accelerate tumor growth.)

cover or bracket myofascial trigger points or constrictions

around the throat to relieve some kinds of irritations

- over nerve plexi for electrical nerve block analgesic treatments

Dermatome and Distal (μA Pads #2) - The parameters for this treatment are the same as local low-volt stimulation (mA Pad #1), except that a fixed polarity is employed, so that one pad of each set stays positive and one stays negative. This creates a flow of electrons from the negative to the positive pad through the targeted body area. The application of directed electrical flows in accord with the body's natural polarities is one of the most powerful ways to relieve pain and promote homeostasis. Some conditions responding well to this protocol:

- Radiculopathies of the arms and legs, such as sciatica, pinched nerve syndromes of the neck leading to pain and numbness down the arm, peripheral neuropathies.
- Elbow and wrist pain, such as tennis elbow, carpal tunnel syndrome, and wrist sprain and strain.
- Ankle strain and strain.
- Low back pain

In most cases, place the positive electrode proximally and the negative electrode distally.

Acute (μA Pads #4) - As the name implies, this setup utilizes somewhat more intense and aggressive parameters than the other microamp presets. Even so, the treatment will be comfortable for most patients, and much gentler than milliamp treatment. This option is used for more acute disorders and muscle tightness when microamp treatment is indicated. This can be a valuable treatment for low back, hip and shoulder pain, especially if preceded by microcurrent electro-acupuncture probe treatments on appropriate meridian points.

Gentle (Cool Down) (μA Pads #5) - This is a treatment that uses the gentlest possible parameters, with minimal intensity, very low frequency, and a sloping waveform. This option is appropriate for hypersensitive patients or a cool down period after intense stimulation. The principle of cool down electrotherapy is explained above. Having a more intense "pain mode" followed by a very gentle "healing mode" has been well established by microamp practitioners as having great therapeutic value.

3. Micro-Interferential (I.F. #1 and 2)

This is a more complex microamp pad setup that involves four pads – two sets of two. An alternating biphasic polarity is used, so positive and negative placements are not an issue. As mentioned above for classic interferential, each set of pads outputs a slightly different frequency rate. When the two electric frequency fields interfere during treatment, additional harmonics are generated which may increase therapeutic efficacy. I have found this treatment to be excellent for kinetic electro-therapeutics, in which microcurrent stimulation is applied with simultaneous exercise, mobilization or myofascial release techniques. A fuller description of these "microcurrent with motion" treatments follows in this chapter.

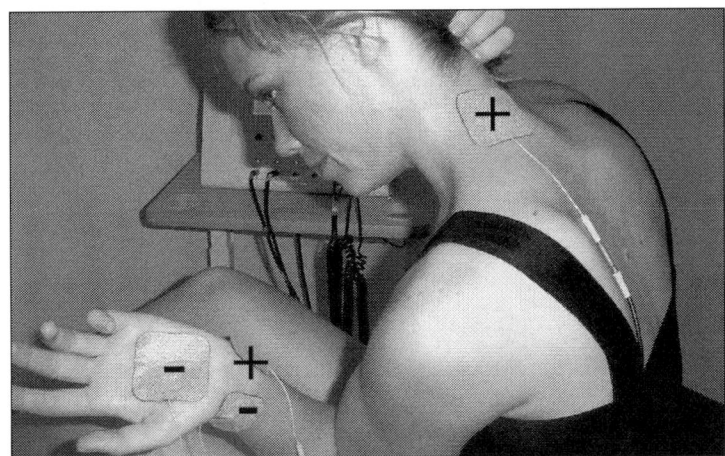

Figure 9.6: Dermatome interferential for carpal tunnel syndrome. Pads bracketing wrist are biphasic, set from neck to hand are polarized

Dermatome and Distal Interferential (I.F. #3) - This treatment is similar to micro-Interferential parameter above, except that of the two sets of pad electrodes utilized, one is polarized and one is biphasic. The polarized set is used with the + electrode proximal to the injury and the – injury on or distal to it. The other, biphasic set is used to locally bracket the affected area. This setup is highly appropriate for extremity disorders. For example, when treating carpal tunnel syndrome (CTS), most practitioners place electrodes only around the wrist for stimulation. This is a far from reliable way to benefit this condition. This is because most cases of CTS are caused by or at least involved with proximal tension and constrictions of the upper arm, shoulder, neck or pectoral areas. Although pain is mostly felt in the wrist and hand, that is not always the causative area of the disorder. For this reason, stimulation of the entire affected quadrant of the body with correct polarity placements is a more comprehensive and effective treatment than just local biphasic stimulation.

4. Kinetic Electro-Therapeutics

Most practitioners apply electro-therapies passively – that is, to a patient sitting or laying still. While this is a good opportunity for the patient to catch up on magazine reading, it is not often the most effective way to promote rehabilitation and re-education of injured bodily areas. Please see Shortcoming #5 in Chapter 6 for a good explanation of the value of microcurrent stimulation with simultaneous exercise and mobilization. I call this practice kinetic electro-therapeutics. Such kinetic therapies work well with microcurrent pad stimulation, especially four-pad interferential placement, with which broader areas of the body are stimulated. This practice is not recommended with milliamp pad stimulation, however, as the muscle twitching and contractions sometimes caused are not conducive to comfortable exercise, and can in some cases cause painful spasms.

Kinetic electro-therapies can involve active or passive movement on the part of the patient. In other words, he can exercise the treated area himself, or the practitioner can move it for him. An example of active therapy would be an athlete with shoulder injury moving his shoulder through range of motion with simultaneous micro-interferential pads bracketing the affected area. An example of passive motion would be an elderly woman with hip pain laying supine on a treatment table. Pads are placed from groin to S-I joint area, and from ASIS to greater trochanter areas, and stimulation is applied as the therapist moves the patient's leg and hip through increasing ranges of motion. Chapter 13 offers details on kinetic electro-therapies.

For most professionals in the United States, kinetic therapeutics with or without simultaneous electrical stimulation are billed under a special CPT code 97530. This code is reimbursed at a higher rate than electrical stimulation due to the increased amount of time required.

Section III

FOUR-STEP PROTOCOL

Chapter 10

FOUR-STEP TREATMENT INTRODUCTION

Basic Principles

In this section, all the elements of diagnosis and treatment described in this book are integrated into one practical system. Having instructed hundreds of acupuncturists, chiropractors, medical physicians and other professionals during my teaching career, I have concluded that each profession offers patients some important aspects of pain and injury management, and yet ignores or minimizes other vital aspects.

> **THE ELEPHANT AND THE FOUR BLIND MEN**
>
> One day an elephant walking through a village stopped in front of a group of four blind men. Each used his hands to feel a part of the elephant. After the elephant walked away, they compared notes with each other. One, who had felt the ear, described the elephant as a huge banana leaf. The next blind man, who had felt the trunk, described it as a thick vine. The next one, who felt the legs, described it as a tree trunk. The final blind man, who felt the elephant's tail, described it as a rope! The four men got into a heated argument about who was right, even though the reality was that they all were partially right. It's just that none of them were seeing the whole picture of what an elephant is.

In the same way as the four blind men in the story, each health specialty usually focuses on just one aspect of what a patient needs. While specialization is necessary in our modern health care system, unfortunately many patients do not receive the complete care they need. Few have the time or money to visit a complete package of different professionals who offer all the needed aspects of treatment. Ideally, a pain and injury patient would receive:

- manipulation to adjust the skeleton when indicated
- bodywork or acupuncture to release myofascial constrictions

- acupuncture to balance the meridians and soft tissues, promote healing and address the root
- drugs, casting or surgery when needed for severe emergency conditions.

The Four-Step protocol integrates many valuable aspects of energy balancing, symptomatic treatment and hands-on input into the physical body. The beauty of this system is that the techniques and skills utilized by each profession can be plugged into the protocol in a balanced way. For example, most emergency medical intervention would be Step Four treatments. The amount of such heroic intervention will certainly be minimized, however, if the first three steps are performed first. In emergency cases in which this is not possible, the other steps of treatment will still be valuable to accelerate recovery if used as soon as is practical after emergency measures are administered.

So many of the patients we see in our modern society present with complex, multifaceted conditions. Many require treatments that address both Root and Branch, as explained in Chapter 5. Even for patients with a relatively simple complaint, such as "tennis elbow", there are often energetic relationships to take into account beyond just the elbow pain itself. Once our consciousness has become aware of the inter-relatedness of all the parts of the body/mind, it becomes increasingly difficult for us as practitioners to be satisfied just relieving a local symptom without looking at the whole picture.

As mentioned earlier, some traditions of acupuncture teach a primarily symptom oriented approach, while others teach students to focus only on Root treatment. Other schools direct practitioners to erect Traditional Chinese Medicine (TCM) diagnoses and choose herbal formulas and point prescriptions to fit specific patterns. Each of these systems will favor the treatment of certain types of patients, and be somewhat less effective for others.

Those of us who have studied acupuncture in the United States have dealt with massive amounts of often confusing and contradictory information. Sources of this information include varying perspectives on TCM, Japanese meridian work and Hara diagnosis, French auricular therapy, Korean hand acupuncture, and Western medicine and physiotherapy. The Four-Step pain mastery protocol is very valuable because it is an effective and well-organized way to bring together these critical elements in a truly elegant manner.

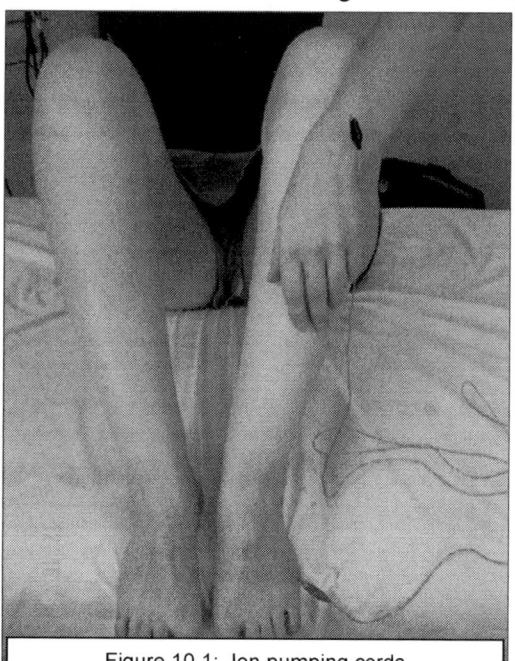

Figure 10.1: Ion pumping cords

Yoshio Manaka of Japan has contributed greatly to the field of acupuncture, perhaps more than any other modern practitioner. Starting during World War II, he innovated ways to speed the healing of military burn victims using metal foils over the burned areas connected with cords to distal acupuncture points. He later added elements of polarity therapy to his acupuncture protocols. Eventually he developed his famous ion-pumping cords -- electrically conductive cords with alligator clips that are connected to pairs of Master acu-points. The red clip contains a diode. This allows a one-way drift of ions through the cord creating a powerful induction of balancing flow through the internal energy systems of the body.

Manaka, and his contemporary Reinhold Voll of Germany, were two of the most innovative acupuncture researchers of the 20th century. Both men worked long and hard to test and verify ancient acupuncture knowledge and techniques through rigorous research. Voll is well known in this regard for his monumental work in re-mapping the meridian systems of the body through painstaking reference to medically diagnosed pathology. Manaka also rigorously tested the clinical validity of many of the principles of traditional acupuncture, including traditional meridian point locations, Back Shu-Transporting points, Luo-Connecting points, Extraordinary Vessels, Mu-Alarm points and much more. He verified that most traditional information based on the classics of acupuncture was correct, although often incorrectly applied.

One of Manaka's greatest contributions was the study of how polarity agents affect the meridian system. This is at the core of the most effective microcurrent electro-acupuncture techniques. Manaka used needles, moxa, magnets, wooden hammers and several types of electrical polarity devices in his research and practice. After a lifetime of such study, Manaka summarized his clinical approach through a Four-Step system that integrates an energetic, whole-body acupuncture with structural balancing and symptomatic treatment. A comprehensive account of Manaka's research and treatment methods can be found in his excellent book Chasing the Dragon's Tail.[150] His work is based on classical Chinese and Japanese medical knowledge, yet also thoroughly grounded in modern scientific principles and research methods. I have modified and amplified this system for use with microcurrent electro-acupuncture.

Manaka taught his students to synthesize information from several diagnostic methods, and then to confirm the correctness of the diagnosis and point selection before treating. This approach is extremely useful because treatment does not proceed until the practitioner is clear and confident in the selected treatment protocol. There are two major styles of patient interaction. One is to decide on a diagnosis and treatment plan, carry it out, and then wait until the patient comes back for his next visit to learn how effective the treatment was. The other is to confirm the usefulness of the treatment several times during the session, frequently checking that it is working and correcting the approach when necessary. With the second, more dynamic approach, it is more likely that the treatment will be successful, and its effectiveness will usually be known before the patient leaves the office. While there are some carry-over effects of treatment that take hours or days to show themselves, there are many immediate indicators of treatment efficacy. These indicators include reduced pressure pain on palpation points, increased range of motion, decreased pain and increased positive energy and emotional affect. This interactive, dynamic approach to treatment is usually practiced by highly successful practitioners of all kinds, including chiropractors, physical therapists, psychotherapists, medical physicians and acupuncturists.

After a lifetime of practicing, testing and researching in the field of acupuncture, Manaka came to many clear conclusions about acupuncture clinical practice. Those that relate to the subject of this chapter are summarized as follows:

- A subtle signal system in the body is at the heart of all life processes. It is more basic and primitive than the complex biological systems that our modern science has studied and explained. Manaka called this the "X-signal" system to signify that it is hidden and unknown to modern science. This X-signal system is primarily informational, and can be thought of as preceding the energy systems of the body.

---

[150] Published by Paradigm Publications, with Kazuko Itaya and Steven Birch

- This signal system cannot be explained through the principles of neuro-physiology because it responds to stimuli that are too subtle to be understood to affect the nervous system. The X-signal system readily responds to stimuli even considered too subtle to have an effect by traditional acupuncture, yet often producing dramatically successful clinical effects.

- The meridian system can be successfully used to influence and adjust the X-signal system, and these effects fit well into and provide an explanation for many classical acupuncture concepts and theories. It also explains and verifies the effects of holographic micro-system effects, such as auricular and Korean hand acupuncture.

- The X-signal system is highly polarity-responsive. For this reason successful adjustment of the body's energy octahedron must be administered with correct use of positive and negative stimuli on treatment points. It can be easily demonstrated with simple experiments that correct polarities on sets of relevant acu-points will immediately reduce pressure pain on sensitive spots, while reversing the polarity will immediately bring back or worsen the pain.

- It requires only very minute stimuli on acu-points to influence the X-signal system and to balance the body. Stimulation above that level, as is induced by most needle acupuncture, moxibustion and electro-therapies, operates on physiologic levels that are different from the X-signal system. As stimulation intensity increases, there is less informational adjustment and more physiologic effects, and vice-versa.

- The two main kinds of acu-points used by Manaka to adjust the octahedral structure of the body were the Master and Coupled points of the Extraordinary meridians, and tonification and sedation points of the principal meridians.

- Alarm (Mu) points on the front of the body are highly useful for evaluating the state of the meridians. They can be diagnosed using palpatory skills or kinesiology, both of which reveal the condition of the X-signal system as expressed through the Organ/meridian being examined.

- There are palpation points over the gastrocnemius muscles of the legs that give accurate indication of which polar meridian pair requires treatment.

- Manaka used the biorhythmic principle of the Chinese Clock, which reveals that during each two-hour period of the 24-hour cycle a different Organ/meridian is at its peak energy, and another at its lowest energy. He taught his students to use appropriate polarity to treat the tonification and sedation points of two indicated meridians *opposite* on the Chinese clock. Manaka called such couples polar pairs[151]. For example, Small Intestine (peak: 1 – 3 PM) and Liver (peak: 1 – 3 AM) are opposites, and so can be treated together for global balancing. In this case one would treat SI 3 (+) and SI 8 (-) and Liv 8 (+) and Liv 2 (-), with both meridians being treated on the side of the body opposite the sore gastrocnemius reaction.

---

[151] Explained in Chapter Eleven

- The energy systems of the body can be visualized as an octahedral structure, with each junction line of the planes of the octahedron representing one of the eight Extraordinary meridians. This structure is intimately related to the X-signal system. Structural distortions of the body, such as torticollis, leg length differences, scoliosis, etc. are due in part to imbalances of this energy geometry, starting during embryonic development. The correct treatment of appropriate acu-points can be used to adjust the energy octahedron, thereby correcting structural imbalances and many internal medical conditions.

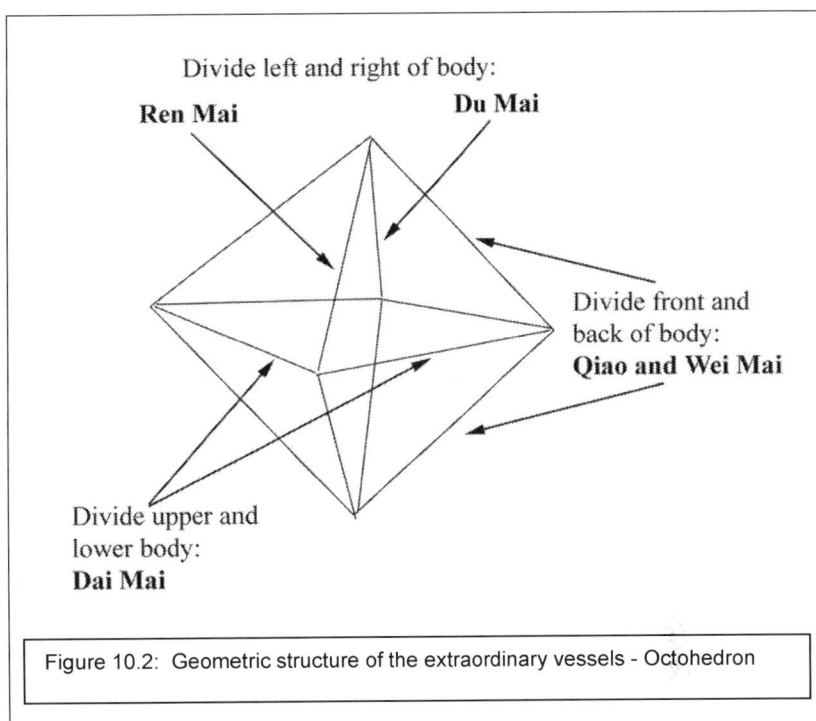

Figure 10.2: Geometric structure of the extraordinary vessels - Octohedron

- The most effective treatment plans include a combination of adjustment of the energy octahedron with direct physical input into the structure of the body, as well as symptomatic treatments where necessary. Manaka developed his Four-Step treatment protocol based on this principle.

Full instructions for applying the above principles follow in the rest of this Section.

In this book, the Four-Step treatment system has been adapted to the use of non-needle microcurrent electro-acupuncture. Subsensationsal microcurrent treatment can be understood to be a valuable intermediary between pure informational influence through the X-signal system and physiologic stimulation. In other words, it is gentle enough to adjust the X-signal system without undue interference, yet also strong enough to have some positive physiologic effects such as gating of pain response and accelerated tissue healing. This is what makes microcurrent electro-acupuncture such a versatile and valuable clinical approach.

THE FOUR STEPS

1. **Step One - Meridian Balancing** (Yin aspect)

    The process of gathering information about the state of the meridian system (the octahedron), administering appropriate treatment, and rechecking to confirm that balance has taken place is what Manaka referred to as Step One of his Four-Step system. To do this, test the Organ/meridian system using one or more diagnostic methods. Then, use data obtained to determine a *pair* of treatment meridians that are most likely to correct the imbalances found during evaluation. Choose either Extraordinary Vessels or polar meridian pairs based on the pattern found during meridian evaluation. Use brief confirmatory methods to prove or disprove meridian selection, and adjust if necessary. Treat, and then briefly recheck diagnostic points to ensure that improvement has happened. If so, go onto Step Two. If not, re-evaluate, choose new meridian strategy and re-treat.

2. **Step Two - Treat Yang**

    Choose Yang meridian points that correspond to the meridians treated in Step One. Select from Back Shu points on the posterior Urinary Bladder channel or other indicated Yang meridians on the extremities. Steps One and Two help create balanced input to the Yin and Yang aspects of the body. Manaka most commonly used needles with moxa burned on the handle (kyotoshin). Alternative microcurrent treatments for Step Two are presented in Chapter 12.

3. **Step Three - Structural Adjustment**

    Most distortions of the physical body are caused by, or exist in conjunction with, Organ/meridian imbalances. In many cases, these exist as left-right imbalances. Once the body octahedron has been adjusted on a meridian/energy level, this indirectly helps adjust the physical. Yet, because the body is much denser than the meridians, it is often necessary to address its distortions directly. This can be accomplished through many methods, including sotai, exercise, yoga, osseous manipulation, myofascial release, electro-massage and many types of physical therapies.

4. **Step Four - Symptomatic Treatment**

    In many cases, administering the first three steps completely resolves the patient's presenting complaint. Some painful or constricted areas frequently remain that require additional intervention. This is often the case with some long-standing complaints or acute injuries. Step Four draws from a wide range of treatment techniques to relieve remaining symptoms, including acupuncture, intradermal needles, moxibustion, electro-therapy, lasers, and much more. Dr. Manaka's favorite method of symptomatic treatment was application of intradermal needles that could stay in place for several days. I also include "homework" the patient does for herself as aspect of Step Four, such as therapeutic exercise or self-acupressure.

These four steps are a framework into which any treatment plan can be fit. Not all patients need all the steps. Some patients, especially children, may experience full resolution from the first one or two steps. Some chiropractors have found that simple microcurrent stimulation of Back Shu points, a Step Two treatment, is a valuable precursor to spinal manipulation. In some cases of acute injuries in otherwise healthy patients, all that may be needed is symptomatic treatment. Yet, even in these cases some Root treatment will often speed their recovery and extend carry-over of improvement.

This Four-Step system provides a clear way to integrate both Root and Branch treatments into a clinical session. In clinical practice, the decision about how to prioritize treatment is a challenge. Should you focus holistically on the overall constitutional issues of the patient to support him in healing himself? Alternatively, is it better to directly open Qi blockages to relieve his symptoms? Experienced practitioners develop a good sense of treatment planning, yet may still have many unclear moments when confronted with challenging patient conditions. Manaka's Four-Step protocol integrates all necessary aspects, and provides a framework to address all of the patients clinical needs.[152]

The first two steps, meridian testing and balancing and Back Shu stimulation, provide the holistic aspect of treatment. These aspects may be determined and applied without any necessity for reference to the patient's symptomatic complaints, although symptoms may be helpful in confirming choice of treatment meridians. In many cases, this holistic approach is all that is needed. Once blockages and imbalances in the flow of Qi through the channels are corrected, the body's regulatory and homeostatic mechanisms may be activated to promote accelerated recovery and healing. This applies to many cases of internal or chronic health conditions, especially in the treatment of children. The second two steps, structural alignment and symptom control treatments, provide direct input to the manifestations of the patient's complaints. Hands-on bodywork or manipulation is often essential in resolving pain and injury. Usually, it is the synergy of energetic balancing with direct structural input that provides the most complete and lasting results. Yet, even after such bodywork, there may still be some remaining areas of pain or dysfunction. Step Four treatments address these remaining symptoms, generally through micro-system stimulation.

I have found this Four-Step system to work very well in my clinical practice, and have used it extensively. Through continuing research with microcurrents, I discovered that low-level polarized stimulation is an effective and convenient method for carrying out or enhancing all four steps of this system. Manaka's original ion pumping cord method is powerful, yet a bit awkward to apply. This is because Japanese needling technique requires very shallow insertions of only a few millimeters. The heavy alligator clips on the ion cords often pull the needles out of the skin. As of the this date California acupuncturists are not permitted to use these cords under their practice act, so this information is of even greater significance to them.

The next chapter details Step One energetic balancing procedures, the most involved aspect of this system.

---

[152] Chapter 5 contains an extensive discussion of Root and Branch treatments

Chapter 11

STEP ONE:

BALANCING THE MERIDIAN SYSTEM

This chapter offers detailed instructions for interpreting meridian data and selecting appropriate treatment to regulate the meridian system. This is recommended as a valuable first priority in patient care. Through this step of treatment the overall presenting energetic pattern can be recognized and brought into balance. The diagnostic methods referred to in this chapter are detailed in Section IV.

Regulating, or balancing the meridian system is a Root treatment. This step can be performed without any reference to the patient's symptomatic complaints. Whether she has come to you for help with elbow pain, stomach ulcers, high blood pressure, migraines or depression, the overall procedure for Step One Root treatment is the same, and is likely to have a beneficial influence.

Most health care practitioners, including some acupuncturists, offer little in the way of Root treatment, and when presented with patient's complaints, immediately start into formulaic symptomatic relief treatments. In the system presented in this book, symptomatic treatments are the fourth and final step, only offered when necessary after Root and systemic treatments have been applied. In the early days of my own acupuncture practice, my approach to pain management was largely symptomatic. My results were quite inconsistent until I started utilizing these Four-Steps, after which I have been able to promptly help most of my patients reduce their pain and dysfunction.

Meridian balancing is an ideal treatment for babies and young children, as their energetic bodies are less dense and physical bodies less constricted than most adults, and as a result many of their illnesses respond well to this step alone. Meridian balancing primarily works on the level of the subtle X-signal system of the patient[153]. Only minute stimulation is required to influence this system. That is why you will be guided to retest significant test points after only one second of microcurrent stimulation. That is enough time to determine the appropriateness of your chosen treatment.

---

[153] See Chapter 10 of this book, or read Chapter 1 of Chasing The Dragon's Tail

Polarized microcurrent probe stimulation works very quickly to balance the meridian system and correct patterns of disharmony, even faster than the ion pumping cords developed by Manaka. This procedure generally takes less than a minute[154]. The use of acupuncture needles and cords for the same purpose requires a 10 – 20 minute treatment. The main difference is that ion cords only conduct the subtle drift of ions from the patient's body and the environment, while microcurrent probe treatment adds an outside energy source, i.e., the microcurrent stimulator.

What is meridian balancing? In a sense, most forms of acupuncture, when appropriately applied, have a regulating effect on the energy systems of the body. Imbalance of the meridians generally accompanies most pain conditions and health disorders, and can be ascertained through any system of meridian evaluation. This includes pulse diagnosis, Hara (abdominal) diagnosis and electronic meridian testing at distal test points. Fluctuations and relative imbalances in the levels of the meridians are normal in healthy people due to the circadian cycles of the body in relation to the Earth and cosmos. Yet when there are extreme differences in readings, left-right differences or other patterns of dysfunction in the meridian system, these indicate health problems that require correction.

There have been many methods of meridian balancing developed. The original electronic system, known as Ryodoraku,[155] used regulatory points to balance each individual meridian that was out of balance. While this is of significant value, contemporary Japanese practitioners such as Manaka have developed more elegant systems that treat the overall pattern of disharmony through just a few Master points. When the pattern is thus resolved, the other meridians generally come into balance without being directly treated.

The key to this system of meridian balancing is to look for pairs of out-of-balance meridians, one with a Master point on the upper extremity and the other with a Master point on the lower extremity. Treatment points from either Extraordinary or principal meridians are selected. The eight Extraordinary Vessels are highly effective because of their strong correlation with the octahedral structure of the body. Many chronic pain and disease conditions are associated with distortions in the physical body that tend to perpetuate the disorder. An example is leg length difference, which is frequently found in patients with hip and low back pain. The meridians of Shaoyang - Gall Bladder and Triple Warmer, are often indicated to correct this imbalance, and may be treated through the Extraordinary or principal meridian systems.

Extraordinary Vessel treatment generally works on a root level due to the embryonic development of these meridians. The use of the eight Extraordinary Vessels for correcting structural imbalances is well established in modern Japanese acupuncture practice.

When Extraordinary Vessel treatment is not indicated for Step One, treatment of polar meridian pairs will usually be effective. These are explained later in this chapter. In my experience, brief microcurrent treatment of either Extraordinary or polar meridian treatment will be effective for balancing the meridian system in 85 – 90% of patients. In the remaining cases I need to dip into my acupuncture knowledge and try creative methods, for examples choosing from Luo-Connecting or Back-Shu points, or through analysis of the complaint through Five Element principles. In some cases of extreme deficiency, moxibustion, nutrition or herbal medicine is required to tonify the patient for a period of time before meridian balancing can be effective. It is more common, however, that meridian balancing will be appropriate and supportive of deficient patients, including those with mental/emotional imbalances.

---

[154] Based on the experience of the author. Results were measured by improvement in meridian balance as read through abdominal and pulse diagnosis, and symptomatic improvement.
[155] See Chapter 17

Step-By-Step Overview

An effective process for meridian balancing is detailed below. The process is summarized in the Manaka Meridian Balancing Chart, which follows in this Chapter. This chart will be referred to in the items below. Further explanations follow in the text after the chart.

1. Use EMT, Alarm point kinesiology, pulse diagnosis or other methods to evaluate the energy of each meridian[156]. Record all readings. It is recommended to use at least two different systems, so the results can be compared and confirmed. EMT and Alarm point kinesiology measure different levels of information. EMT indicates what is happening on the more superficial meridian level, while Alarm point kinesiology is more indicative of Organ function. For this reason, it is unlikely that all readings will agree between the two systems. When they do agree, however, this is a strong and reliable diagnostic indication.

2. Palpate the gastrocnemius according to instructions in Chapter 18. Note most tender leg/zone.

3. Refer to your knowledge of the symptomatology of the Extraordinary Vessels in helping confirm which ones may be affected. A reference chart can be found at the end of this chapter.

4. Based on the intake information, symptoms and your other perceptions, determine the patient's **Key Imbalance**. The key imbalance is the Organ/meridian function that is out of homeostasis, and is most impacting their chief complaint. This is analogous to the primary diagnosis arrived at through TCM diagnosis, such as Kidney Yin deficiency, Liver Fire Rising, Shaoyang disturbance, etc.

5. After you have determined on the key imbalance, examine the meridian testing results and look for another significantly abnormal reading(s) that may be paired with the key imbalance meridian, either in the Extraordinary meridian or polar meridian pair charts below. Each pair includes treatment points on one upper extremity and one lower extremity meridian. Further explanation of this inductive process follows.

6. Once you have selected the most indicated meridian pair, palpate indicated confirmation points for that pair that are listed in the third column of the chart. If some are tender to pressure, this is a good confirmation that your selection was correct. If none are, it is worth re-evaluating your choice.

7. Look in the fourth column of the chart for indicated treatment points and polarities. If Extraordinary meridians are being treated, Master and Coupled points are selected. If polar meridian pairs are used, tonification and sedation points are used. The Extraordinary meridians will be used about 70% of the time, and Manaka recommended beginning students of this method to concentrate on their usage at first.

8. Use polarized microcurrent probe treatment[157] to give a brief, 1 second stimulation to the selected treatment points with the indicated polarities[158]. For example, + probe on Lu 7 and − probe on K 6 for treatment of Ren-Yinchaio Extraordinary Vessels.

9. Immediately recheck one or two of the most significant abnormal meridian(s) from your testing to see if the readings have improved. Make sure you recheck the key imbalance

---

[156] Instructions for these diagnostic methods are found in Section IV
[157] Acupuncture needles and Manaka ion-pumping cords may be used as well for this step. Place the red clip of the cords on the needle that is inserted into the point that requires + polarity, and the black clip on the point that requires − polarity. Treatment time with ion-pumping cords is about 10 times longer than is required with polarized microcurrent probe therapy.
[158] For Acutron Mentor, use probe preset #2

meridian test point. If it is clearly improved, you are on the right track and can proceed with treatment. If they do not improve, or only improve marginally, the treatment will have to be altered. Extraordinary vessel treatment polarities may be reversed if the suggested polarity from the chart does not improve the readings. *The suggested polarities for polar meridian pair treatment may not be reversed.* If reversing polarity does not improve abnormal readings, re-evaluate the disordered meridians to select another treatment approach, and follow steps 4 - 9 again from this list.

10. Once you find a meridian pair that, when treated for one second, does clearly improve the readings from step 8, you are ready to treat. This is simply done by treating all the indicated treatment points (from the fourth column of the chart) for about 20 – 40 seconds with polarized probe electrodes in the same way as the confirmatory stimulation that improved the readings.

The following table and the ones on the next page give guidance for whole-body meridian balancing based on recognition of the Key Imbalance. A convenient intake chart for use with this process can be found after the Index at the end of this book.

Point Selection Based On Key Imbalance

Key Imbalance	Extraordinary Vessel Confluent Points	Polar Meridian Pairs
Kidneys	Lu 7 + Ki 6 or Pc 6 + Sp 4	Kidney/Large Intestine
Liver	Pc 6 + Sp 4 or Pc 6 + Lv 3	Liver/Small Intestine
Spleen/Pancreas	Pc 6 + Sp 4	Spleen/Triple Warmer
Lungs	Lu 7 + Ki 6	Lungs/Urinary Bladder
Heart	Pc 6 + Sp 4	Heart/Gall Bladder
Gall Bladder	TW 5 + GB 41	Heart/Gall Bladder
Triple Warmer	TW 5 + GB 41	Spleen/Triple Warmer
Urinary Bladder	SI 3 + UB 62	Lung/Urinary Bladder
Stomach or Pericardium	Pc 6 + Sp 4	Pericardium/Stomach
Large Intestine	Pc 6 + Sp 4	Kidney/Large Intestine
Small Intestine	Pc 6 + Sp 4	Liver/Small Intestine

Figure 11.2 MANAKA MERIDIAN BALANCING METHOD

I. Extraordinary Vessels

Reactive Meridians	Extraordinary Vessel Pairs	Confirmatory Palpation Points	Treatment Points	Polarity
Kidney Lung	Ren (Conception) Vessel/ Yinchaio	Lu 1, K16, St 11	Lu 7 + K 6 - Treat bilaterally	Positive (Red I.P.) Negative (Black I.P.)
Small Intestine Urinary Bladder	Du (Governing) Vessel/ Yangchaio	Ren 3 & 4, St 26	SI 3 + UB 62 - Treat bilaterally	Positive (Red) Negative (Black)
Gall Bladder Triple Warmer	Dai (Belt) Vessel/ Yangwei	St 25, GB 24, Ren 4	TW 5 - GB 41 + Usually treat left or side of abdominal reaction	Negative (Black) Positive (Red)
Spleen, Pericardium, Liver, Kidney	Chong (Penetrating) Vessel/ Yinwei	Ren 10, Ren 17, Ren 22, Lv 13, Lv 14	P 6 – Sp 4 or Lv 3 + Usually treat right side	Negative (Black) Positive (Red)

For Extraordinary Vessels, start with indicated polarity and re-check. Polarity may be reversed if not balancing. For Polar Meridian Pairs (below), do not reverse listed polarities, treat all points on same side as most pronounced abdominal signs, and usually opposite to most sore gastrocnemius palpation points (see Chapter 17). I.P. = Manaka's ion-pumping cords.

II. Polar Meridian Pairs (by Chinese Clock)

Polar Meridian Pairs	Confirmatory Palpation Points	Treatment Points
Spleen Triple Warmer	Lv 13, St 25, Ren 10, Gastroc zone A	Sp 2 +, Sp 5 – TW 3+, TW 10 -
Kidney Large Intestine	K 16, St 27, GB 25, Gastroc zone B	K 7+, K1- LI 11+, LI 2-
Liver Small Intestine	Lv 14, St 26, Ren 4, Gastroc zone C	Lv 8+, Lv 2- SI 3+, SI 8-
Pericardium Stomach	Ren 12, area from P 7- P 3, UB 13 Gastroc zone D	P 9+, P 7- St 41+, St 44-
Lung Urinary Bladder	Lu 1, Lu 2, Ren 3, UB 13, Gastroc zone E	Lu 9+, Lu 5- UB 67+, UB 65-
Heart Gall Bladder	Ren 14, K 23, GB 24, area anterior to ASIS, Gastroc zone F	H 9+, H7- GB 43+, GB 38-

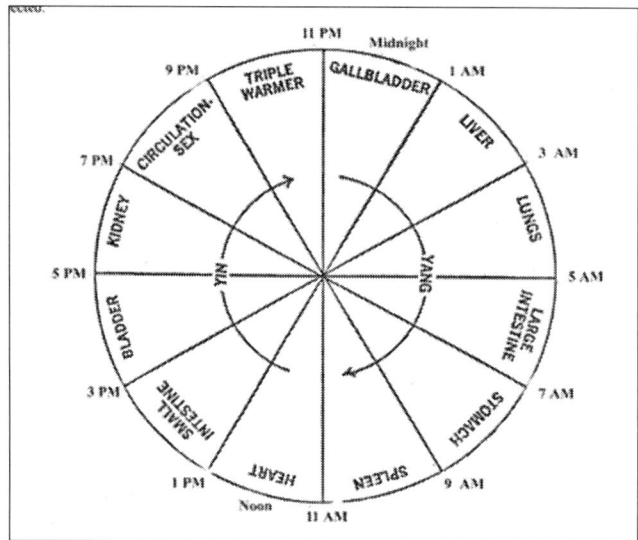

Figure 11.3 Chinese Clock (Basis of Polar Meridian Pair relationships)

Key to abbreviations for charts on previous page:

LU- Lung, LI- Large Intestine, ST- Stomach, SP- Spleen, H- Heart, SI- Small Intestine, UB- Urinary Bladder, K- Kidney, P- Pericardium, TW- Triple Warmer, GB- Gall Bladder, LIV- Liver, ASIS- Anterior Superior Iliac Spine, I.P.- Ion Pumping Cords, Gastroc. – Gastrocnemius palpation points, refer to Chapter 17

Notes:

1. Red clip of ion pumping cord corresponds to positive pole of microcurrent stimulator
2. Use electronic meridian evaluation, abdominal palpation, or kinesiology to test meridian
3. Always confirm positive reaction after treating each set of points before proceeding

More on Choosing Treatment Meridians and Points

The process of selecting appropriate treatment meridians from diagnostic data requires some additional explanation. This is an inductive process greatly facilitated by the above charts. The first priority is to determine the Key Imbalance in the Organ/meridian system. This is the function most significant to the patient's condition. This function, when corrected, will generally improve most of the other imbalanced meridians automatically. It will usually show a very weak O Ring test, abnormal EMT readings, and correlate strongly with the patient's symptomatic presentation. It is the proper treatment of the Key Imbalance that saves us from having to balance each meridian individually. You can visualize this as a complex knot in a stretchy fabric. Once the knot is released, all the other fibers are allowed to spring back into their proper places.

Once the Key Imbalance is ascertained, the second priority is to see how that imbalanced meridian may be paired with another imbalanced meridian as indicated on the above charts. For example, if Kidney is found to be the most significant single imbalanced function both charts would be referenced. The Extraordinary Vessels chart will show it can be paired with Lung to treat the Ren / Yinchaio Extraordinary Vessels or with Pericardium, Spleen or Liver to treat the Chong / Yinwei channel system. Using the Polar Meridian Pair chart, it may be paired with Large Intestine to treat the Kidney-Large Intestine polar meridian pair.

So, if your patient has chronic fatigue and low back pain, and you know from intake that his main treatment priority is Kidney, the first thing to do is think about the other abnormal readings. Is Large Intestine also showing a problem?[159] If not, is Lung? If neither of them, may there be a common pattern with Pericardium or Spleen? When first working with the chart, it will take frequent study to choose the indicated meridian pairs to be treated. Once you have practiced this system for some time, it will be easy to commit these relationships to memory and your treatments will become more intuitive. In summary, the overall aim is to find a pair of abnormal meridians that indicate either an Extraordinary Vessel or polar meridian pair treatment that matches the patient's presentations. The Key Imbalanced meridian should be one of the selections.

Maintaining the discipline of confirming your choice of treatment points will greatly improve your clinical skills. This can be easily done by palpating the confirmation points listed for each meridian pair in the third column of the chart. It is not necessary for all these points to be sore. Even one or two that are clearly sore provides a confirmation. The final confirmation, as explained above, is to actually treat the indicated treatment points for one second, and then go back and repeat your same diagnostic methods to recheck the test point of the Key Imbalanced meridian(s). This will show whether your choice of treatment points was correct.

In my practice, I generally just retest the Key Imbalance test point, trying various treatment strategies until that test point dramatically improves.

CASE STUDY - KIDNEY INSUFFICIENCY

For example, I recently encountered a patient with weak Kidney readings showing up on the abdomen, EMT and pulse. Although there were other imbalanced readings, I focused on what it would take to correct the Kidney. I tried treating through the Ren-Yinchaio combination (Lu 7+ and K 6-) for one second, but this did not correct the reading. I then tried using the same treatment points, but reversing the polarity. This also did not bring about a strong Kidney reading. I then tried treating it through the Chong-Yinwei combination (P 6- and Sp 4+). This also did not help, with either polarity placement. Next, I gave a brief treatment with the Kidney-Large Intestine polar pair. This one worked like a charm, and the Kidney reading on the abdomen, pulse and electronic measurement all came into balance. I checked this patient several hours later, and it was still holding. Trying all these combinations and rechecking took only 5 minutes.

It is also valuable to refer to the pattern of symptoms your patient is presenting in choosing the meridian pair to treat. In this system, the patient's symptoms are used as another confirmatory tool rather than the primary source of data. A useful table of Extraordinary Vessel and polar meridian pair symptoms is given at the end of this chapter.

---

[159] The Kidney-Large Intestine polar meridian pair is often indicated for low back pain associated with Kidney imbalances.

Abdominal reactions that are used to choose patterns to treat are well summarized in the diagrams on the next page.

Treatment Laterality

You will also need to decide which sides of the body on which to stimulate the indicated treatment points. This is highly significant in the correction of the X-signal system of the body octahedron, as distortions often manifest through right-left imbalances. It is not always appropriate to stimulate the points bilaterally, as is often done in TCM acupuncture technique.

Manaka's research and experience suggest the following guidelines for choosing treatment laterality for treatment of Extraordinary Vessels:

1. When treating Lu 7 and K 6 together (Ren/Yinchaio), treat bilaterally.

2. When treating SI 3 and UB 62 together (Du/Yangchaio), treat bilaterally.

3. When treating GB 41 and TW 5 together (Dai/Yangwei), in most cases treat on the left side only. This is not always the case. The deciding factor is to treat the side of the abdomen with the most sore and reactive palpation points.

4. When treating P 6 and Sp 4 together (Chong/Yinwei), in most cases treat on the right side only

Figure 11.4 – Abdominal Diagnostic Patterns

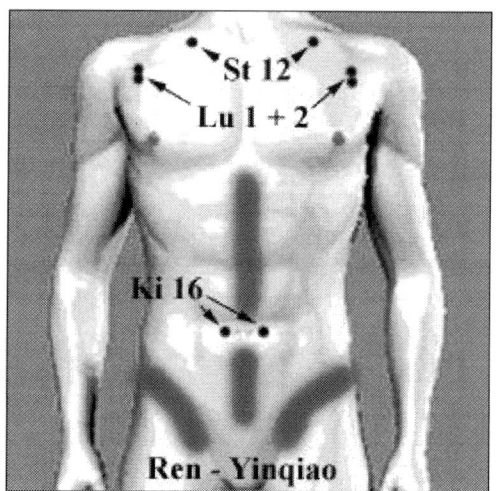
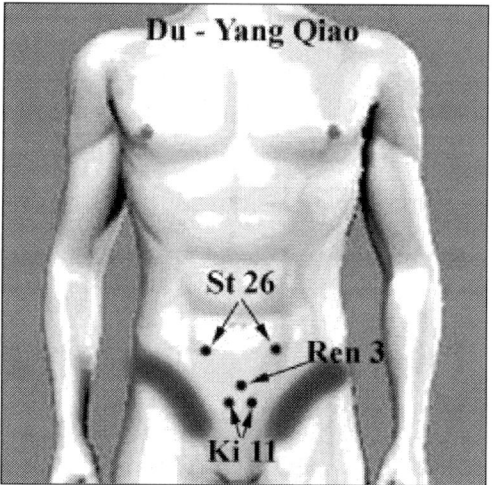
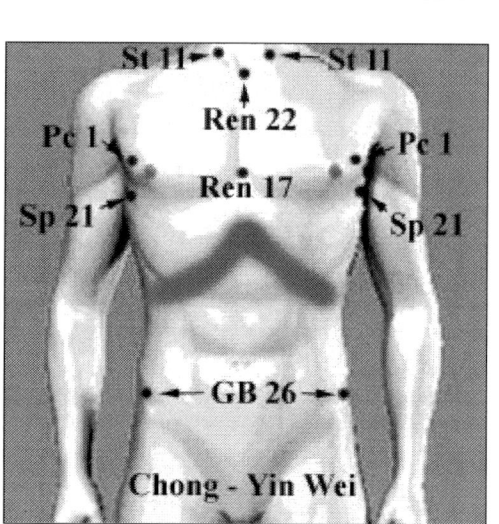
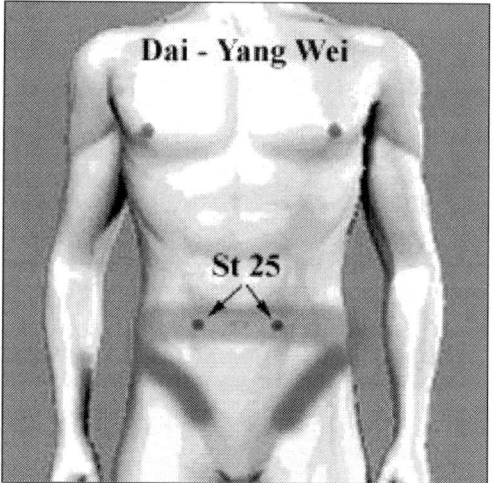

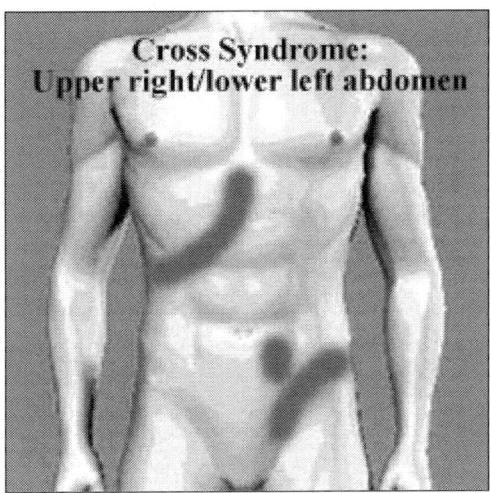

5. When treating Manaka's Cross Syndrome (see below), treat GB 41 and TW 5 on the left side, and P 6 and Sp 4 on the right side

These guidelines are based on the most commonly observed abdominal reaction patterns. In most cases abdominal reactions are bilateral for items 1 and 2, and only one sided for items 3 - 5. There are exceptions to these guidelines, of course. The best key is abdominal reactions. When reactive abdominal diagnostic points are equal on both sides for items 3 and 4, they may be treated bilaterally. If items 1 and 2 only show abdominal reactions on one side, they may be treated on that side only. Those presentations are not common, however.

In the treatment of polar meridian pairs, laterality is selected through reference to the gastrocnemius palpation test. Treat all points on the side *opposite* to the most tender gastrocnemius points. For example, if the left leg Spleen-Triple Warmer zone A is the sorest, and is more sore than the same zone on the right leg, treat Sp 2 and 5 and TW 3 and 10, all on the right side of the body.

Master Points and Polarity

As mentioned in many other places in this book, one of the most important and powerful aspects of microcurrent electro-acupuncture is the selection of proper treatment polarity. Nowhere is this more important than in the Step One treatments presented in this chapter. The polarity indications in the chart above are based on the most common clinical presentations. In the case of Extraordinary Vessel indicated polarities may be reversed. The explanation for this is interesting.

Of the Eight Extraordinary Vessels, only two, the Ren and Du, have their own discrete acu-points. The other six Vessels have some acu-points in common with the pathways of certain principal meridians. The Master points for the Extraordinary Vessels however, including Ren and Du, are usually not even on their trajectories. These are special Master points called confluence, or jiaohui points, and are acu-points on the principal meridians that have a powerful regulating effect on the Extraordinary Vessels. The treatments presented here involve the treatment of two such points, which are often referred to as the Master and Coupled points of each Vessel. For example, when treating the Du (Governing) Vessel, the Master point is SI 3 and the Coupled point is UB 62. When treating the Yangchaio Vessel, UB 62 would be the Master point and SI 3 the Coupled point.

When treating Extraordinary Vessels with microcurrent electro-acupuncture, the Confluent-jiaohui point stimulated with the negative probe will be the Master point, and the point stimulated with the positive probe (or red ion cord clip) will be the Coupled point. Therefore, when treating SI 3 with positive and UB 62 with negative, you will primarily be treating the Yangchaio Vessel, and secondarily the Du Vessel. If you reverse the polarity and treat SI 3 with negative and UB 62 with positive, you will primarily be treating the Du. Using Manaka's recommendations, it is clear that it is much more common for patients to require treatment as follows:

Manaka's Recommended Polarities	Primarily Treats:	Secondarily Treats:
UB 62 (-), SI 3 (+)	Yangchaio	Du
TW 5 (-), GB 41 (+)	Yangwei	Dai
K 6 (-), Lu 7 (+)	Yinchaio	Ren
P 6 (-), Sp 4 (+)	Yinwei	Chong

This information seems to indicate that the larger Vessels with more overall energy, all of which are in the second column, require correction less frequently. The Du is the "sea of all Yang meridians" and the Ren the "sea of all Yin meridians". Similarly, the Dai and Chong contain more overall energy and have greater spheres of influence than their counterparts Yangwei and Yinwei. Therefore we are usually treating the relatively smaller and less energetic Vessels to correct the distortions of the body's energy octahedron. This is analogous to the fact that small, accessory muscles are more commonly responsible for pain and dysfunction than larger, more powerful muscles. In whiplash injuries, for example, it is more common for the more delicate scalene and SCM muscles to be damaged than the larger, more powerful trapezius.

If, after administering the recommended polarities the diagnostic indicators do not improve, it is advisable to try reversing polarities and re-testing. If this procedure corrects the imbalance, then this shows that it is the larger Extraordinary Vessel that needs treatment (i.e., the Du, Dai, Ren or Chong). In my experience, this is indicated in less than 35% of the patients I have treated.

Other Step One Treatments

Extraordinary Vessels are the most commonly selected treatment in Step One, and are the easiest aspect for a beginner to this method to learn. Polar meridian pairs are next common. These systems will be effective for at least 85% of all Step One treatments. In the remaining cases, it is necessary to draw on other energetic meridian relationships to achieve global body balancing. An excellent treatment of additional meridian relationships that can be used for Step One treatments can be found in Manaka's book Chasing The Dragon's Tail, Chapter Nine.

In my clinical experience, I have used the following acupuncture principles to balance the meridian system when use of Extraordinary Master points or polar meridian pairs did not work:

1. Source Points

One point on each Yin meridian strongly tonifies its associated Organ due to direct connection to Original (Yuan) Qi[160]. These Source points may also be used in diagnosis, as they often show visible changes when the associated Organ is diseased. Although the Yang meridians also have Source points, they are not as useful for regulation as the Source points on the Yin channels. When a patient does not respond to Step One treatments through the Extraordinary Vessels or polar meridian pairs, Source point stimulation may be effective to bring up deficient Qi in the function being treated. This type of treatment is especially valuable when treating the Kidney, Spleen and Lungs.

To treat a Source point, either needle with tonifying technique or moxibustion, or apply a microcurrent negative probe to the point and the positive probe to Ren 6 (Qihai) on the lower abdomen. This is a powerful point called the "Sea of Qi" which is directly connected to the Original Qi that the Source points draw upon. Alternatively, the patient may simply hold a grounding hand mass to complete the circuit.

2. Five Element Relationships

The Five Elements, or Five Phases, is a system of correspondences between Organs, acupoints and many human and earthly phenomena. A table of Five Element correspondences follows in this chapter.

The Five Elements are translated as Fire, Earth, Metal, Water and Wood, each referring to an essential quality of creative Source energy, which gives rise to an internal Organ, emotion, personality type, direction, color and much more. These correspondences offer many valuable diagnostic insights, such as reddish skin hues showing a Fire[161] imbalance, and a groaning voice revealing Water[162] imbalances. This system of acupuncture diagnostics lends itself well to evaluation and treatment of mental, emotional and spiritual conditions due to the many consciousness-based indicators. There are five points on each principal meridian, each of which corresponds to one of the Five Elements. The use of these Five Element points provides another energy-balancing acupuncture system. The aspect of this system most useful for Step One treatments is the understanding of how the Organs affect each other. There are two primary relationships: the Generation (Mother-Son) and Control (Ko) cycles. The Generation cycle is the way each Organ feeds Qi to another specific Organ. This is illustrated in the diagrams on the following page.

---

[160] Original Qi is an aspect of the highly refined Essence in the body that a person is born with, and is supplemented by eating and breathing. It is concentrated in the Kidneys, and helps to catalyze all Organ functions.
[161] Fire Element = Heart, Small Intestine, Triple Warmer and Pericardium
[162] Water Element = Kidney and Urinary Bladder

Generation Cycle

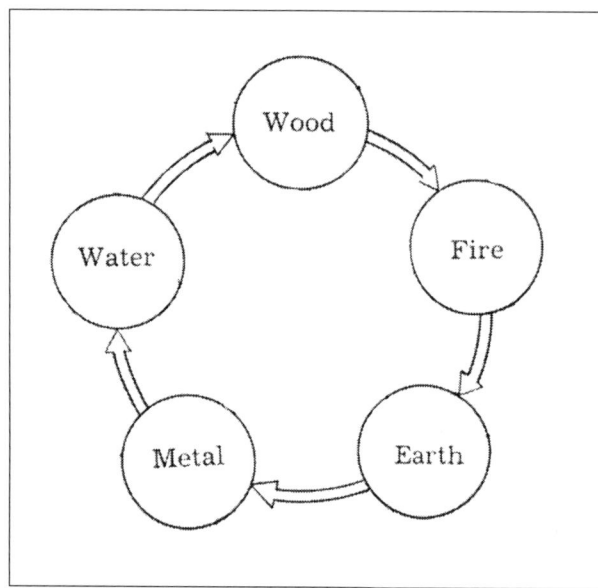

FIRE is mother of EARTH
EARTH is mother of METAL
METAL is mother of WATER
WATER is mother of WOOD
WOOD is mother of FIRE

Figure 11.5: Generation Cycle

The other relationship is the Control cycle, which is how each Organ inhibits the Qi of another specific Organ (see next page).

Control (Ko) Cycle

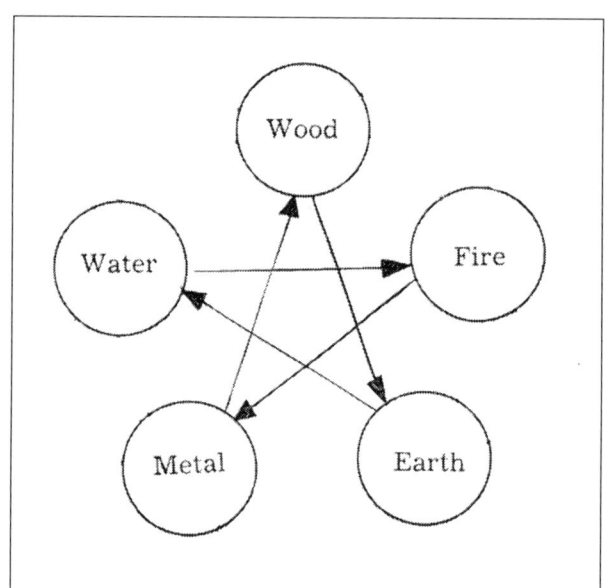

FIRE inhibits METAL
EARTH inhibits WATER
METAL inhibits WOOD
WATER inhibits FIRE
WOOD inhibits EARTH

Figure 11.6: Control Cycle

> **CHECKS AND BALANCES - THE GENERATION AND CONTROL CYCLES IN ACTION**
>
> The Generation and Control system of checks and balances is essential in maintaining homeostasis[163]. There are many ways to understand the application of these relationships. For example, if a patient expresses anger excessively, it creates an excess of Wood (Liver/Gall Bladder), and inhibits the energy of Earth (Spleen-Stomach) through the Control cycle. This can lead to indigestion or stomach ulcers. Yet, the emotion of grief, corresponding to Metal (Lung-Large Intestine) can inhibit anger. So, "giving grief" may tend to keep your angry friends in line! On the other hand, if a patient has digestive weaknesses (Earth), you can help her by fortifying her Fire element, the "Mother" of Earth. This can be accomplished by stimulating the Earth point on her Heart or Pericardium channels. If the digestive problems are due to excess in Wood (as from too much anger, rich fatty foods, or toxins), you can also sedate (weaken) the Liver or Gall Bladder to prevent it from suppressing the digestive system through the Control cycle. These are examples of the Generation and Control cycles in action.

The Five Elements in Step One Treatments

An understanding of these cycles can be used to balance the meridian system for Step One treatments. As mentioned above, I often look to the Five Elements when a clear pattern cannot be found through the Extraordinary Vessels or polar meridian pairs.

Let us look further at our example of the patient with Kidney Qi deficiency, which was determined to be the primary focus of treatment. Using the Manaka Meridian Balancing chart to determine an effective treatment, we first looked at the Extraordinary Vessel section to see if the Kidney could be treated through the Ren/Yinchaio Vessels or possibly through the Chong/Yinwei. A concurrent finding of imbalance in the Lung, or soreness upon palpation at St 11, K 16 or Lu 1, would indicate the former, while findings in Spleen, Liver or Pericardium would suggest the latter. If none of these indicators is found to be imbalanced however, we can then look at the second part of the chart, Polar Meridian Pairs. There we see that Kidney can also be treated through its polar relationship with the Large Intestine. To confirm this, there would need to be weak O Ring test or tender palpation points at St 27, or a positive response at the Kidney/Large Intestine gastrocnemius palpation point. If these signs are unclear, it is possible to just briefly treat some of the indicated treatment points for a second or so and then go back and retest the Kidney to see if the strategy worked. Sometimes this is what is necessary.

If after trying all these steps, however, the Kidney reading still won't come up, we are "back to the drawing board" and need to find an alternative method. In these situations, we may turn to the Law of the Five Elements. Kidney is of the Water element, so we may look at its mother, Metal. If there is an abundance of Qi in the Lungs, we may draw some of this resource to the Kidneys by treating the Metal point of the Kidneys, K 7, or by treating the Water point of the

---

[163] The Extraordinary Vessels offer another method of homeostasis to the principal meridian system. It is unclear how much the regulatory aspects of Extraordinary Vessels and Five Element relationships overlaps.

Lungs, Lu 5. Either of these points can draw Qi from the Lungs to the Kidneys. What about the Earth element, which controls or inhibits Water? If there is excess in Earth, such as from too much sugary or rich foods, or from too much worry and mental over-activity, this may be suppressing the Kidneys too much. This can be alleviated most directly through being kinder to the Spleen through dietary improvements and/or harmonizing the mind through meditation, tai chi or "getting a life."

Emotional Balancing with the Five Elements

Each Element, and the Organs associated with it, generates a specific movement of Qi that is experienced as an emotion. Just as the sensation of blocked Qi and Blood causes the perception of pain, emotions are felt because of the characteristic movement of Qi generated by each Organ. Each emotion has an appropriate level of expression. Anger, grief, fear, introspection and joy are all healthy parts of life. Yet, when any specific movement of Qi is prolonged and overemphasized it brings about an unhealthy persistence of emotions that can lead to physical and mental health disorders. The Generation and Control cycles of the Five Elements may be used to help balance unhealthy emotional states. Based on the understanding that Water controls Fire, Wood controls Earth, Fire controls Metal, Earth controls Water, and Metal controls Wood, emotional balancing can be supported by treating the meridian point on the Organ's channel that corresponds to the Control element. The following chart illustrates these principles:

FIGURE 11.7: FIVE ELEMENTS AND EMOTIONS

ELEMENT	ORGANS	QI MOVEMENT	EMOTION	EMOTIONAL IMBALANCE	CONTROL EXCESS EMOTION WITH:
Fire	Ht, Pc, SI, TW	Expand	Joy	Mania, hyper, party animal	H 3, P 3, TW 2, SI 2 (water points)
Earth	Sp, St	Condense	Introspection	Worry, obsession	Sp 1, St 43 (wood points)
Metal	Lu, LI	Disperse	Grief	Prolonged grief, empty Qi	Lu 10, LI 5 (fire points)
Water	KI, UB	Descend	Fear	Prolonged fear, paranoia	K 3, UB 40 (earth points)
Wood	Lv, GB	Ascend	Anger	Rage, violence, depression	Lv 4, GB 44 (metal points)

Five Element emotional balancing can be a powerful adjunct to counseling and psychotherapy. The principles of the movements of Qi associated with emotional states are important understandings.

The suggestions for controlling excess emotion originally came from Dr. Nguyen Van Nghi of France, a pioneer in the acupuncture field. The treatments are performed with needle sedating technique on the specified points. Polarized microcurrent electro-acupuncture may be used as well. A suggestion for use is to place the positive probe on the specified point and the negative probe on the Source point of the same channel.

Emotions can be based on excess or deficient energy states, which may bear on the appropriate treatment. The emotional imbalances of mania and hyper states (Fire) and rage and violence (Wood) are excess in most cases. All the other imbalances can be of excess as well, but may also be of deficiency. For example, grief that arises from a recent loss is generally an excess condition, and part of healthy human emotion that only requires support, not treatment. Yet, if the person stays in a grieving state for a very long time, the draining, dispersing effect of grief will seriously weaken the Lungs, causing deficiency and possibly lung disease. The same is true for the emotions of the Spleen and Kidneys. In these cases of Organ deficiency caused by long-term emotional states, it may be more appropriate to simply tonify the Organ rather than use the Five-Element control point listed in the above chart. Tonification can be achieved by tonifying the Source point of the Organ and the tonification point of its mother Organ. Further analysis of the other Organ relationships through the Control cycle may be required as well.

FIVE ELEMENT CORRESPONDENCES

CORRESPONDENCES	WOOD	FIRE	EARTH	METAL	WATER
Yin Organ (Zang)	Liver	Heart, Pericardium	Spleen	Lungs	Kidneys
Yang Organ (Fu)	Gall Bladder	Triple Warmer, Small Intestine	Stomach	Large Intestine	Urinary Bladder
Emotion	Anger	Joy	Introspection	Grief, sadness	Fear
Sense Organ	Eyes	Tongue	Mouth	Nose	Ears
Body Tissue	Tendons	Blood Vessels	Muscles	Skin and hair	Bone
Vocal Sound	Shouting	Laughter	Singing	Crying	Groaning
Taste	Sour	Bitter	Sweet	Pungent	Salty
Weather Factor	Wind	Heat	Dampness	Dryness	Cold
Stage of Development	Birth	Growth	Transformation	Harvest	Storage
Orientation	East	South	Middle	West	North
Season	Spring	Summer	Late Summer	Autumn	Winter
Yin-Yang	Lesser Yang	Greater Yang	Center	Lesser Yin	Greater Yin
Number	8	7	5	9	6
Color	Green	Red	Yellow-Orange	White	Black-Dark Blue

Figure 41.8: Five Element Correspondences

Other Meridian Relationships

Other energetic pathways that may be used to balance the meridian system are beyond the scope of this book. The following acupuncture systems may be drawn upon for this purpose:

- Luo-Connecting points
- Micro-system points of the ear, hand and other areas
- Mu-Shu technique (see Chapter 12)
- Open points according to Chinese astrology and meridian color therapy[164]
- Chakra therapy and balancing[165]

Extraordinary Vessel Symptomatology and Points

1. **Ren Mai** (Conception Vessel)/**Yinchaio** (Yin Heel Vessel):

- Gynecological problems, lung problems, kidney Qi deficiency, ear, nose and throat problems, toothache, asthma (harder to breathe in), hemorrhoids, neurosis, urinary difficulties, intestinal problems, cold feet, insomnia, sciatica down the back of the leg, high blood pressure, kidney disease, cystitis, whiplash injury, cold lumbar area, Meniere's syndrome, tinnitus in older, deficient patients, stiff shoulder, deficiency headaches
- Body Regions Influenced and Coalescent Acu-Points:

    Ren: Abdomen, thorax, lungs, throat, and face. <u>Points</u>: Ren 1 – 24

    Yinchaio: Inner aspect of legs, abdomen, and eyes. <u>Points</u>: K 2, 6, 8, St 12, St 9, UB 1

2. **Chong** (Penetrating Vessel)/**Yinwei** (Yin Linking Vessel):

- Heart problems and chest pain with anxiety, palpitations, shortness of breath, neurosis, intercostal neuralgia, herpes zoster and post-herpetic neuralgia, stomach disorders, gynecological problems, cold feet, liver and gallbladder energetic and physical disorders, anus disease, strained back with digestive or GYN problems, some kinds of knee pain, sciatica that shoots down to the big toe or down the inside of the leg (Spleen channel), stomach or duodenal ulcer, many kinds of depressive/anxiety complexes
- Body Regions Influenced and Coalescent Acu-Points:

    Chong: Abdomen, uterus, chest, heart. <u>Points</u>: St 30, Ren 1, K 11, 12, 13, 14, 15, 16, 17, 18, 19, 20, 21

    Yinwei: Chest, heart. <u>Points</u>: K 9, Sp 13, 15, and 16, Lv 14, Ren 22 and 23

---

[164] An excellent discussion and resource charts on these subjects can be found in <u>Chasing the Dragon's Tail</u>, Chapter Nine.
[165] The author offers trainings on this subject. When the client journeys within for the purpose of shifting energetic relationships with deeply held old issues (samskaras), the release of energy that often spontaneously occurs balances the entire meridian system.

3. **Du** (Governing Vessel)/**Yangchaio** (Yang Heel Vessel):

   - Most musculoskeletal problems of the upper and lower back, arm and elbow cramps and spasms, numbness of arms and legs, finger spasms, tension of arms and legs, shaking of arms and legs, epilepsy, low back pain, spinal pain and injuries, neck stiffness and pain, torticollis, occipital headaches, some kinds of shoulder pain, some kinds of deafness, eyes red and painful, glaucoma, tinnitus, Meniere's syndrome, dizziness, epistaxis, insanity, joint pain, excessive sweating, early stages (Taiyang stage) of wind-cold invasion (cold and flu)

   - Body Regions Influenced and Coalescent Acu-Points:

     Du: Back, spine, back of neck and head. <u>Points</u>: Du 1 – 28

     Yangchaio: Lateral aspect of legs, back, neck, head, eyes. Points: UB 62, 61 and 59, GB 29, SI 10, LI 15 and 16, St 4, 3 and 1, UB 1 and GB 20

4. **Dai** (Girdle Vessel)/**Yangwei** (Yang Linking Vessel):

   - Sciatica that runs down side of leg (Gall Bladder channel), rib pain, herpes zoster and post-herpetic neuralgia, tinnitus in stronger patients, trigeminal neuralgia or acute TMJ pain, stiff shoulders, whiplash, leg length imbalances, toes curved over and clawed, backache, most one sided problems, menstrual and lower abdominal pain and problems, achy low back, excessive sweating, tiredness, some ear and eye problems

   - Body Regions Influenced and Coalescent Acu-Points:

     Dai: Waist, hips, genitals. Points: GB 26, 27, and 28, Du 4 (according to some sources)

     Yangwei: Lateral aspect of body, legs, neck, head, ears. Points: UB 63, GB 35, SI 10, TW 15, GB 21, St 8, GB 13, 14, 15, 16, 17, 18, 19 and 20, Du 15 and 16.

Chapter 12

STEP TWO: YANG MERIDIAN TREATMENTS

Revisiting Yin and Yang

Steps One and Two of the Four-Step protocol address the Yin and Yang energetic and physical aspects of the patient. In this case, the term Yin is used to describe those aspects that are more materialized and structural, i.e. more physically manifested, as well as the anterior and left-sided aspects of the body. Yin also references that which is more internal and deep, pertaining to vital Organs, Blood, Fluids, and Essence. Yang, on the other hand, refers to those aspects of the body that are less material, and more superficial, posterior or right-sided. In this light, Yang refers to the energy that infuses and vivifies the substantial Yin aspects. To clarify this relationship, Blood, being a physical substance, is more Yin, while Qi, being a non-physical energetic substance, is more Yang. Without Yang, the Blood cannot circulate and perform its physiological functions; without the physical substance, Yang is not manifested.

Step One meridian balancing work presented in the last chapter is primarily dealing with the more Yin or structural aspects of the body. These procedures mainly affect the balance of Qi in the meridian system to improve Organ functions and help correct structural distortions. This activity influences both Yin and Yang of course, yet the Yin structural effect is more pronounced. In Japan, meridian balancing through the Extraordinary Vessels is a primary treatment used to correct leg length differences, torticollis and other structural imbalances. This is because the Extraordinary vessels are the closest link to the body's original geometry.

To provide a balanced approach, such treatments may be followed by stimulation of the Yang or energetic aspects of the body. This is most commonly done through direct stimulation of Back Shu points associated with the meridians treated in Step One. Back Shu points are Yang because they are on the Yang Urinary Bladder channel, and are located on the back - the most Yang aspect of the body. These points also have a direct effect on the autonomic nervous system through stimulation of the spinal ganglia. The nervous system and its activity is more Yang in relation to Organ and fluid function.

Back Shu Points

The following chart lists the Back Shu points on the Urinary Bladder meridian, including its outer line:

BACK SHU POINTS

Back Shu Point (1 ½ - 2 cun Lateral To Midline/ Du Channel)	Outer UB Line (About 3 cun Lateral To Midline/Du Channel)	Sphere of Influence of Outer UB Shu	Spinal Level (lateral to and below the spinous process of:)
UB 13 (Fei Shu)	UB 42 (Po Hu)	Lung - Corporeal Spirit- sadness, grief, asthma	T 3
UB 14 (Jue Yin Shu)	UB 43 (Gao Huang Shu)	Pericardium - Whole body Qi + essence, connective tissues, chronic disease	T 4
UB 15 (Xin Shu)	UB 44 (Shen Tang)	Heart - Housing the Mind, anxiety, insomnia, depression	T 5
UB 18 (Gan Shu)	UB 47 (Hun Men)	Liver - Rooting Ethereal Soul for grounding, depression, unresolved resentment/anger	T 9
UB 19 (Dan Shu)	UB 48 (Yang Gang)	Gall Bladder - Indecision	T10
UB 20 (Pi Shu)	UB 49 (Yi She)	Spleen - Obsession, memory, concentration, mental clarity	T11
UB 21 (Wei Shu)	UB 50 (Wei Cang)	Stomach - Nurturing, mothering	T12
UB 22 (San Jiao Shu)	UB 51 (Huang Men)	Triple Warmer - Chronic disease, tightness below heart, breast disease, conducts Kidney Qi up	L 1
UB 23 (Shen Shu)	UB 52 (Zhi Shi)	Kidney - Fortify will and personal power, depression/apathy to heal self, back pain	L 2
UB 25 (Da Chang Shu)		Large Intestine	L 5
UB 27 (Xiao Chang Shu)		Small Intestine	At level of 1st sacral foramen
UB 28 (Pang Guang Shu)	UB53 (Bao Huang)	Urinary Bladder - Urinary problems, spreads Qi to genitals, sexual issues	At level of 2nd sacral foramen

Figure 12.1: Back Shu Points

Kyutoshin Treatment Technique

For Step Two treatments, Manaka mainly used moxa[166] burned on the handles of acupuncture needles imbedded into the Back Shu points. This practice is called kyutoshin, which translates to "moxa on handle of needle". This puts pure Yang energies into the Yang aspect of the body.

---

[166] Moxa is the dried, processed leaves of the species of mugwort plant called *artemesia vulgaris*. It is burned to produce radiant heat, as well as other electromagnetic emanations, into acupuncture points and dysfunctional body regions. The practice of burning moxa for therapeutic purposes is called *moxibustion*.

Other Yang meridian points may be used as well. In addition to Back Shu points, Manaka sometimes directly treated tender gastrocnemius found during evaluation or other Yang meridian points on the extremities. The most suitable form of moxa for this purpose is the "semi-pure" grade, or wakakusa, as it is known in Japan. This type, which sticks together strongly, is well suited for keeping the moxa ball on the needle handle as it burns. 1 ½" needles are inserted ½ - ¾" into the points – shallower on the upper back and deeper on the lower back. The semi-pure moxa is formed into a ball about ½ - ¾" in diameter, and then broken into two halves. The two halves of the ball are then pressed together onto the handle of the inserted needle so that the top of the handle is in the center of the ball. If you use the correct form of moxa, and follow this procedure, the moxa should not fall down during treatment. Experiment on inanimate objects before trying this on a patient. Pieces of fruit or veggies work well for practice.

While the moxa is burning, it is essential to stay with your patient to monitor her comfort. I suggest having some skin shields handy, so they can be slipped under the needle if the heat is too much for that patient. Simple shields can be made from thin cardboard squares with slits cut into them. It is also vital to have an ashtray and tongs nearby to rescue the moxa if necessary. Manaka recommended burning two moxa balls on each treated Shu point. He avoided stimulating the upper thoracic Shu points with needles and moxa on thin patients without much upper back musculature to avoid pneumothorax complications. This caution would be applicable when treatment of the Back Shu points of the Lung, Pericardium and Heart were called for. In these cases, he would substitute a different lower thoracic, lumbar or sacral Shu point for treatment. He commonly substituted UB 23 and/or UB 25 for the upper thoracic points since all Extraordinary vessels are intimately connected with the Kidney region. When he did use kyutoshin on the upper back for patients with sufficiently thick paraspinal muscles, it was with ½" insertions and smaller moxa balls.

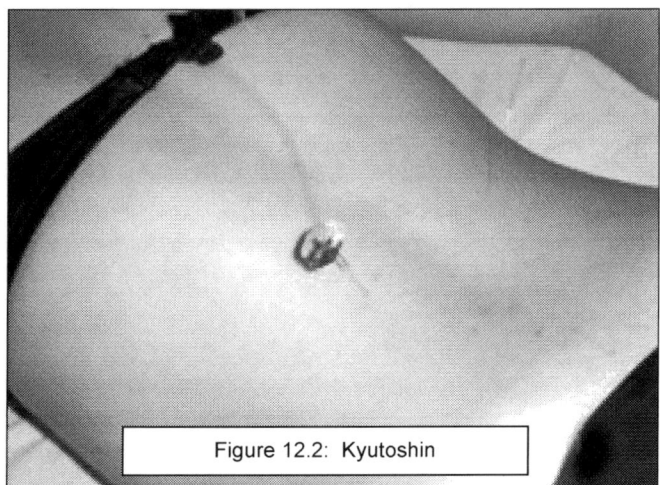

Figure 12.2: Kyutoshin

As an alternative to moxa, polarized microcurrent probe stimulation can also be used for StepTwo, as explained later in this chapter. When microcurrent stimulation of Back Shu points is used instead of needles and moxa, there is no danger of puncturing the lungs or heart, so that is not a consideration. It is possible, however, that electrical stimulation through the thoracic region, even gentle microcurrents, can pose a hazard to some cardiac disease patients. For this reason, it may be wise to follow Manaka's cautions for this method as well.

Back Shu Point Selection

The main principle for Step Two treatments is to choose Back Shu points that correspond to the diagnostic findings and treatment points from Step One. Some considerations are:

- the most significant imbalanced Organ/meridians
- the actual meridians treated in Step One
- tenderness and reactivity on palpation

Example of a typical Step Two treatment:

If the Extraordinary Vessel Master points SI 3 and UB 62 were indicated and treated in Step One, then the Back Shu points for Small Intestine and Urinary Bladder (UB 27 and UB 28) could be the corresponding points to be treated. If the Extraordinary Vessel Master points P 6 and SP 4 were treated, Back Shu points for Pericardium, Spleen, Liver or Kidneys could be chosen. Pericardium and Spleen may be chosen because those meridians were actually treated in Step One. Liver would be included if it was a focus of the treatment, and because this point combination is frequently chosen for treatment of the Liver. Kidney can be considered because the Chong Mai, one of the Vessels treated by this combination, is intimately connected with Kidney energetics, and has many coalescent points with the Kidney meridian. It is best to be both logical and intuitive in your choice of Shu points for this purpose, as well as being guided by palpation.

Outer line shu points

The outer line Shu UB points can be used when they are more tender and reactive than the inner line Shu points. For example, if Liver is a key focus, and UB 47 is tenderer than UB 18, you can choose to treat it with, or instead of, UB 18. You can also consider these points when the patient's complaint involves a high degree of emotional and spiritual issues, as the outer bladder line addresses the "spirit" level. This is revealed by the names and meanings of many of the points:

- *Po Hu* (UB 42, level with UB 13, Shu point of the Lungs) – "Door of the Corporeal Soul"

    Po refers to the most physical aspect of the soul, that which is intimately involved with how deeply a person breathes, and issues of emotional giving and receiving. This is also the aspect of the soul most connected with physical pain and itching, so its usefulness for pain management is profound.

- *Shen Tang* (UB 44, level with UB 15, Shu point of the Heart) – "Mind Hall"

    Shen is the vital force of the mind, the light that shines forth from a healthy person's face and eyes. When *Shen* is disturbed, there is anxiety, insomnia, depression and, in advanced cases, mental illness.

- *Hun Men* (UB 47, level with UB 18, Shu point of the Liver) – "Door of the Ethereal Soul"

    Hun is the closest Chinese medical equivalent to the Judeo-Christian concept of the soul – a spiritual essence that motivates and anchors us on the Earth. Disconnection from *Hun* can make a person feel aimless, ungrounded, depressed and purposeless.

- *Yi She* (UB 49, level with UB 20, Shu point of the Spleen) – "Thought Shelter"

    Yi is the mental aspect of the Spleen. While *Shen* is the vital force of the mind, *Yi* gives the ability to organize thinking and mental processing. Patients with *Yi* disorders can tend to be obsessive and troubled by a racing mind. On the other hand, they can have trouble concentrating and thinking clearly.

- *Zhi Shi* (UB 52, level with UB 23, Shu point of the Kidneys) – "Chamber of the Will"

    Zhi is an aspect of the Will, that which motivates and is the source of creativity. This point is valuable for low back pain due to Kidney deficiency as well as reinforcing the Will aspect in a patient to lift some types of depression and feelings of fear and powerlessness.

The following table gives examples of choosing Back Shu points that correspond to meridians employed for Step One energy balancing. Choose Shu points by indication and/or sensitivity to palpation. When the chart says to consider points in parentheses, these are points that can be substituted for upper thoracic points when contraindicated for the reasons given above.

STEP ONE TREATMENT POINTS AND RELATED BACK SHU POINTS

STEP ONE TREATMENT POINTS	RELATED BACK SHU POINTS
Lu 7 + K 6	UB 3 or 52 + UB 13 or 42 (or consider UB 22, 25 or 28)
SI 3 + UB 62	UB 27 + UB 28 or 53
TW 5 + GB 41	UB 22 or 51 + UB 19 or 48
P 6 + Sp 4	UB 18 or 47, 20 or 49 + UB 14 or 43 (or consider UB 22, 23, 25)
Sp/TW polar pair	UB 20 or 49 + UB 22 or 51
KI/LI "	UB 23 or 52 + UB 25
Lv/SI "	UB 18 or 47 + UB 28 or 53
Pc/St "	UB 21 or 50 + UB 14 or 43 (or consider UB 22, 23 or 25)
Lu/UB "	UB 28 or 53 + UB 13 or 42 (or consider GV 12, UB 22, 23 or 25)
Ht/GB "	UB 19 or 46 + UB 15 or 44 (or consider UB 20, 22 or 23)
Cross-syndrome[167]	UB 18 or 47 + choose from UB 20, 22 or 27 or their outer line points)

Figure 12.3: Step One Treatment and Related Back Shu Points

Other Step Two Treatment Points

As part of Step Two, you can also palpate the gastrocnemius points after Step One, and if still sore, treat them as well[168]. In cases of back pain with tight back muscles, you can also treat any of the points UB 40, 55, 56, 57, or 58 that are sore. You can add one of these final options to the treatment of Back Shu points, not both gastrocnemius and lower UB points. Any other sore or reactive points on the Yang meridians can be treated during this step as well. Kyutoshin, needling alone, or microcurrent probe treatments can be used. Electro-massage may be applicable.

Select one to three significant points for needle treatment. More may be treated with microcurrent treatment. By careful palpation of the Large Intestine, Small Intestine, Triple Warmer, Stomach, Gall Bladder, Urinary Bladder And Du (Governing Vessel) Channels, you may find some very reactive points that are energetically tied to the primary complaint. These can be combined with appropriate Back Shu points. When applying microcurrent for this purpose, I use polarized probe set-up and treat the Yang points in pairs, with the positive (+) probe on a proximal point and the negative (–) probe on a distal point. I use my understanding of the energetic relationships and a bit of intuition.

---

[167] This is a treatment of Pc 6 and Sp 4 on the right side and TW 5 and GB 41 on the left side, usually indicated for patients with coldness and back pain with digestive and/or GYN disorders.
[168] See Chapter 17

Tender channel points may be selected, or specific source, Luo or Transporting points may be utilized when there is a clear energetic reason to use them. For examples, when treating elbow pain along the large intestine channel, you could treat the source point of the Stomach, the Yangming related function, or the Luo point of the Lung, the Yin-Yang relative. Chapter 8, which covers the treatment of the Great Loops, describes more of these energetic meridian relationships.

Microcurrent Mu-Shu Technique

Many acupuncturists and other physicians wishing to practice the Four-Step protocol cannot or will not use needles and burning moxa for legal or logistical reasons. Use of moxa requires a good ventilation system, or at least signs in your office that "No, the staff is not smoking marijuana!" Due to this potential limitation, I have experimented with ways to use microcurrent stimulation for Step Two procedures. I have found that the microcurrent Mu-Shu technique described in Chapter 7 is an effective way to treat the Back Shu points. I would rate moxa's effectiveness somewhat higher than microcurrent for this purpose, but would estimate that polarized microcurrent Mu-Shu method gives at least 70% of the effectiveness of kyutoshin. It is much quicker and easier, and so is a good alternative for practitioners who either do not use moxa in their practice.

My extensive experience has revealed that the placement of the negative (-) pole of the stimulator on the Back Shu point with the positive (+) on the corresponding Front Mu point is most beneficial. This makes sense energetically, as the negative pole of microcurrent is more stimulating and tonifying, similar to moxa. According to one of my mentors, the late Dr. Nguyen Van Nghi, Back Shu points generally require tonification. Front Mu (Alarm) points, on the other hand, often register excess of the Organs, and so positive stimulation, which is more sedating, is often more appropriate. To confirm the correct polarity approach, stimulate the appropriate Mu-Shu points using different polarity combinations and verify the result. For example, test the primary imbalanced points and treat the patient with the negative (trigger) probe on the Front Mu point and the positive probe on the Back Shu point. Re-test the points. Then, reverse the polarity, treat and test again. By re-testing the primary imbalanced points after each application and observing the difference you will see that one approach will improve the balance readings while the other will degrade the balance readings. This can be confirmed using O-ring kinesiology, pulse diagnosis or abdominal palpation. The table of Mu-Shu point combinations from Chapter 7 is copied on the next page for convenience.

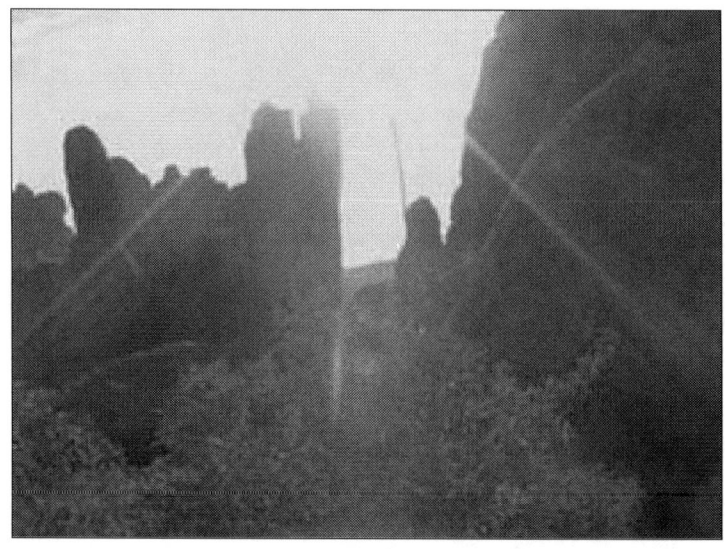

FIGURE 12.4 MU - SHU POINT COMBINATIONS

ORGAN TO BE TREATED	MU POINT: + PROBE	SHU POINT: - PROBE	COMMENTS
Lung	Lu 1	UB 13	Use caution with cardiac/elderly patients with this combination
Pericardium	*Ren 17*	*UB 14*	**Do not pass current through heart** – substitute Kidney Mu-Shu
Heart	*Ren 14*	*UB 15*	**Do not pass current through heart** – substitute Kidney Mu-Shu
Liver	Liv 14	UB 18	Use Manaka Liver 14- in soft tissue below R costal angle
Gall Bladder	GB 24	UB 19	
Spleen	Liv 13	UB 20	In this case the TCM Spleen Mu works better
Stomach	Ren 12	UB 21	
Triple Warmer	St 25/Ren 5	UB 22	Either Manaka or TCM Mu point will work, test to select
Kidney	Ki 16	UB 23	Manaka Mu point better here
Large Intestine	St 25/27	UB 25	Either Manaka or TCM Mu point will work, test to select
Small Intestine	St 26/Ren 4	UB 27	Either Manaka or TCM Mu point will work, test to select
Urinary Bladder	Ren 3/Ki 12	UB 28	

MU-SHU TECHNIQUE AND THE HEART

There is an important caution/contraindication to observe then performing microcurrent Mu-Shu method. When passing microcurrents through the Mu-Shu combinations of the Pericardium and Heart, electrical currents will pass directly through the region of the heart organ. While these tiny currents are unlikely to have any negative effect on healthy people it is an unacceptable risk for patients with cardiac disease, pacemakers or in the frail or elderly. To be on the safe side it is best to avoid utilizing electrical Mu-Shu method through these points. When the patient's evaluation calls for treatment of the Heart and Pericardium functions in Step Two, substitute treatment of the Kidney or other lower back functions. The Kidney is intimately related to Pericardium through the Ministerial Life Gate Fire, and to the Heart through the Shaoyin Great Loop circuit. For example, if the points treated in Step One were Pc 6 and Sp 4, you could choose the Mu-Shu combinations of the Spleen and Kidney for Step Two.

Step Two treatment completes the global energetic balancing of the meridians and Organs that was started with Step One treatment of the Extraordinary Vessels or polar meridian pairs. By focusing on tonifying appropriate Yang meridian points, the balancing of the meridians is stabilized, energized, and further grounded. For Step Two treatment technique, choose from moxa on the handle of needles (kyutoshin) or polarized microcurrent stimulation. The primary focus of treatment is Back Shu points, although these can be augmented with diagnostic points on the gastrocnemius that are still tender after Step One. Another appropriate alternative is treating a few well-chosen points on any Yang meridians that are indicated according to any valid acupuncture approach.

Steps One and Two may, in many cases, completely clear up the patient's complaints, especially for pediatric patients. In this case, you need to decide if hands-on bodywork (Step Three) or symptomatic treatments (Step Four) are necessary to promote longer carry-over of relief. Patients with deeply ingrained patterns of tension and imbalance in their bodies will generally benefit from these additional steps, while some hypersensitive patients may be aggravated by too much intervention in a single treatment session. This is why your awareness of individual patients is of the greatest importance. Monitor their reactions closely, observing changes in diagnostic indicators, ease of movement, energy levels and affect. Kinesiology is often helpful in checking for how much, and what kind of therapy, to administer.

Chapter 13

Step Three:

Microcurrents, Bodywork and Manipulation

Overview

Step Three of the Four-Step protocol can include a wide range of techniques and methods of direct, hands-on input to adjust the structure and function of the physical body. All these methods are categorized as "bodywork" in this book and include:

1. <u>Western-derived methods</u>:
- Massage
- Deep-tissue work
- Myofascial release
- Rolfing and its offshoots
- Strain-counterstrain and other proprioceptive techniques
- Active exercise, isometrics
- Assisted (passive) exercise by therapist or exercise machines
- Chiropractic or osteopathic manipulation
- Visceral manipulation
- Electro-massage

2. <u>Eastern-derived methods</u>:
- Shiatsu

- Sotai
- Tuina
- Thai massage
- Acupressure

The common thread to all these techniques is that a practitioner applies direct, hands-on input into the physical body with the aim of adjusting myofascial, neuromuscular or osseous imbalances. Most acupuncturists rely on needles, moxa or herbs to adjust Qi and Blood for releasing soft tissue blocks and imbalances. While this is of vital importance as a Root treatment, the response of the dense physical body may be much slower than its energetic response to acupuncture. This is because prolonged neuromuscular imbalances create changes and in tissues, such as adhesions, chronic muscle shortening, poor blood and lymph circulation and biases such as postural distortions[169]. The physical body and nervous system also holds patterns of imbalance in a form of memory. In their book <u>The Challenge of Pain</u>,[170] Melzack and Wall describe how "loops" develop in the nervous systems of some chronic pain patients that perpetuate pain even when the original injury to the tissues is healed. While acupuncture and microcurrent therapies can resolve these conditions in many cases, the body often requires direct, hands-on physical input to open and re-educate the affected areas. The power of human touch in a healing program can never be understated.

For further valuable insights on the relationship between acupuncture and bodywork, I recommend the book <u>Acupuncture Physical Medicine</u> by Mark Seem.[171] The author makes a convincing case that most of the external and internal effects of acupuncture are a result of the release of relatively superficial areas of myofascial tension and constriction through use of needles or other methods. Neuromuscular re-education is the practice of assisting injured and post-surgical patients to regain normal use of their bodies. This is an important priority for physical and occupational therapists. I believe that acupuncturists should also gain some of these skills to best serve our patients. This is the aim of Step Three treatments.

Microcurrents, Exercise and Proprioception

As mentioned in earlier chapters, the old model of electrotherapy looks something like a patient lying still on a treatment table, usually being over-stimulated by milliamp currents. This may be appropriate in some cases for the acute stage of injuries, when movement must be restricted and inflammation sedated. Once the acute stage has passed, however, the highest priority in most cases is rehabilitation and neuromuscular re-education of the injured areas. Interactive, dynamic approaches are far more effective for these aims than passive electrotherapy[172]. There are several important advantages to an interactive approach.

The most apparent advantage is that motion is the way the body/mind is innately programmed to calibrate our neuromuscular system, and its relationship with the central nervous system. As we move with gravity pulling on us, our remarkable proprioceptive systems are constantly responding and adjusting the balance of muscular tone throughout our bodies. In my view, this is intimately related with Qi flow through the meridians.[173] Proprioception is the feedback

---

[169] For discussion of biases, see Chapter 3
[170] Melzack and Wall, <u>The Challenge of Pain</u>, Basic Books, 1973
[171] Published by Blue Poppy Press
[172] Please review Chapter 6 for further explanation of this point
[173] The connection of proprioception to the balance of Qi flow is the opinion of the author

system between the peripheral neuromuscular systems of the body and the central nervous system. Proprioception enables the muscles to grossly and subtly adjust their individual tone, or degree of tension, as well as coordinating interacting muscle systems to work together to facilitate smooth and graceful movement.

The addition of microcurrent stimulation to areas of the body in motion can significantly accelerate and improve the results of rehabilitative exercise. There are several likely reasons for this:

- The patient feels less pain and stiffness, and so can expand his range of motion more easily with less resistance and discomfort.
- Microcurrent stimulation increases circulation of Qi and Blood through the area, reducing energetic blockage. This facilitates longer carry-over of the improved range of motion.
- Levels of available ATP in the muscular cells may be increased, facilitating muscle relaxation and increase of available energy.
- It is likely that the addition of low-level currents enhances the process of proprioception, so that re-education can be accomplished with less effort on the part of the therapist and patient.

Another advantage of the interactive approach of microcurrents with motion is that the practitioner can monitor the patient's response. In doing so he can continually adjust the treatment approach until maximum results are obtained.

MICROCURRENTS IN MOTION - FROZEN SHOULDER

A patient came to me with a frozen shoulder condition. This man could only abduct his arm about 90 degrees. First, I stimulated his shoulder with a four-pad microcurrent interferential placement and asked him to try to extend his range of motion by abducting his arm. After observing him for no more than 30 seconds, I could tell that this approach was not helping much. So I removed the pads and applied probe electrodes by placing one probe on the center of the restricted part of the lateral shoulder, and the other distally on the arm, around acu-point LI 11.

I then asked him to again try to repeatedly abduct the shoulder. I also used my hand holding the probe at this shoulder to apply electro-massage to the muscles of his shoulder. With this second approach, he was able to gradually increase his arm's range of motion almost to full range of 180 degrees.

The total treatment time was about 4 minutes. I give this example to show that the first treatment approach tried may not be the most effective one, and some experimentation may be necessary to provide the best results.

Step Three Treatment Techniques

The basic principle of Step Three treatments is to have the patient actively or passively mobilize or exercise the injured or affected area while simultaneous microcurrent stimulation is applied. Manaka mainly relied on the practice of sotai, which is a Japanese bodywork system. For details on this practice, the reader is referred to Chasing The Dragon's Tail, Chapter Ten. Some applications of sotai with microcurrent stimulation are given below.

Almost any form of physical therapy or manipulation may be employed in this phase of treatment. The techniques that are most effective are those that support and adjust healthy proprioception. It is best to start with any skills you already possess in bodywork or manipulation for Step Three, adding microcurrent stimulation as described below. First, see how much improvement is brought about by these methods and then experiment with new techniques. This chapter is not intended to provide complete training in hands-on bodywork skills; but mainly to give practical examples of how kinetic therapies may be combined with simultaneous microcurrent stimulation for accelerated resolution of myofascial disorders.

It is important to know which specific muscles are involved in pain and dysfunction syndromes. Each muscle has trigger points (TP's) that tend to appear in predictable spots. These TP's have been well mapped out by Travell and Simons.[174] Any successful therapy must address release of TP's, and there are local and distal strategies for doing so[175]. Trigger points have different electrical characteristics than the healthy, surrounding tissue, and generally have lower electrical resistance, and therefore, greater conductivity. For this reason GSR testing with your microcurrent device can help to locate trigger points, and the application of appropriate currents can help release them. As explained in Chapter 2, the fascial network of the body is electrically conductive with piezoelectric properties. When this vital network is functioning well, subtle energy signals freely move throughout the body, and all of our movements generate additional charge to help power the system.

Because our fascial network is also a semiconductor, subtle energy signals are transmitted without much loss of energy across large expanses of the body. For example, in the case of frontal headache, when one microcurrent probe is placed on the forehead and the other on the foot at acupoint St 44, conductivity readings can be just as high as if the probes were a few inches apart. You can easily verify this for yourself.

Travell and Simon offered many techniques for releasing TP's, mostly involving local applications of dry-needling (similar to acupuncture), pressure, and spray and stretch[176]. Combining such local treatments with appropriate distal acu-points generally improves the results. Adding the element of simultaneous active motion provides an even more dynamic and effective treatment. This is the essence of Step Three treatments.

A simple principle for combining the principles of trigger point release with microcurrent electro-acupuncture is to identify which meridian intersects the TP's to be treated. Treat the area in 2 – 3 stages. First, use a biphasic probe treatment (Circling the Dragon), connecting the TP with adjacent points of tenderness and anatomical significance. Next, change the polarity of the treatment probes from biphasic to polarized, and place the positive (+) probe on the trigger point, and the negative (–) probe on a major distal point on the same or related meridian as the one that runs through the TP.

---

[174] Travell and Simons, Myofascial Pain and Dysfunction, The Trigger Point Manual Vol. I & II, William and Wilkins

[175] Please see Treatment Formulary, Part I for diagrams of common trigger points

[176] The practice of spraying an analgesic agent over a painful body region so it may be stretched beyond previous limitations caused by pain

For example, for pain of the shoulder involving the levator scapulae muscle, the positive probe can be placed on the TP in that muscle (around acu-points SI 14 – 15) and the negative probe on SI 3 on the hand. You can then stimulate while the patient shrugs his shoulder or attempts a limited rowing motion. During the acute stage of injury, the motion aspect will have to be reduced or eliminated depending on the presentation.

For more extensive or chronic injuries, it may also be helpful to follow these two steps with microcurrent pad treatment to bathe the entire region in gentle current. When these methods fail to release the TP, more aggressive electro-therapy may be locally focused on it, pinching the TP between probe tips.[177]

Sotai

The aim of this aspect of sotai is to restore neuromuscular balance and full range of motion to the neck, torso and low back. The basic principle here is to find a limb or torso movement with restricted motion, and to stimulate a key acu-point or set of points while the patient moves the affected part. This movement is done on the out-breath. In most cases

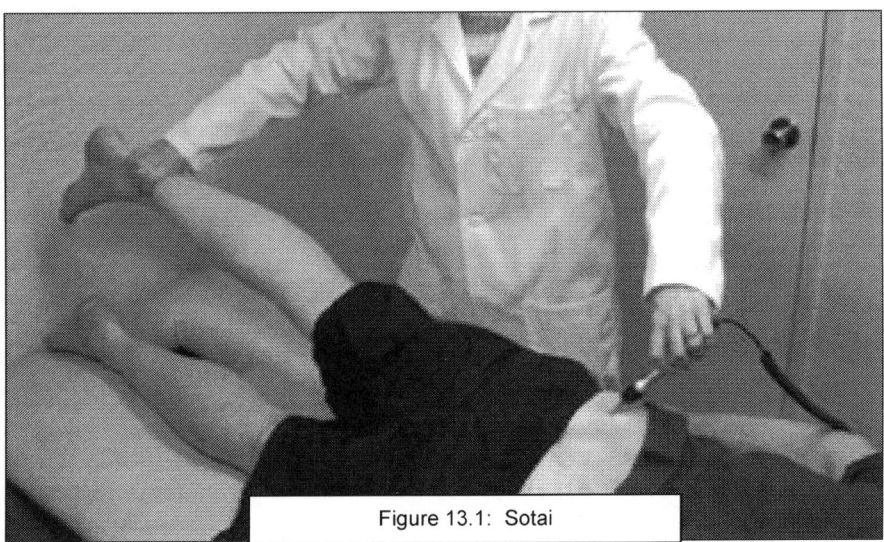

Figure 13.1: Sotai

the therapeutic movement will be in the direction that is opposite from that which is restricted, and on the side of the body with less restriction. When the patient's movement reaches its maximum, some resistance is applied by the therapist for her to move against while a few seconds of stimulation on the acu-point is applied. The patient is then instructed to totally relax her whole body. This procedure has powerful proprioceptive adjusting effects.

For example, in cases of lower back stiffness, have the patient lie prone on a treatment table. Try to touch her heels to her buttocks. The stiffness will often not allow both heels to touch. Next, palpate the bladder meridian of the lower back and legs, looking for very tight zones. Any very tight spot or trigger point in the area may be chosen. The side of the body that is looser (less restricted) is then treated by asking the patient to straight raise (extend) her whole leg as high as possible, pressing against your hand. You then raise her leg slightly higher, a little beyond her comfortable range of motion, while she holds her breath, simultaneously applying stimulation to the selected tight point. After a few seconds, ask the patient to drop her leg while you catch it and gently lower it to the table. Stop the stimulation.

Stimulation may be applied on the tight point with direct moxa cones, fire needle[178] or microcurrent probe stimulation. Applying any of these methods during the assisted exercise of sotai requires skillful coordination. Microcurrent stimulation is the easiest method to apply, and

---

[177] The Acutron Mentor probe preset #3 "Acute" is specifically programmed for this purpose

[178] Fire needle is the practice of heating an acupuncture needle red hot in the flame of an alcohol or gas burner, and then briefly inserting and removing it in tight muscular points. It works by relaxing the tendino-muscular meridians, and is especially effective in cases of cold-induced pain.

very effective. For this purpose, choose relatively aggressive treatment parameters. I suggest a modulated frequency of 80 – 130 Hz at about 150 µA, using the negative probe for treatment.[179] Plug in the brass hand mass and ask the patient to hold it in her hand, generally on the side of her body opposite to the acu-point being stimulated[180]. Press and release the probe trigger switch to stimulate the chosen point or points while you use your other hand to guide the leg on the looser side as described above. A well-chosen auricular point on the tighter side of the body may also be used for this procedure. I refer you to Manaka's book for further details on his use of sotai for Step Three treatment.[181]

Electro-massage

There are two main ways to administer electrically-enhanced therapeutic touch. One is by running microcurrents through the hands of the therapist into the patient; the other is through special electro-conductive gloves that transmit the current to the patient without passing through the hands of the therapist. While both methods are valuable, I prefer skin-to-skin contact electro-massage, as this allows for more sensitive palpation and influx of subtle healing energies that the gloves would block. If set up and performed correctly, there is no hazard to the therapist as long as this technique is not practiced too extensively. I would not recommend running microcurrents through your hands more than a couple of hours a day at the most. If longer periods are needed, the conductive gloves may be used. The most important factor in set-up is to make sure that no currents flow between your hands. It is incorrect to place one electrode on one hand and the other of the same channel on the other hand. This will treat you, and not the patient. For each output channel of the stimulator used, place one pad on the patient and the other on the back of one of your hands. Two methods of electro-massage are described below.

Interferential electro-massage

This is the most versatile and useful set-up, as you can freely work on the patient with both of your hands. Set-up your device for microcurrent interferential.

Most commonly used to treat:

- Adhesions and scar tissue: use cross-fiber friction massage
- Lymphatic stasis: use draining lymphatic massage
- Trigger points and myofascial knots: use manual pressure and draining massage
- Whiplash and other specific muscle disorders: apply pressure to origins and insertions of affected muscles
- Extremity joint pain, such as carpal tunnel and tennis elbow: use polarized electro-massage with negative pads on your hands, and positive pads on the patient over the symptomatic region. Use your hands to massage and stimulate distal points according to the principle of the Great Loops (see Chapter 8).

Time required: 10 - 15 minutes

Set-up: Acutron Mentor: I.F. #2 (with modification)

---

[179] Probe preset #3 (Acute) on the Acutron Mentor is ideal for this purpose. Modify polarity to negative.
[180] For patients with cardiac problems, avoid passing currents across the chest, therefore either forego electrical treatment or ground the patient on the same side if the condition permits
[181] Chasing the Dragon's Tail, Chapter 10, pgs 197-202

Other devices:

Intensity: 400-600 µA. Current needs to be much higher than with pads. This is turned up after starting treatment

Frequency: 80 – 130 Hz for acute constrictions, 0.6 – 10 Hz for chronic or deficient areas

Waveform: Square wave for most patients, Slope wave for very sensitive patients

Modulation: A ramping Hz is best if available

Polarity: Biphasic for most applications, polarized if working along extremities

Channels: Use two channels, four pads total, with out-of-phase interferential set-up if available

Steps:

1. Moisten the area of the body to be massaged with tap water or saline solution. A plant sprayer is ideal for this purpose. Electrically conductive gels may also be used, but can tend to get on your microcurrent device as you touch the controls. This is why I prefer tap water, which is plenty conductive in most cities. If your tap water comes from a well or some other pure source, you will need to add salt to the water prior to use.

2. Attach electro-pads to end of patient leads and plug into Channels A and B. For Channel A place one pad on patient's body, and the other on the back of one of your hands. For Channel B, place one pad on the patient's body and the other on the back of your other hand. Arrange the pads so that, when you touch the patient, the pathways of current flow between each set of pads will intersect each other in the target tissues to be treated. (see diagrams).

3. Press the start button of your device and turn up the current intensity to 300 – 600 µA. You should feel a tingling feeling in your fingers as you touch the patient, but it should be gentle and comfortable. The patient will probably not feel much unless she is very sensitive.

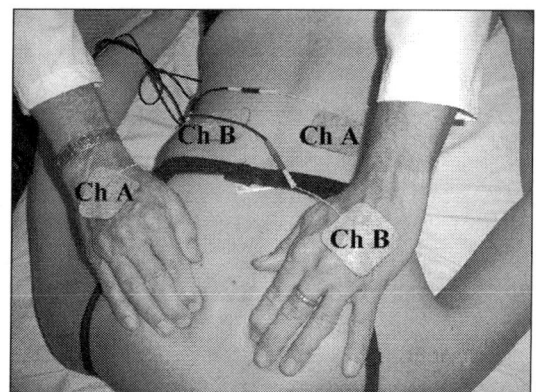 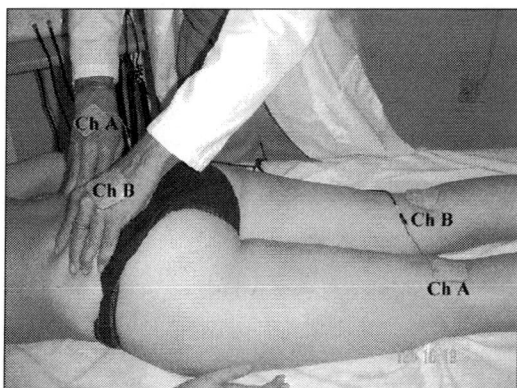

Figures 13.2: Electro-massage - upper and lower back regions

4. If your device has conductivity monitoring, the indicator should rise up to the 80 – 100% level in conductivity test mode.

Quick electro-massage using probes

This method is a fast way to apply electro-massage in the midst of a probe treatment.

Steps:

1. Select and moisten the target treatment area of the body.
2. Set probe timer control to 30 seconds or more, or simply activate a series of 6 second treatment cycles.
3. Using one of your hands, touch the counter probe tip to an area adjacent to the target treatment site, or on a distal or proximal acu-point.
4. Grasp the trigger probe in the palm of your other hand so that its metal tip is pinched between your 3rd and 4th fingers, making an electrical contact with your hand.
5. Press the trigger button to activate treatment, and use the free fingers of your hand holding the trigger probe to massage the affected area. The pathway of current will flow between your massaging fingers and the counter probe.

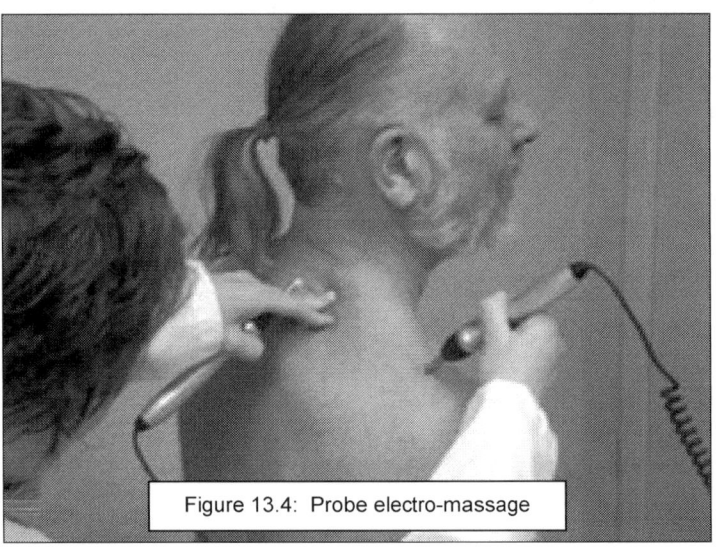
Figure 13.4: Probe electro-massage

Stretching, Yoga and Microcurrents

Stretching is one of the most therapeutic and natural therapies to both prevent and treat pain. Lack of stretching is a major predisposing factor in many forms of chronic pain, including low back pain, neck pain and fibromyalgia. Systematic stretching is a primary physical therapy prescribed for back pain patients. When I had a severe herniated disk problem in my lower back several years ago, it was a program of stretching and microcurrent interferential treatment that saved me from surgery and continued pain.

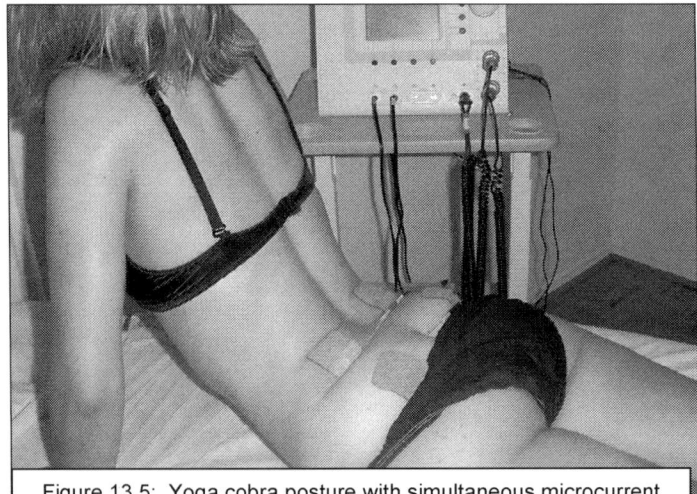
Figure 13.5: Yoga cobra posture with simultaneous microcurrent IF

I recommend such a combination for a wide range of myofascial pain disorders. Such therapy is an excellent Step Three treatment, and I frequently ask patients to perform stretches at home in between treatment sessions.

Step Three for chiropractors and bodyworkers

The main focus of chiropractic physicians and bodyworkers are treatments to correct structural distortions. In the chiropractic profession there are two main streams – the "straights" and the "mixers". Straight chiropractors are those who only manipulate the spine, choosing not to directly treat the soft tissues with adjunctive treatments. Mixers are those who combine aspects of physical, electro or meridian therapies with manipulation. Mixer chiropractors are a step closer to practicing the Four-Step protocol than the straights, as they are combining some form of energy stimulation with bodywork. Osseous manipulation is also practiced by many doctors of osteopathy (D.O.'s) in the United States. Osseous manipulation has been practiced in various forms since ancient times. Manipulation is one of the Eight Branches of traditional Chinese medicine. The combination of this skill with meridian balancing and therapeutic movement provide a masterful and comprehensive treatment style.

It is best to perform most meridian testing and balancing (Step One) and Yang channel treatment (Step Two) prior to manipulation (Step Three). By first relaxing and balancing the soft tissues, spinal distortions will release more easily, and adjustments will tend to hold longer. Patients will also be more likely to accept manipulation more easily.

This also holds true for soft tissue bodyworkers, such as those practicing Rolfing, MFR, deep tissue work and other styles. These professionals can also utilize electro-massage with great benefit, as its use can reduce the amount of time and effort expended. Soft tissue constrictions will release more readily when microcurrent is applied, with or without massage. In fact, several physical therapists and bodyworkers have told me that practicing electro-massage has reduced overuse pain in their own hands and wrists. If, after practicing Steps One, Two and Three, the patient still has some residual areas of pain, additional brief techniques can be applied to "clean up" and release the remaining symptoms. These "Step Four" treatments will be addressed in the next chapter.

Chapter 14

Step Four: Symptomatic and Take-Home Treatments

It is appropriate that symptomatic treatments are dealt with in the final chapter of this Section. In sharp contrast with most books about electro-therapy and pain management, most of the information contained herein is not just about relieving painful symptoms in isolated parts of the body. It is more concerned with the knowledge and tools for working with electromedical interventions in a truly holistic manner. Yet we do live in dense physical bodies, and treatment of its painful symptoms remains an important priority in health care. After all, this is largely what motivates our patients to come to us, and what they primarily pay us for.

Anyone who has practiced this protocol has observed that the first one to three steps are often sufficient to relieve the presenting symptom, and that no further interventions are needed. This is especially true of pediatric care and conditions based on deficiency. Step Three treatments, combining therapeutic massage, manipulation or mobilization with microcurrent (or other) stimulation address symptom relief quite powerfully in itself. In fact, many of the Step Three treatments actually combine aspects of Step Three and Four. Additional symptomatic intervention is still often necessary for many of our patients, however, even after they have received well-chosen holistic treatment.

There are several reasons for this:

- Many modern patients present with multiple areas and levels of dysfunction. Effective and focused acupuncture treatments require recognizing the diagnostic patterns the patient is presenting, and prioritizing treatment of the most significant pattern. Even if the treatment is well chosen and effectively administered, there may be remaining painful or dysfunctional areas of the body. These could be due to injuries that are not directly related to the main complaint being treated. For examples, a patient with fatigue who also had a stiff neck, a gynecology patient who had an old tennis injury that was still painful, an athlete with sciatica also asking you to help her with her smashed finger. How many times have your patients asked you, at the end of a successful session, if you could also help with a similar complaint? Fortunately, microcurrent stimulation offers many ways to deal with such remaining symptoms quickly and easily.

- During many emergencies, symptomatic treatment is all that can be given. This is often true in cases of acute pain and recent injury. It will be necessary to relieve enough pain for the patient to be able to relax, breathe and start the recovery process. As long as the patient's body is tense and contracted, circulation of blood, lymph and vital energy are impaired. Inflammatory conditions also greatly reduce local circulation and cause release of prostaglandins and bradykinins that maintain pain. Milli and microcurrent electro-acupuncture treatments can rapidly reduce acute pain and inflammation.

- The healing process of many, if not most, pain patients must include action they take of their own volition to help themselves. There is no medicine, or technique the greatest doctor can perform, that will replace this. Often a lack of self-care and self-love originally leads your patient to her chronic pain condition or disease. Lasting improvement in her chief complaint will depend on a balance of professional care and self-motivation to take charge of her life and help himself. Some of the methods expressed in this chapter lend themselves well to home care.

- Patients with chronic pain complaints need an extended period to relax and re-educate areas they have been favoring and guarding. This cannot be fully accomplished during office visits. Giving these patients a way to stimulate key acu-points in conjunction with therapeutic exercise on their own will significantly speed their progress.

This chapter will be divided into two parts, one dealing with symptomatic treatments that can be administered in office, and the second with take-home treatments and other self-administered methods. Please also see the Treatment Formulary section of this book for specific protocols.

SYMPTOMATIC TREATMENTS

Symptomatic treatments are appropriate during episodes of acute injury or intense pain. Sprained ankles, back or neck strain, acute headaches, fractures and concussions are common examples. The first priorities after injuries are to stop any bleeding, check for shock or stopped breathing, and to immobilize broken bones. Once those life-threatening issues are addressed, electro-acupuncture treatment can proceed to relieve pain, reduce inflammation and restore circulation to the injured area.

As mentioned above, acute pain, inflammation, muscle spasm and edema can greatly reduce blood and lymph circulation to the affected area. In these cases, it may be appropriate to use milliamp stimulation to "force" the body to relax its tension and to stimulate local muscles to pump out excess fluids. This can help restore proper circulation, which carries off toxic waste products, thereby promoting healing.

There are also times when a highly invasive "nerve block" effect that milliamp electro-stimulation can provide is appropriate. Although the "nerve block" mechanism is poorly understood, it is likely that it breaks a looping of pain signals between the injury and the central nervous system that sometimes leads to chronic pain -- in effect a pattern interrupt. In these cases, therefore, milliamps can act to *override* out of control electrically based nervous system activity in the body.

Milliamp electro-therapy may therefore be indicated for acute injuries when the priorities are to stop pain and promote macro circulation to open the passageways for healing. Once you perceive that the patient is more relaxed and mobile, gentler microcurrent treatments become more appropriate, as such currents are superior for directly accelerating cellular and tissue healing, and balancing meridian energetics.

To summarize, milliamp treatments are useful for relaxing the body and opening the way for healing, while microamps directly accelerate healing. Some of the most severe cases of acute pain that are fixed and stabbing may be associated with blood stasis. In such cases, a few drops of the stagnant blood must be bled out to allow the body to restore circulation of fresh, healthy blood. When bleeding technique is indicated, other acupuncture and microcurrent interventions will usually not be very effective.

The Priorities of Treatment and Techniques

Inflammation and swelling:

Western medicine and first aid methods prescribe ice over the inflamed area as first aid. Chinese Medicine, paradoxically, more often calls for use of hot-natured herbal liniments to create counter-irritation and increased circulation in inflamed areas. Both approaches have value. Ice, which is more readily available in emergencies, can be successfully used for initial acute treatment for most patients. Patients with Yang deficiency and cold constitutions cannot tolerate extended use of ice, however. For such patients use ice only until acute pain and swelling has started to decline, then follow with warm or hot applications.

Techniques:

- *Ice Electrotherapy*

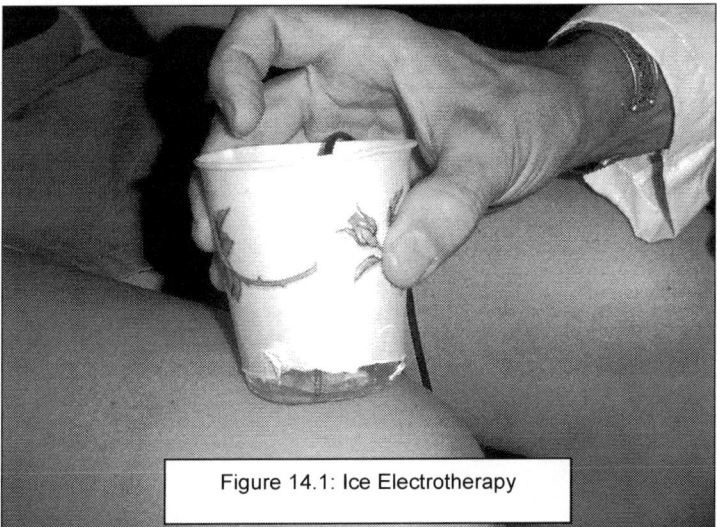
Figure 14.1: Ice Electrotherapy

This is an innovative treatment offered by Dr. Thomas Wing, performed as follows: Fill small wax paper cups with water containing some dissolved salt. Locate the cables from your microcurrent device that are used to stimulate pad electrodes. Each cable has two metal pins at its termination that plug into pads. Drape each pin into one of the paper cups so that its tip is near the center of the water in it. Put the cups in the freezer compartment of a refrigerator and allow the cups to freeze.

When ready for treatment, set up your stimulator for the appropriate current -- milliamp or microamp depending on the presentation. Tear off the bottom of the cups so that about an inch of ice protrudes. You can hold the ice electrodes by the remaining part of the cup to protect your fingers. Start current, and liberally apply the electrified ice to the inflamed area with both cups so you are completing the circuit.[182] This technique offers the dual

---

[182] The Acutron Mentor, MENS and some other devices have conductance monitors that let you confirm that adequate conductivity exists between the ice cups. Treatment is working as long as conductivity during treatment is at least 30% on the scale.

advantages of ice and electrical stimulation. A TENS pad frozen in the cups with attached leads hanging out is an alternative to using device lead wires.

- *Milliamp Edema Reduction*

The aim of this technique is to literally pump pooled fluids out of swollen areas. Each muscle has nerve bundles in it called motor points. Electrical stimulation on motor points creates the strongest muscle contractions. Locate the motor points on the muscles in the swollen or edematous area. Set up your stimulator for milliamp current with pulsed waveform and pulse duration of at least 200 μS. Set frequency to about 1 Hz.[183] Place pad electrodes directly over the indicated motor points. You may need two channels powering two sets of pads to adequately stimulate a large edematous area. Start current, and gradually turn up current intensity until you can see a noticeable pulsing contraction in the area. If you do not see pulsing all around the swollen area, try moving the pads to other locations, perhaps motor points on other local muscles. Once the affected area is pulsing, continue treatment for 10 – 20 minutes. Monitor your patient carefully, and immediately discontinue treatment if he reports increased pain or other discomfort. Using the same pad placements, follow milliamp treatment with another 10 minutes of low-frequency microcurrent treatment.

Acute Pain Due To Blocked Qi

Acute pain is generally due to one or two factors – blocked Qi or stagnant Blood. Qi is blocked any time there is pain. When it is blocked suddenly, as is the case with acute injury, the blocked Qi often turns into heat. Fluids may also be blocked, causing swelling. Pain is the sensation of the blockage of Qi. When the pain is fixed and stabbing, Blood has become blocked.

Techniques:

Great Loops technique

This technique, which was explained in Chapter 8, can be very effective for treating acute pain. The principle is that the positive microcurrent probe is reducing electrical charge at the injured area, while the negative probe is supplementing a distal point that can help restore energy circulation through the affected meridian. Auricular or Korean hand micro-system points can also be used as distal points (see below).

- *Auricular Micro-Macro Technique*

A variation of the Great Loops technique, this utilizes micro-system points as the distal point instead of a point on the principal meridians. Set up your microcurrent device for polarized probe stimulation, at intensity of 25 – 50μA.[184] Place the + probe directly on the most painful injured point, or alternatively, ask

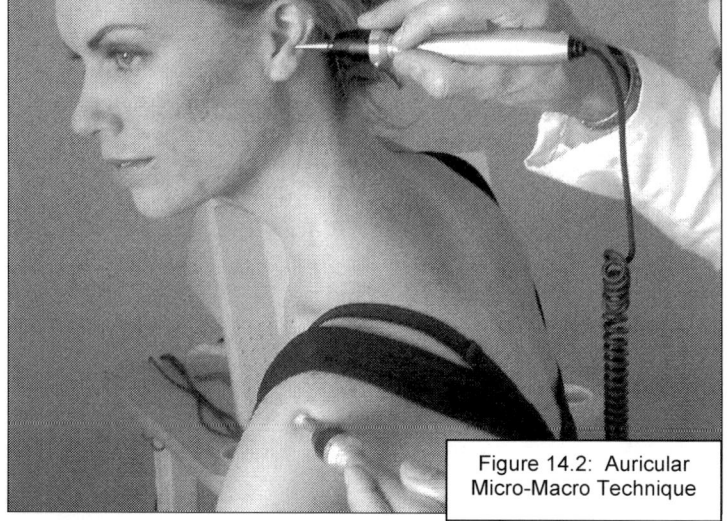

Figure 14.2: Auricular Micro-Macro Technique

---
[183] Use Acutron Mentor mA pad preset #1
[184] Use Acutron Mentor probe preset #2

the patient to hold it there herself. This frees you up to use both hands to locate and treat the micro-system point. Using a 2mm auricular probe tip and the device point searching feature, locate an ear or Korean hand point that corresponds to the injured area. For example, if the patient is presenting with acute pain in the right shoulder, ask her to hold the cotton probe tip of the positive (+) probe on the most painful point in that area. You can then use the auricular tip on the negative (–) probe to search in the Shoulder area of the right ear.

You should find a point in that area that reads significantly higher than those around it. Press the start button on the probe and treat for 15 – 20 seconds. Ask your patient to try to move the shoulder, and note if there is any reduced pain. You can then use other combinations of local shoulder points and ear or hand points to continue treatment. This technique can also be combined with Great Loops treatments using principal meridian distal points.

- *Classic Interferential*

Please see Chapter 9 for details on this popular intense electro-therapeutic treatment. Most patients will benefit more from local and distal acupuncture meridian strategies for pain relief. However, in some acute cases involving muscle spasm, edema and severe pain, Classic Interferential or I.F. combination treatment[185] can be a fast and effective way to stop pain and relax tense muscles.

Acute Pain Due To Blood Stasis

No discussion of the treatment of pain is complete without addressing the subject of blood stasis. Pain is the experience of the blockage or retardation of the free flow of Qi and Blood in the body. As previously stated, balancing or supplementing the electrical aspect of Qi, or unblocking its free flow are effective methods of pain control. "Qi is the commander of Blood" according to Chinese medical theory, so when Qi is constrained for any extended period, Blood in that area also starts to lose its free flow and becomes static. Blood stasis is more common in elderly patients, in women, and those that are overweight and sedentary. It should also be considered with patients who have had acute trauma, even if a long time ago.

When Blood stasis is a significant factor in a painful condition the following symptoms can be present:

- Pain is focused on a specific spot, is stabbing, biting and persistent. This is contrast with pain due to Qi constraint, which comes and goes, and often moves around.
- When affecting the low back, patients are often twisted with pain and may not be mobile.
- There are often dark veins in the painful area or distally on the same or related meridian.
- Tongue is purple, sometimes with purple spots, pulse is choppy or wiry.
- Patient's face looks dark, lips purplish.
- Patient often has fixed abdominal masses that can be palpated.

There is often heat associated with the painful area, although this is not always the case with elderly or frail people with underlying vacuity.

The primary treatment for blood stasis is bleeding techniques, in which superficial veins and spider nevi are pricked with a sterile lancet or prismatic needle to let out a few drops of blood. Bleeding is done on or around the area of stabbing pain, or on related distal acu-points. Distal

---

[185] A sequence of milliamp and microamp interferential treatment. I.F. preset #5 on the Acutron Mentor.

bleeding is usually done on the same meridian on which the painful area lies, on energetically related meridians, or points of special effect. Bleeding technique can be very effective for acute stabbing pain, high fever without Yin deficiency, acute itching, numbness and tingling in the extremities, varicosities, hot sore throat and headaches behind the eyes. In cases of advanced blood stasis, the blood released will look dark or purplish. The vein will often change appearance after being bled, and look less dark and distended.

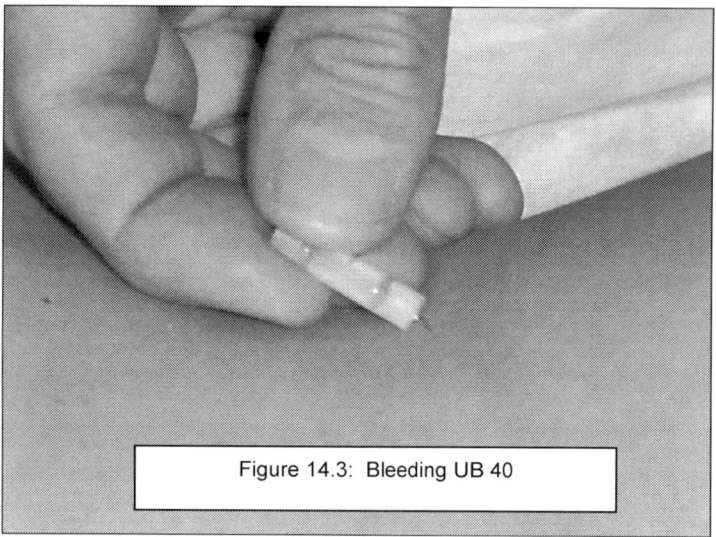

Figure 14.3: Bleeding UB 40

Microcurrent treatment is not directly effective for pain due to blood stasis, yet may help resolve chronic cases or prevent it through the mobilization of Qi. It is an excellent follow-up to bleeding treatment, however. As mentioned above, it is often the stasis of Qi that eventually leads to stasis of Blood. By improving the free flow of Qi, it is easier for the body to absorb and resolve Blood stasis. I would suggest following any bleeding treatment with microcurrent pad stimulation to the affected area to soothe the tissues, enhance healing, and to smooth the flow of Qi. Step One meridian balancing should be administered to patients with chronic pain due to blood stasis to address the root of their condition.

Techniques:

- *Bleeding For Acute Pain, General*

Look for dark or distended veins or spider nevi in the area of the stabbing pain. Using sterile technique, prick with a lancet or prismatic needle to let out a few drops of blood. Palpate down the meridian to see if there are any such veins on its distal regions. If so, bleed these also. Alternatively, you can bleed the distal point only and follow with use of polarized microcurrent probes, with the + probe on the painful area and the − probe on an indicated distal point. In any case, finish treatment by applying a few minutes of microcurrent stimulation or moxa stick over the area that was bled.

- *Bleeding For Acute Low Back Injury*

Look for a distended or purplish vein on the back of the knees near acu-point Weizhong (UB 40). Prick it with a lancet to let out a few drops of blood. This point may also be bled for dysmenorrhea with clots.

- *Bleeding For Headaches Due To Blood Stasis and Excess Heat*

Prick points according to area of headache. Du 20 and Lv 1 for pain on top of the head, St 8 (or dark vein in region) for frontal pain, *Taiyang* and tender GB points on temple for temporal or parietal pain, UB 67 for occipital pain. Distal SI meridian points may also be used for occipital pain if they coincide with dark veins. There are also three points on the midline of the sacrum below S3, S4 and S5 collectively called Chong Xiao that are highly effective when bled for severe occipital pain.[186]

- *Bleeding For Excess Headache Associated With High Blood Pressure, Arteriosclerosis, Yang Dizziness and Hemiplegia*

Bleed a series of points on the upper back collectively called *Wu Ling*. These points are described in the book Master Tong's Acupunture.[187] They are arranged in five vertical lines. The middle line is on the midline of the spine starting below C7 at acu-point Du 14, and includes each depression between the spinous processes of each vertebral segment down to T10. There are two outer lines. The first is four finger-widths lateral to the midline on each side, with one point lateral to each of the midline points down to the level of T8. The second outer line is four finger-widths lateral to the first one, with points lateral to the levels of T1 to T7. The placement of points on each line is symmetrical. The area should be cleansed with alcohol prior to pricking, and each point pressed before bleeding. The entire area must be thoroughly cleaned after bleeding to prevent infection. Light moxa stick treatment or microcurrent interferential treatment throughout the entire region after bleeding will be beneficial to smooth the flow of Qi and sooth the patient. See Miriam Lee's book for more details on this valuable treatment.

HOME TREATMENTS

There are limits to how much can be accomplished in a clinical setting, no matter how skilled the practitioner. Once a painful bias (see Chapter 3) has become deeply programmed into a patient's neuromuscular systems, it may take a repeated or continual counter-bias to rebalance it. Patients can do this by continuing their treatment at home.

Nutrition and Herbal Medicine

The method most commonly employed by acupuncturists for home treatment is the use of nutritional or herbal medicines prescribed to match the patient's pattern. Chinese herbal medicine is a form of heteropathy. This term refers to giving substances that act as a counter-bias to the disease or pain condition. For example, for hot conditions, give cold herbs such as Coptis or Gardenia. For damp conditions, give drying herbs, etc. Diet and herbal therapies are particularly vital for patients with deficient or toxic conditions that underlie and prolong pain and organic dysfunction.

Although beyond the scope of this book, dietary counseling is often of great importance in healing programs. This is particularly relevant for patients with digestive, metabolic, allergic and energy deficient conditions.

Hydration and Minerals

Two essential factors must be addressed here. The first is sufficient intake of pure water by your patients. The entire healing process depends on proper hydration. Acupuncture, microcurrent therapies, nutrition and exercise will all be very limited in effectiveness in dehydrated patients. Interestingly, patients who drink a lot of soft drinks, coffee and alcoholic beverages may still be dehydrated, as these substances can act as diuretics. It is only pure

---

[186] As described in Master Tong's Acupuncture, translated by Miriam Lee, Blue Poppy Press, pg 158
[187] ibid, pgs 148-149

water and moderate quantities of fruit and vegetable juices that serve to properly hydrate patients. Even some herb teas have diuretic properties, although the ones most commonly used for beverage purposes such as peppermint, chamomile, hibiscus and rose hips do not. Many elderly patients are in the habit of drinking little or no water. It is vital that you enlist your patient's cooperation in drinking a quart or more of spring or purified water each day.

Minerals are the substrate of the body's innate bio-electric systems. Most major diseases of our society are associated with mineral deficiencies. No progress in acupuncture or microcurrent treatment is likely for patients with severe mineral deficiencies. It is remarkable how many affluent and well-fed people in the United States suffer from lack of vital minerals. This is due to over- consumption of processed foods, the demineralization of our soils and drinking waters and increasingly chemicalized agricultural practices. Even those of us that take mineral supplements may be deficient, as few people can efficiently absorb minerals in pill form through the gut. I suggest the use of liquid colloidal mineral solutions, which are much more easily absorbed. It is important to use a product that has had heavy metals removed from it.[188]

Whenever you have a patient who is not responding well to appropriate treatment, I suggest that you check on her water and mineral intake, and help her increase these to levels that support full bio-electric functioning.

Therapeutic Exercise

Corrective or strengthening exercises are excellent methods for improving the effectiveness of a course of clinical treatments. Many painful conditions, especially neck and back pain, are due in part to poor tone and balance of the musculature supporting those areas. Teaching patients how to systematically strengthen and stretch the muscles of the injured area or whole body is a vital part of a treatment regimen. The subject of simultaneous exercise and microcurrent stimulation has already been discussed in Chapter 13.

A complete treatment of therapeutic exercises is also beyond the scope of this book, but I do want to state that Hatha Yoga is one of the finest methods I know to both treat and prevent recurrent or chronic pain. Most of us have sedentary lives relative to our ancestors, and consequently our muscles and tendons are often chronically tense and shortened. This predisposes us to injury when trauma occurs or simply from too much sitting at a desk. A good yoga regime allows you to systematically stretch and tone all the major muscles and tendons of the body. This prevents pain and injury, massages the internal organs, enhances circulation of Qi and Blood, and makes the emotions more cheerful. For patients who are injured, there are specific Yoga postures and movements that will, over time, correct most or all of their physical imbalances. There is a book and video from Marshall Govindan that shows the specific health and healing benefits of each posture.[189] I also recommend the excellent self-help exercise books by Robin Mackenzie called <u>Treat Your Own Neck</u> and <u>Treat Your Own Back</u>.[190]

Intradermal Needles and Ion Pellets

Auricular and/or Korean hand points that correspond to the painful area may be stimulated with devices called intradermal needles or ion pellets. These are ideal take-home treatments, as they can be easily and quickly applied before the patient leaves your office. The patient should be instructed to rub the devices several times a day to counter accommodation, and to remove

---

[188] The product I use is Liquid Minerals, distributed by Remington Health Products, Fort Worth, Texas, ph: (888) 333-4256
[189] <u>Babaji's Kriya Hatha Yoga Publications</u>, tel. (450) 297-0258, fax (450) 297-3957
[190] May be ordered from OPTP, Minneapolis, MN, ph: (800) 367-7393.

them immediately if significant pain or inflammation starts in the site. A mild sensation of aching or slight soreness is usual.

Instructions for applying intradermal needles:

- Select point(s) for application, and disinfect thoroughly with alcohol.

- Cut a tiny (about 4-5 mm) square of adhesive tape, and use forceps to apply it right next to the point. Precut squares of tape can be purchased from some acupuncture supply companies.

- Grasp the handle of the needle with the forceps, and slide the shaft into the point obliquely, so that the head is close to parallel with the skin, and right over the square of tape. When placing into body points, place needle in line with creases so it moves minimally with body movement.

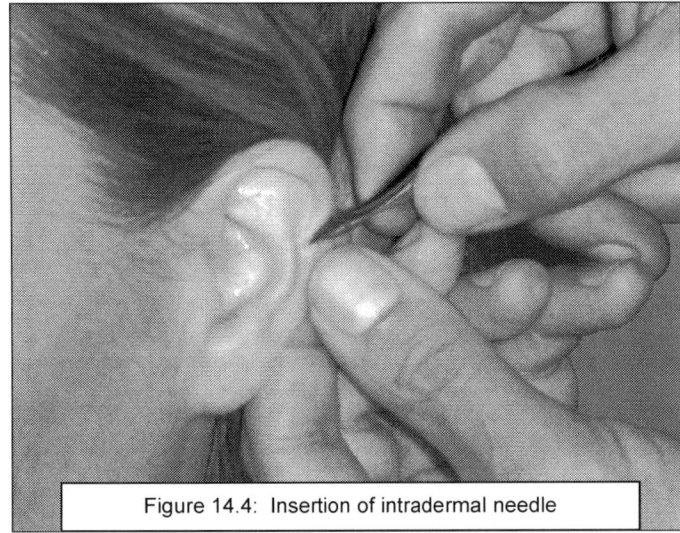

Figure 14.4: Insertion of intradermal needle

- Take another square of adhesive tape, and place it to cover the needle head.

- When you or the patient is ready to remove the needle, this arrangement makes it easy. Just grasp the tape with forceps or fingers, and pull the whole assembly out.

There are two main sizes of intradermal needles, 3 mm and 6 mm. Use the 3 mm size for auricular and hand points. The larger size can be used for applications to ah shi points on fleshy areas of the body. There is one caution in the use of intradermal needles. In hot and humid climates there is a greater risk of infection when a needle is left inserted into the skin in this way. In such locales, it is better to use ion pellets (see below).

Ion pellets are placed in a similar manner to intradermal needles, except that there is no penetration. These are tiny metal balls that are made of steel, and usually plated with silver or gold. They come with their own patch of adhesive tape attached, and can be easily placed with forceps. Gold pellets are placed on points to be supplemented, silver over points to be reduced. For pain control, silver pellets are usually more applicable, although these can be combined with gold placements over related points to be supplemented. For example, in placing ion pellets in the ear for low back pain, silver can be placed over points for the low back and lumbar spine, with gold pellets placed on systemic points such as Shenmen or Subcortex (Thalamus). The penetration of intradermal needles provides a stronger effect than ion pellets, and so were favored by Manaka for his Step Four treatments. Ion pellets are better, however, for children, people easily prone to infection such as those who are HIV+ or with other immune system impairment, and in climates that are hot and damp.

Exercise and Intradermals

In Chapter 13 several varieties of treatment were detailed that combine movement or mobilization with simultaneous acu-point stimulation. This principle is also valuable for home therapy. Apply intradermals or ion pellets to points on your patient that correspond to the injured or painful area, and simply instruct him to rub them while he is stretching or exercising the affected area. This practice is a powerful way to accelerate re-education through a maximum counter-bias effect. For example, if your patient has a bias toward tight low back muscles, he can go a long way by stretching them while rubbing a hand or ear intradermal associated with that body region. This brings added Qi and Blood to the area, as does the exercise. It also helps the central nervous system in its attempts to rebalance and augment neuromuscular functioning of the area through proprioception and meridian balancing.[191]

Three-Point Treatment

One of Manaka's favorite Step Four treatments was placement of intradermals in three related places – a trigger or ah shi point over the site of pain, an ear point and a Korean hand point. All three points help adjust the hologram of the body from different levels, and together provide a powerful synergistic effect. As mentioned above, this practice can also be done in office with microcurrent probe treatment.

TAKING CHARGE

What we do is called the "healing arts" because there is a large role for creativity and intuition in assisting our patients. In assessing and treating a patient, we must make several decisions that guide us. Do we treat the Root or the Branch first? Which acu-points? How do we weigh an underlying Kidney or Spleen deficiency pattern? Do we refer the patient to other practitioners? In my practice, one of the factors I focus on the most is the patient's consciousness. I ask myself what is underlying the main complaint that brought her to my office. What is she really asking for? Does she really just want symptomatic relief, or is the symptom more a marker for a life transition she is having a hard time with? Ultimately, the healing journey is about our patients taking charge of their own lives and embracing more life-affirming, self-loving attitudes and actions. When a patient comes to me, I check to see how ready she is to move out of old, stuck patterns and expand into these qualities.

We have all heard amazing stories about people who have healed supposedly terminal diseases and have made great athletic accomplishments despite disabling bodily conditions. These show the power of the human spirit when unleashed from fear and self-doubt. I am making this point here because supporting our patients in "taking charge" is the most important gift we can give them, and is the ultimate take-home treatment. Our armamentarium of devices and techniques, including those detailed in this book, are for intervention at critical times to give our patients a space free from pain and dysfunction. This provides the opportunity or launching pad as it were, to move ahead on their healing journeys. Of course there are those that seem to want to be "professional patients", and want to give their own precious power of self-healing away to doctors and healers. It is always my intention to guide my patients toward taking this power back and fully using it.

I feel that the approaches explained in this and the previous chapter can be empowering to patients, as their participation is required for much of it. Microcurrent electro-acupuncture is one of the most valuable innovations in modern acupuncture, and is an excellent transition between direct energetic healing and the healing interventions recognized by the Western health care professions. The gentle nature of microcurrent and its healing acceleration potential make it a relatively non-invasive and highly effective tool to help patients heal

---

[191] Probably aspects of the same phenomenon.

themselves. Yet, even these techniques must eventually fall away once they have outlived their usefulness in the healing process. It is our duty as healing professionals to return our patients, as soon as possible, to reliance on their own innate potential for growth and regeneration of body, mind, emotions and Spirit. By blessing and letting go of those that come to us in this way, we are actively entering into the rich network of those that serve the upliftment and healing of our Earth and the life upon it.

Section IV

MERIDIAN DIAGNOSTICS

INTRODUCTION

When performing the Four-Step protocol described in the last Section most detailed diagnostic work takes place during Step One. This step includes most intake work, which is then synthesized to arrive at choice of a Root treatment. This necessitates the use of one, or preferably several, energetic diagnostic methods. Most acupuncturists have received training in Chinese pulse and tongue diagnosis, and some are skilled in abdominal (hara) evaluation. Some chiropractors have learned to use forms of kinesiology, or muscle testing, to evaluate the energetic balance of the body's muscles and organs.

The science of acupuncture is a regulatory input-output system. Diagnosis and treatment are equally important. Simply applying cookbook formulas of acu-points according to symptomatic necessity is far short of the true art of acupuncture. For best results, it is recommended to base treatment selection on specific diagnostic findings, and to also use additional confirmatory methods, such as palpation test points, pulse diagnosis or electronic meridian testing (EMT).

Chinese acupuncture traditionally utilizes palpation of the pulses at the radial arteries as a major method for reading the condition and balance of the Organs and meridians. This is determined through the strength, speed, depth and qualities of the pulse. In its advanced form, this form of diagnosis requires subjective skills that can only be properly learned by a collaboration between a student and teacher, as they feel pulses together and then compare notes. Although basic level pulse diagnosis is not difficult, few acupuncturists in the United States have fully mastered this technique.

Researchers in California have recently constructed a device that uses pressure sensors on the radial arteries that feed pulse waveform data into a computer analysis system, which then furnishes images of the pulse.[192] The different waveform patterns have been correlated with the pulse qualities of TCM. This system has facilitated the learning process for students studying pulse diagnosis, and has provided an objective way to confirm the various pulse qualities.

It is a serious clinical limitation, however, to rely on only one form of meridian diagnosis. Traditional acupuncture diagnostic methods can be subjective and equivocal, and lack of confidence on the part of practitioners often leads to faulty treatments. In my opinion, it is far better to know and practice several forms of energetic evaluation that can be used for comparison. If more than one method points to the same diagnosis, thereby providing a positive confirmation, then practitioner confidence is greatly augmented and treatment is more likely to accurate and effective.

The following chapters contain instructions for three powerful and effective diagnostic methods for meridian/Organ diagnosis – Alarm Point Kinesiology, gastrocnemius palpation and Electronic Meridian Testing (EMT). All of these systems originated in Japan – the first two from Yoshio Manaka and his colleagues, and the latter from Yosio Nakatani. Nakatani's system is called Ryodoraku, which has been refined in Germany and the U.S. since its introduction in the 1950's. Of these two system, the easier one to practice, in my opinion, is Alarm Point Kinesiology.

---

[192] as reported in California Journal of Oriental Medicine, Fall 1999

Organs and Meridians

These three diagnostic systems give information about both meridians and Organs. It is not always clear, however, which level is really being read. I will present my best understanding here.

Each **Organ** is composed of a physical structure with biochemical functions as well as an energetic orb of influence in the body. In other words, from the TCM perspective, Organs include the organs as defined by Western medicine as well as additional functional aspects described in TCM.

A **meridian** is an energetic pathway through the fascial or circulatory networks of the body that connect the Organs, the skin surface and the autonomic nervous system. Although most principal meridians are named after specific Organs, in many cases the association is not very direct. For example, the indications for treatment of acu-points on the Small Intestine meridian have little direct relationship to the Organ. Yet according to traditional meridian pathway charts, an internal pathway of this channel does connect with the Small Intestine Organ. Meridians have five Command, or Master points at their extremity, on and distal to the elbows and knees. The most distal point, the Jing or Ting point lies near the bed of the fingernail or toenail, and is the most superficial level of the meridian. The rest of the Command points, moving proximally, are the Ying, Shu, Jing and He or Ho points.

According to the book "Essentials of Chinese Acupuncture[193]":

> Jing-Well is the place where the *qi* of the channel starts to bubble. Ying-Spring is where the *qi* starts to flourish. Shu-Stream is where the *qi* flourishes. Jing-River is where the *qi* of the channel increases in abundance. Finally, He-Sea represents the confluence of rivers in the sea, where the *qi* of the channel is the most flourishing.

These images suggest an energetic deepening of the pathway as we move proximally through the Command points. The He or Ho points, which are located near the elbows or knees, are the places where the meridian connects to the associated Organ most directly. Source points also connect directly to the Organ.

Abdominal, or Hara diagnosis involves careful palpation and sensing of zones on the abdomen. In this practice superficial tissues over many of the physical organs themselves are palpated, and so this practice would seem to give more direct organ information than that of the meridians. Yet many Japanese practitioners palpating the abdomen, including Manaka, have used this information to diagnose the meridians. Which level is actually being felt? It would appear that there is a strong correlation between physical organs, Organs[194] and meridians.

In the practice of electronic meridian testing, the test points being measured are on the distal extremities, and so this would appear to be addressing the meridian level more than the Organs. Yet EMT can be used to diagnose Organ function as well. It is my experience that the choice of test points in EMT has a bearing on which level of information is being accessed. I believe that test points on or near the terminal Jing points near the fingernail or toenail beds[195] are more appropriate for myofascial pain treatment, as they most closely measure the

---

[193] Foreign Languages Press, Beijing, China 1980
[194] Again, drawing a distinction between the TCM and Western definition of the organs.
[195] Including BFD points mentioned later in this text

meridians, while Source points on the wrists and ankles are more appropriate for internal medical disease treatments, as they more closely measure the status of the Organs.

According to the Nan Jing[196] the Source energy of the body wells up at the Source points. From an embryological viewpoint, the wrists and ankles are connected to the Source Qi that is reflected in the abdomen (hara). Wrists and ankles also energetically correlate with the second chakra, which is certainly associated with Source Qi. Manaka observed that palpation (Mu) points on the abdomen that are latent (not sore on palpation even with Organ pathology) can become active when the wrist and/or ankles are moved. This reveals one more link between exercise and internal health.

It is not clear where the meridians end and the Organs begin in our diagnostic methods. There is a continuum between these orbs, yet distinct differences as well. A patient with Crohn's disease affecting the small intestine organ may not have any imbalanced readings on the Small Intestine meridian. A patient with weak readings on the Kidney meridian may not have any signs or symptoms of renal disease. Yet there is a definite overlap in most cases. This is due to the Law of Resonance. One end of an energetic spectrum may be used to sense or affect the other end, again, like the low C note on a piano causing the other C notes to vibrate when it is struck. Fortunately, balancing the meridians system does have powerful beneficial effects on the Organs, and herbal or nutritional healing of the Organs can help balance the meridians.

I have found that the *intention* of the practitioner has a great bearing on acupuncture diagnosis and treatment. Whichever level, Organ or meridian, that you are focusing on, will tend to reveal itself through testing.

---

[196] A classic of Chinese Medicine

Chapter 15

ALARM POINT KINESIOLOGY DIAGNOSIS

Chinese acupuncturists generally rely on pulse and tongue methods for diagnosis, while Japanese practitioners favor abdominal (Hara) diagnosis. Manaka and other leading Japanese researchers have used a form of kinesiology to confirm and validate Hara diagnosis. Experience has shown that kinesiology is one of the easiest and most consistently reproducible form of energetic diagnosis, and can be mastered within a short time. For this reason, kinesiology is taught at many of my seminars.

Kinesiology is the science of testing indicator muscles to obtain information about the body. A strong response of an indicator muscle shows a positive energetic state of the tested body part, while a weak response indicates a blockage or disconnection. This is a generalization that does not apply to all cases, yet is sufficient for the explanation at this point. Kinesiology is based on the Law of Resonance, in that specific muscles have an energetic connection with certain bodily structures, while some muscles are markers for the energetic integrity of the whole body. The systems of Applied Kinesiology and Touch For Health utilize many different muscles throughout the body, each of which is an indicator for a specific internal organ or other structure. These systems are complex, and beyond the scope of this book.

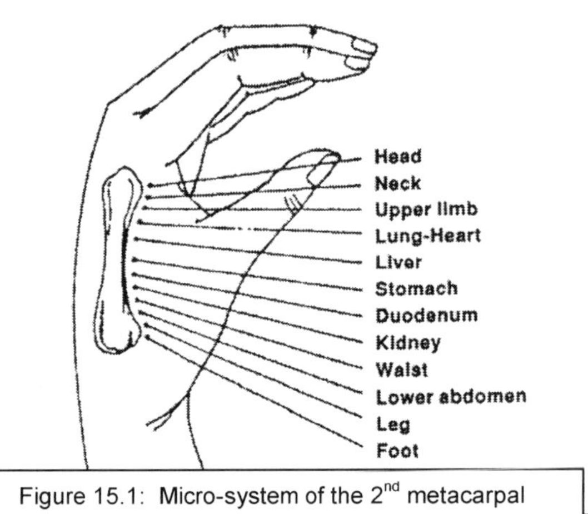

Fortunately, a very simple system called O Ring testing, developed by Yosio Omura of New York, can give us all the information we need to effectively diagnose the meridian system. Manaka adapted Omura's system for evaluation of the Front Mu-Alarm points. This simply consists of having the patient touch the various Alarm points to be tested on her own body in turn while the practitioner tests the strength of indicator muscles of the other hand. A complete energetic evaluation can then be quickly obtained. This is based on the principle of therapy localization. When the patient touches an Alarm point on her body that energetically connects to a dysfunctional Organ/meridian, this briefly puts the focus of the body/mind consciousness on that function. If there is an energetic imbalance there, this causes the indicator muscles of her hand to "blow out", or go weak.

Figure 15.1: Micro-system of the 2nd metacarpal

O Ring evaluation utilizes the muscles of the patient's hands for testing by having her touch the tips of her thumb and middle finger together while the practitioner tries to separate them. This test reflects the energetic reaction of the whole body. This can be understood by the nature of the region of the second metacarpal bone area. The area between acu-points LI 3 and Ling Ku[197] is a powerful micro-system that connects to and can treat any part of the body. It has been used for with electro-acupuncture for anesthetic purposes in Chinese hospitals.

Because this region connects to the whole body, the O Ring test can be used as a general indicator of whole-body energetic response. When O Ring testing is impractical, such as in cases of hand arthritis when the patient cannot muster much strength in her hands, an alternative whole body test is the forward arm raise, also explained below[198].

An important factor in kinesiology is called "clearing the patient". It is usually necessary to prepare the patient for muscle testing to ensure true and accurate results. Clearing would not be necessary for patients who are clear, calm and well grounded, but this is obviously not often the case! Most people, especially those in pain or illness, exhibit various distortions in their etheric and emotional bodies, which are forms of coping mechanisms. These are especially pronounced in individuals who are "in their heads" or experiencing emotional distress. These forms of cloaking the true energetic picture are in fact a form of self-protection to prevent others from seeing or harming them. In order to allow accurate energetic testing the patient must reduce his defenses, at least temporarily.

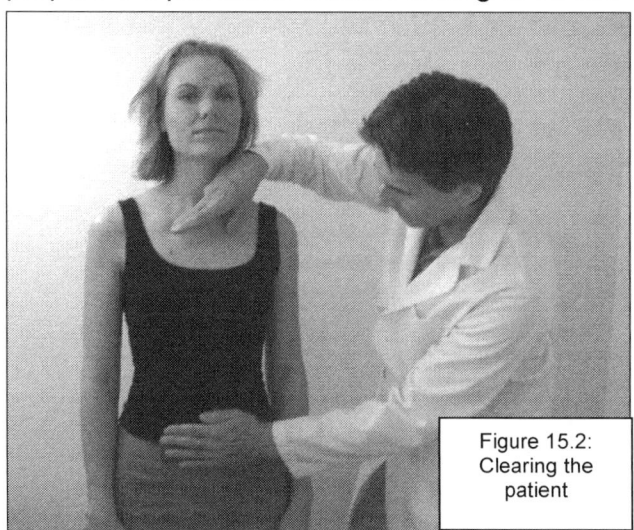

Figure 15.2: Clearing the patient

One strong form of energetic distortion is called "switching". This is a form of rebellious Qi[199] in which many normal energetic flows are going in the wrong direction (the word wrong is not used as a judgment, but to indicate that it is abnormal or counterproductive). A switched patient cannot be accurately tested. Instructions for O Ring and shoulder raise kinesiology are outlined below.

O Ring Kinesiology Instructions

Clearing the patient – Ask your patient to sit or stand in a comfortable position. Stand at his side. Ask him to start breathing into his lower abdomen so that the lower abdomen expands with each in-breath. Ask his permission to place your hand on his lower abdomen (your right hand if you are standing on his right side, or vice versa). If permission is given, place your hand there and your other hand on his upper chest. Spread your thumb and middle finger of that hand into a "U" shape and start bilaterally rubbing his K 27 points, which are just below the center of the clavicles. With one hand rubbing his K 27 points and the other gently touching his Hara, observe and tune into his energy. When you get a sense that it has settled down somewhat and is more centered in the lower abdomen, this step is complete.

---

[197] Ling Ku is an extra point on the dorsal aspect of the hand, at the junction of the 1st and 2nd metacarpal bones.
[198] 2nd metacarpal diagram from article "Postoperative Pain- Clinical Study on the Use of the 2nd Metacarpal...", AJA Vol. 20, #2, 1992
[199] Rebellious Qi is a condition in which Qi is moving in uncustomary directions, due to weakness of Source Qi of the abdomen or repressed emotions. It primarily affects the head and neck area with annoying to dangerous symptoms.

If you sense his energy is still unbalanced (too much up in his head or chest), again encourage him to relax and let his breathing swell his lower abdomen more fully so his energy can drop. You might say something like "Now just let yourself drop down into your lower body." In the rare cases that this procedure does not help the patient to relax, you can try asking him to concentrate on tightening and relaxing his legs and feet alternately. You can also help pull the Qi downward by rubbing his feet at Liv 3 and K 1.

1. *Baseline test* – After clearing the patient, perform the O "Ring" test as follows:

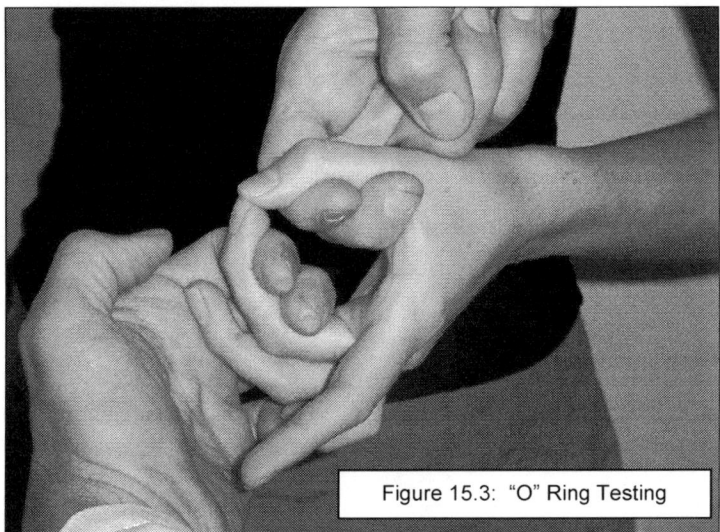

Figure 15.3: "O" Ring Testing

A. Choose one of the patient's hands for testing. (It doesn't matter which one.) Ask her to hold her hand toward you with her palm facing upwards and arm relaxed.

B. Ask her to touch the tips of her thumb and middle fingers together to produce a circle. Make sure she is not touching the pads of her fingers flatly together. Only the very tips should be touching to form a circle with the hand. Also, make sure her other fingers are not touching the thumb and middle fingers.

C. Position yourself so you are centered and well grounded. With your feet spread and flat on the floor and your elbows splayed outward, hook the 2nd and 3rd fingers of each of your hands in though the O created by the patient's hand. Do this in such a way that you can smoothly use all the strength of your arms, if necessary, to pull her fingertips apart.

D. Ask the patient to hold her fingertips together while you pull them apart. Don't use the word "resist" to your patient. It may communicate to her subconscious to not cooperate with the test. Simply say "hold" each time you pull her fingers apart. Smoothly start separating her fingers, starting with minimal strength. Do not suddenly jerk the fingertips apart! Gradually increase your strength until her fingers *slightly* separate. If the patient is much stronger than you, you can suggest to her that she only use "3/4" of her strength for the test. Experiment with this relationship until you are comfortable with performing the O Ring test. When you are testing an individual much stronger than you, he can also use his thumb and pinky for the test to make it easier for you.

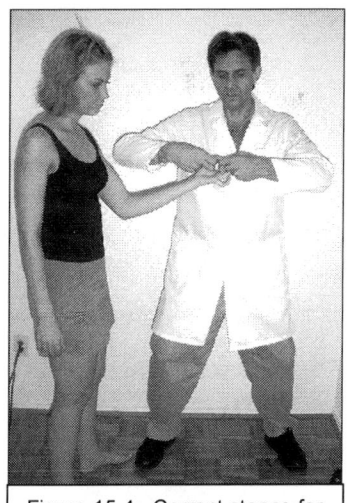

Figure 15.4: Correct stance for O Ring testing

E. Determine how much strength it takes for you to start separating the patient's fingertips. You can now compare this baseline to his strength after the following steps.

2. *Zip up – zip down test* -- It is useless to start testing the patient until you are certain of the meaning of the strong or weak muscle indicators. This step will establish this very clearly.

A. Stand at the patient's side, as before. Place one hand on her upper back to connect and support. Slightly cup your other hand and place it, palm up, at about the level of the pubic symphysis of the lower abdomen. Place your hand just in front, but not touching, the patient's belly.

B. As you breathe in deeply, steadily raise your hand in front of the patient's Ren channel, stopping at the level of the throat. Project intention to raise the Qi of the Ren channel over which you are moving your hand. This is "zipping up" the patient.

C. Now repeat the O Ring test. Is it the same? Stronger? Weaker? Because an upward movement of your hand over the Ren channel boosts the channel, the Seas of all Yin meridians, this should yield a strong muscle test.

D. Now perform the zip down test. Keeping your free hand on her upper back, place your moving hand at the throat level, with your hand slightly cupped with palm down. As you breathe out forcefully and slightly bend your knees, move your hand swiftly down, a few inches in front of the Ren channel back to the pubic symphysis. Project strong intention to pull down the Qi.

E. Retest the indicator muscle. What changed? If performed correctly with the patient properly cleared, this should weaken the O Ring significantly.

F. Don't forget to finish the test by zipping the patient back up. Otherwise she may not have a very good day!

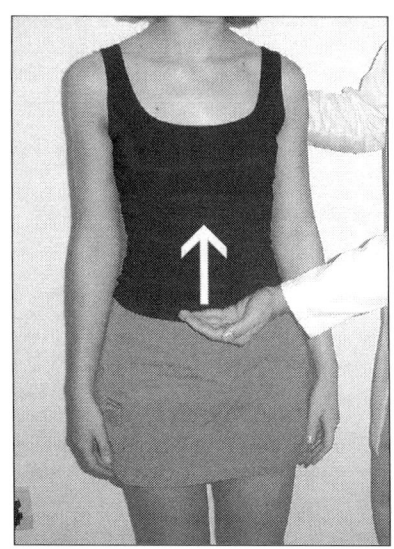 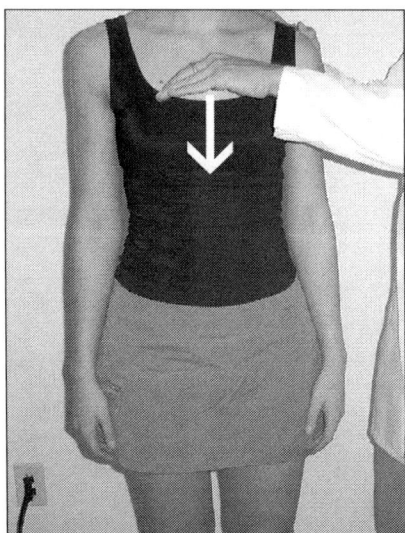

Figure 15.5: "Zip Up" and "Zip Down"

Now you know that a strong O Ring reading indicates positive energetic integrity, and a weak test shows a negative energetic condition. In the case of negative energetic condition, the weakening factor was the temporary counter-flow of the Ren channel you induced by "zipping down" your patient. A "yes", or strong muscle test, results when a stimulus to the body supports or enhances its overall energy quality and circulation. A "no", or weak muscle response, results when a stimulus in some way weakens, scatters or disrupts normal Qi quality and circulation.

You are now ready to evaluate the patient's Alarm points, test allergic substances, indicated herbs, or any other test requiring a "yes" or "no" answer from the body. There is no limit to how this test can be employed – use your imagination. I have found that I can simply say or clearly think of a substance, acu-point or condition and elicit an accurate O Ring test for the benefit to the patient. It is better to have the patient touch the Alarm point or hold actual substances to be tested when you are first learning this technique, however.

If you have trouble with the zip up and zip down tests, and can't elicit a clear strong and weak reaction, then it is necessary to either clear the patient more completely, or clarify your own intention. Performing this test is a form of Qi Gong, in that you, the practitioner, must be able to project your energy and clear intention to the patient. You may want to try breathing out more forcefully and drop your body a little more dramatically as you zip down the patient, in other words, drop your own Qi more. Realize that you cannot hurt the patient by doing this as long as you finish by zipping them back up. If you have a subtle concern that you may hurt the patient by zipping them down, you will not project a clear intention.

Arm Raise Kinesiology

Most of the above steps also apply to this test. The only difference is the part of the body being used for testing.

Clear the patient as explained above.

To get a baseline test, follow these steps:

A. Ask the patient to stretch her arm straight out in front of her chest with palm facing down and fingers outstretched. Place your free hand on her upper back and your testing hand lightly touching the back of her outstretched wrist. Ask her to hold the arm up (not to "resist") while you GENTLY press downward on the back of her wrist. All you need is a slight downward force until you feel the muscle start to give and the arm begin to lower. In fact, the less downward pressure you can use for testing the better. Practice tuning into the subtlety of feeling the muscle give with minimal force. Eventually you will be able to feel the test on a more energetic level and less on a gross physical level. The same principle applies to O Ring testing. Repeat the test a few times until you are clear as to her baseline strength. Ask her to "hold" each time you press down on her arm. When you are done, allow her to drop her arm and rest it.

B. Perform zip up-zip down test as explained in O Ring test instructions above. Repeat arm raise test after zip up and zip down steps. Once you have clearly seen the strong and weak responses, you are ready to test the patient.

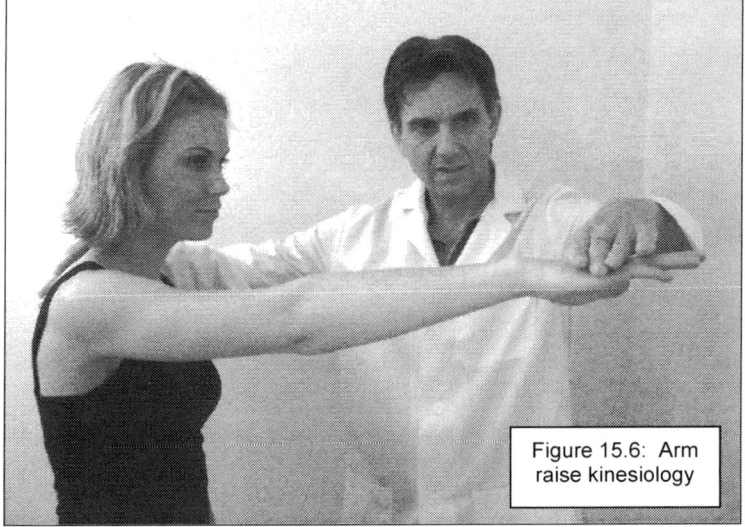

Figure 15.6: Arm raise kinesiology

Alarm Point Kinesiology

Manaka applied the O Ring test to energetic evaluation of Alarm/Mu points. In this text I primarily use the term "Alarm" to describe these points. As mentioned above, Alarm-Mu points primarily give direct information about the Organs. Modern Japanese practitioners and researchers also consider Hara (abdominal) diagnosis, which overlaps with Alarm point testing, to give information about the meridian system as well. Because it is utilizing test points on the extremity of the meridians themselves, Electronic Meridian Testing (EMT) primarily gives information about the meridians. Therefore performing and comparing both methods is highly comprehensive, as any Organ/meridian indicators that show up in both systems is guaranteed to be highly significant. I recommend that you try this in your clinical practice.

FIGURE 15.7: TCM AND MANAKA MU/ALARM POINT COMPARISON

ORGAN	TCM Mu Point	Manaka Mu Points
Lungs	Lu 1	Lu 1
Pericardium	Ren 17	Pc 1, Ren 17
Heart	Ren 14/Ren 15	Ren 14/Ren 15
Stomach	Ren 12	Ren 12 – St 21 area
Gall Bladder	GB 24	GB 24, ASIS (around GB 29)
Spleen	Liv 13	Sp 21 – GB 26 axillary line
Liver	Liv 14	Soft tissue just below angle of right costal region
Kidney	GB 25	K 16
Triple Warner	Ren 5	St 25
Small Intestine	Ren 4	Slightly medial to St 26
Large Intestine	St 25	Slightly lateral to St 27

CHAPTER FIFTEEN – ALARM POINT KINESIOLOGY DIAGNOSIS 201

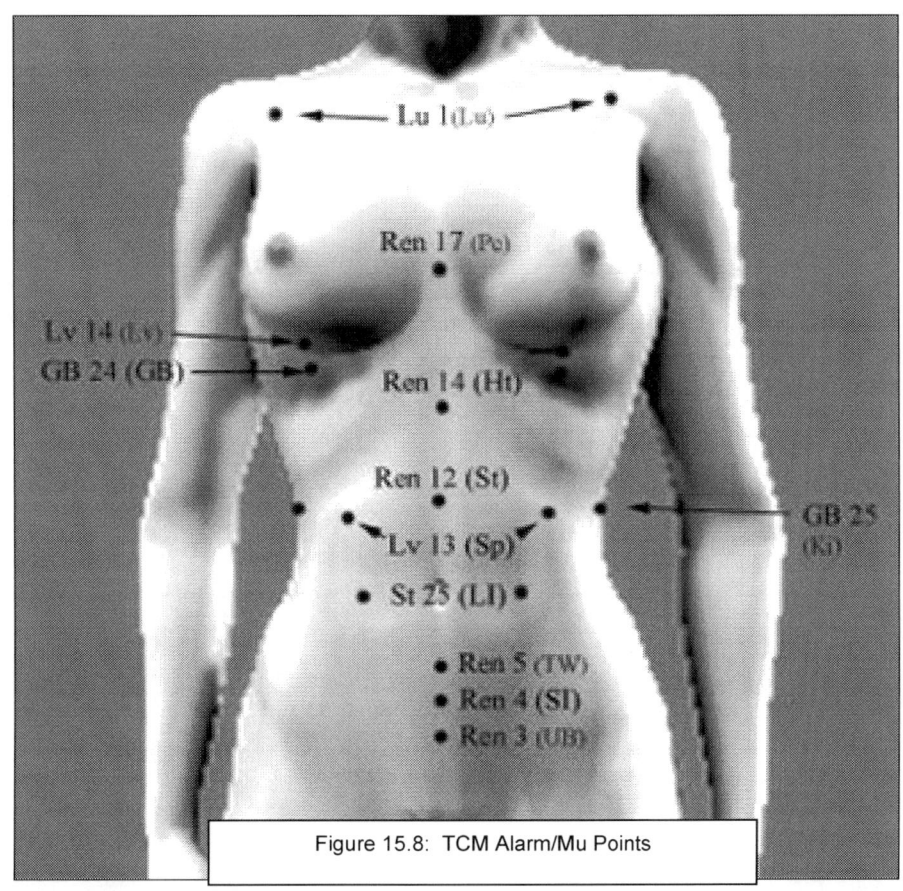

Figure 15.8: TCM Alarm/Mu Points

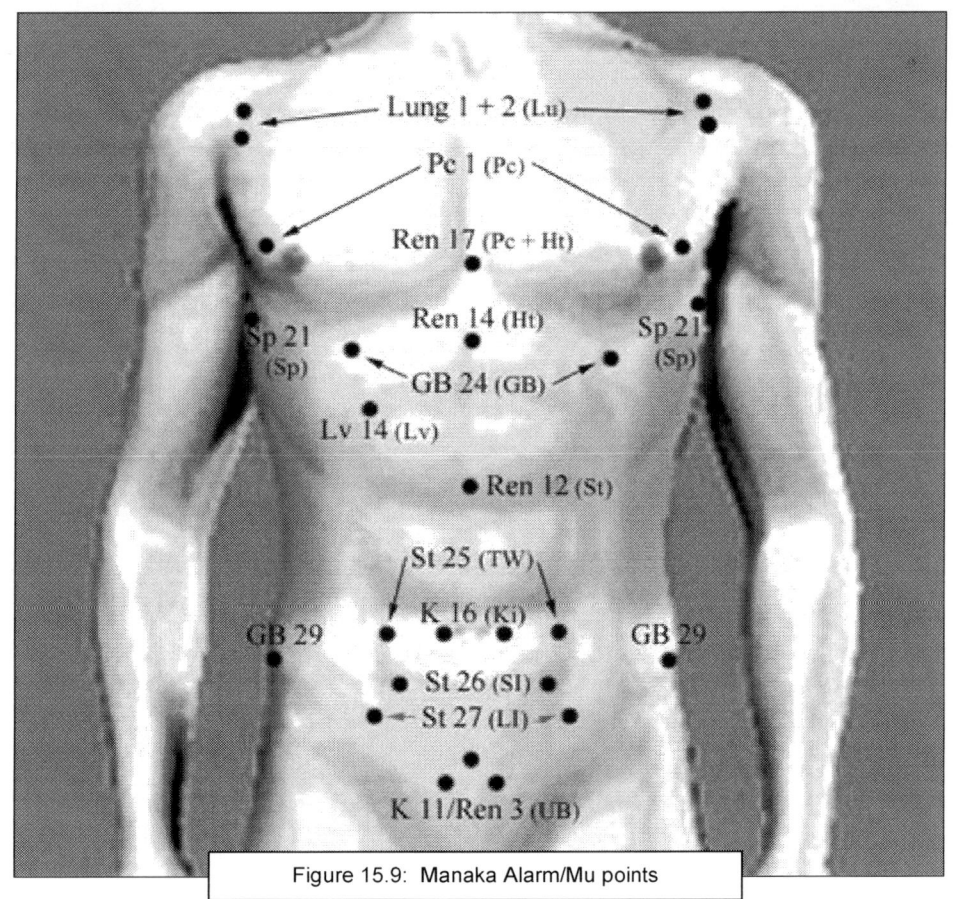

Figure 15.9: Manaka Alarm/Mu points

Mu/Alarm point selection guidelines

Manaka's research led him to conclude that the abdominal TCM Mu points were only accurate when a patient was standing or moving, while the chest points were accurate in all cases. The abdominal Mu points were actually in different locations when the patient was lying supine on a treatment table. For palpation purposes, Manaka used the TCM points only when a patient was sitting up or standing, and his points when patients were lying down. He mostly used the TCM Mu points for the kinesiology procedure described in this chapter. In my practice, I have used both point systems freely for this purpose, and have found that they both work. I usually check both systems, and look for confirmations between them.

PUTTING IT TOGETHER: STEP-BY-STEP PROCEDURE FOR ALARM POINT KINESIOLOGY TESTING

1. Help patient to find comfortable position laying face up on a treatment table. Place a bolster under her knees to help relax her abdomen and reduce back strain. It is also possible to perform this test with the patient sitting up, but Alarm point location is less accurate in that position.

2. Clear the patient and perform zip up-zip down test as described above. This can be done prior to her lying down or while on the table. Once you have established clear strong-weak reactions and determined the baseline strength of her O Ring muscles you are ready to proceed.

3. Explain how the test works to your patient. Tell her that you will guide her pointing finger to touch some test points on the front of her body while you test the strength of her other hand. She only needs to touch lightly on the test points, not press into them. Touching through light natural fiber clothing is okay, as each Alarm point projects a field that extends through most materials.[200] You will be simply saying the word "hold" to her when you are ready to test her O Ring - that is the signal for her to hold her thumb and middle fingers together on her test hand while you attempt to pull them apart. Tell her that you will explain the test results at the conclusion of the test, not during it, as knowing which Organ is being tested may bias her responses.

4. Use the patient's hand closest to you for O Ring testing, with palm facing upward. Ask her to hold her other hand above her chest, with her index finger pointing toward herself. Ask her to hold all her other fingers curled back so only the index finger is extended.

5. Guide her pointing finger to lightly rest on the first test point. I usually start with right Lu 1. While she is touching the point, test the O Ring on her other test hand. Note the strength in comparison with the baseline reading. Try to use as little of your own strength as possible in detecting the "give" point of the patient's test hand. Kinesiology works best with tuned-in subtlety rather than force.

6. Continue by guiding her pointing finger to touch each Alarm point, testing each time. The order I generally use is Lung, Pericardium, Heart, Gall Bladder, Liver, Spleen, Stomach, Triple Warmer, Kidney, Small Intestine, Large Intestine, ASIS[201], and finally Urinary

---

[200] This may not work with polyester and some other synthetic fabrics

[201] Just anterior to the Anterior Superior Iliac Spine. Tests for Gall Bladder channel as it relates to pelvic region and Dai Mai, or Belt channel

Bladder. All Alarm points except Pericardium, Heart, Stomach, Urinary Bladder and Liver are tested bilaterally. The first four of these are on the Ren channel on the midline of the body. Liver is usually just tested on the right side, in the soft tissue below the center of the costal angle.

7. Indicate test results for strong and weak Mu point O Ring readings on a simple intake form.

8. Once you have gathered data about all the Mu points, you are ready to analyze the pattern revealed, so proper treatment can be applied. The first priority after gathering diagnostic data is to determine the Key Imbalance. That will be the Organ/meridian complex that is at the Root of the patient's condition. The Key Imbalance is recognized through an inductive process of O Ring testing and other diagnostic methods, the complaints and symptoms of the patient, and confirmatory tests. Once the Key Imbalance is determined and confirmed, the next step is to choose the best way to treat that function. In the system taught in this book, this is best done through treatment of the Extraordinary Vessels or polar meridian pairs. (See Chapter 11).

Chapter 16

ELECTRONIC MERIDIAN TESTING

Introduction

When some practitioners are first introduced to the practice of electronic meridian testing (EMT), it is a stretch for them to understand how slight changes in electrical skin resistance on the big toe can reveal accurate information about the Liver, or how an Extraordinary Vessel diagnosis can be arrived at from electrically measuring a few points on the hands and feet. Meridian electro-diagnosis has been successfully utilized, however, since the 1950's.

There are many electro-diagnostic methods in common use in our modern medical system. These include electro-cardiogram (EKG), electro-encephalogram (EEG), electro-myography (EMG), plesthysmography, magnetic resonance (MRI), and galvanic skin response (GSR) testing. Electronic meridian testing is a system originated in Japan that uses electrical changes on the skin over acu-points to diagnose the condition of the meridian system.

There has been much experimental evidence that the skin surface can reflect pathology and changes in the internal organs (viscero-cutaneous reflex),[202] and conversely, that stimulation of the skin can cause effects in the organs (cutaneo-viscero reflex). Through experimenting with spinal cord removal in animals, researchers have observed that these reflexes do not operate primarily through the spinal cord, but through peripheral aspects of the autonomic nervous system. This reveals that much of the effects of acupuncture are not due to the gating principle as proposed by some Western scientists[203], for the action of the gate theory only operates through the central nervous system.

Practitioners of auricular therapy use observation of discoloration and nodules on the ear to diagnose pathologies in the organs and structures of the body. Many other cutaneous therapies such as cupping, *gwasha*, plum blossom needle and acupressure also work in part through the relationship between the skin, superficial fascia and the viscera and other deeper tissues.

If you have read this far in this book, it should be obvious by now that electrical activity is intimately associated with all life processes. Skin changes in response to visceral events are no exception. In most cases of discoloration of the ear, formation of myofascial trigger points,

---

[202] A summary of this research can be found in the book Acupuncture – The Ancient Chinese Art of Healing and How It Works Scientifically by Felix Mann, Chapter One
[203] See Chapter Five

or other cutaneous changes, there are also measurable changes in electrical conductivity at those sites. Acupuncture point detection devices work on this principle.

So what is conductivity? It is the ability of a substance to allow the passage of electrons when an electrical current is applied to it. Resistance, also called impedance, is the opposite of conductivity. Therefore the greater the conductivity of a substance, the less its resistance, and vice versa. The more resistance a substance has, the more electrical voltage is required to pass a current through it. This is the summed up in Ohm's Law:

$$\text{Electrical Current = Voltage divided by Resistance } (I = V/R)$$

Skin is, by its nature, an electrical resistor. This is necessary for our survival. We are bombarded by many energy waves in our environment, including sunlight, climatic extremes, wind, and in modern times, many kinds of intrusive electro-magnetic fields and microwave transmissions. Our skin is the first line of defense against vulnerability to these influences. While skin resistance is a great benefit to our health, it can be an obstacle to therapeutic electrical stimulation. Many stimulator designs have been created to overcome skin resistance in order to deliver therapeutic currents deep into the body. This has usually involved using high-intensity milliamp currents delivered at high frequencies, as in the case of classic interferential devices. Yet, such invasive currents are not always necessary. Through the viscero-cutaneous reflex, the electrical resistance of many therapeutically useful skin points are significantly lowered. These can be considered "open" points. Over such points even gentle microcurrents can deeply penetrate to affect the viscera.

Many of these open points are useful in electro-diagnosis, and are utilized in the systems of Ryodoraku and EAV discussed in this chapter. In accordance with the principles of TCM, the Command, or Five-Element, points on the distal extremities are most diagnostically useful.

One of the meridian diagnostic systems I learned in acupuncture school was the Akabane system. In this system, lighted incense is passed over the Jing points at the base of the finger and toe nails until the patient says it is "hot". By counting how many passes of the incense are necessary to get the "hot" reaction, and comparing the counts on different meridian end points, a diagnosis can be carried out of the entire system. Because Akabane testing is messy, uncomfortable to the patient and time consuming, I looked for other ways to accomplish the same end. I found that electronic meridian testing was a much quicker and more accurate and comfortable system.

One of the most valuable contributions of EMT is the ability to determine diagnostic patterns from a set of meridian readings. Extensive information on interpreting EMT patterns follows in this chapter. Please see the Treatment Formulary, Section III, for some examples of treatment protocols developed by Voll.

Is Electronic Meridian Testing For Real?

EMT is still a controversial topic in contemporary acupuncture circles. Few acupuncturists currently use it, and most are skeptical about its accuracy. As mentioned above, it is often hard to understand how superficial measurements of electrical conductivity can index the condition of deep meridians and Organs. Following are some essential considerations concerning EMT:

Measurement Technique

The first consideration is measurement technique. Readings taken at test points can vary tremendously depending on factors such as exact point location, degree of pressure, and wetness of the test probe. Many would-be EMT practitioners have become discouraged after obtaining wildly changing readings that do not make any clinical sense. I felt the same way when starting to practice EMT. Doubts that my readings were accurate overshadowed all else, and I was on the verge of giving up on this practice. Yet I persevered and continued to test many patients. I either explained to them that I was learning a new procedure, or just acted confident and professional in spite of my trepidations! Eventually I "got" it, and developed a clear confidence in my measurement technique.

Just like any other procedure that involves sets of complex motor-sensory responses, EMT testing skills take some time to develop. These skills must be developed on two levels. The first is mental and kinesthetic familiarity with correct techniques, which are explained in detail below. The second is the ability to energetically "connect" with your patient beyond the logical mind. I believe that all energetic testing and evaluation involves some kind of direct consciousness connection between tester and client. This is true of pulse diagnosis, abdominal palpation and kinesiology, as well as verbal intakes and examinations. EMT is no exception. This does not make EMT any less "scientific", it just involves several types of science, including that of subtle energy communication[204].

In my classes, most students rapidly learn correct measurement techniques utilizing EMT and O Ring kinesiology. The hardest part for some is releasing their own mental blocks concerning energetic testing. It is my opinion that many of these mental blocks held by modern healers are the result of unpleasant experiences with misuse or misunderstanding of spiritual energy and power in the past. Such impressions[205] create resistance to the easy free flow of subtle information from patient to tester. It is usually not difficult to release mental resistance about this subject once it is understood that these skills are now only being used for healing and service to our clients.

Precision

The advantage of EMT over many other types of energetic testing is the precision of the readings. Because a 0 – 100 scale is utilized, it is possible to gauge the degree of Excess or Deficiency of a meridian. This is much harder to determine with other methods. It is also possible to track indicator drops, which reveal organic degeneration and allergic conditions. Once test skills are developed, it is quick and easy to create a chart, or graph, of the meridian readings for a patient at a specific time and date. One of the greatest benefits for modern practitioners is that readings can be displayed on a computer monitor and printed out for "hard" evidence of improvement. Software is available to facilitate this process.[206]

Confirmation of Readings by Comparison

Although there is a necessary learning curve with EMT, it is not difficult to master. Once we become confident in our results, the next question concerns the validity of the readings obtained. First of all, it is apparent and easily observed that conductivity readings on the "test points" for EMT do reveal readings that vary from one another, and vary from time to time. For example, the reading at the Biologically Functional Diagnostic (BFD) point (explained below) on

---

[204] See Chapter Two for more about this
[205] Negative impressions from past experience are called *samskaras* in Sanskrit language
[206] Information on this software can be found in the Resource section of this book

the medial side of the little toe may be lower in the afternoon than in the morning, and may be lower on some days than others.

The best and most direct way to confirm that EMT information is meaningful is to compare it to other, known methods of energetic evaluation in the same session. Whether you are most comfortable with Chinese pulse diagnosis, hara palpation, kinesiology or even medical laboratory results, it can be used as a comparison. For example, pulse diagnosis may reveal rapid and weak qualities, and the patient may exhibit a red face and tongue, heat sensations and nervousness. These are signs of a yin deficiency pattern according to TCM. If EMT is performed in the same session, we observe whether the readings confirm this impression. Most yin deficiency patients exhibit EMT readings that are lower (weaker) on some or all of the foot meridian test points, and higher or high with indicator drops on some or all of the hand meridian test points. The Kidney reading in particular is often abnormally high or low. These readings do support a pattern of yin deficiency, as the vital, yin Organs are largely represented on the foot test points, while the hand test points more represent the more superficial energies of the body. A compendium of EMT patterns is presented at the end of this chapter. These are very valuable in interpreting EMT graphs in terms of TCM diagnostics. In the seminars that I teach we often compare the results of EMT, Alarm point kinesiology and pulse diagnosis to reveal the confirmations the methods offer each other.

Ryodoraku

Nakatani developed the first well-documented system of EMT in Japan in the 1950's. The term "ryodoraku" means good electro-permeable point. Nakatani and his colleagues charted many points that reproducibly demonstrated changes in accordance with internal pathologies. These ryodoraku points have a high degree of correlation with traditional points of the principal meridian system, although many traditional acu-points do not exhibit ryodoraku characteristics.

According to this body of research, these points have about 30% greater conductivity than the surrounding skin. They can be measured with an ohmmeter device to read out the degree of excess or deficiency in each meridian. Nakatani advocated the use of Source acu-points on the wrists and ankles for testing.[207] TCM tonification and sedation points are used for treating the meridians with high or low readings. He also advocated using one regulatory point on each meridian for treatment as a simpler approach. These are points approximately in the middle of the meridian pathway of the distal extremity.

In the Ryodoraku system, the correct reading of a test point occurs about 3/4 second after initial contact with the measuring electrode, and each test point is about 1 cm in diameter. Japanese research concurs with Felix Mann in stating that EMT works through reflex systems of the autonomic nervous system. As explained earlier, the autonomic nervous system interfaces with the endocrine hormonal system in regulating most visceral functions.

Electroacupuncture According to Voll (EAV)

Dr. Reinhold Voll and his medical colleagues expanded on Nakatani's work in the 1960's and 1970's. They charted a comprehensive meridian system based on empirical acu-points that showed abnormal readings in response to known medical pathologies. They proposed the existence of "new" meridians on the sides of fingers and toes without charted meridians in TCM such as the Allergy, Neural, Skin and Fatty Degeneration Vessels. Dr. Voll, who was

---

[207] The location of the Large Intestine and Kidney test points differ from TCM source points in Ryodoraku. LI 5 is used as a test point, as is a point at an indentation near K 4.

diagnosed with terminal bladder cancer in the 1950's, lived over 30 more years. He attributed this to his practice of balancing the terminal points of each of his own meridians each morning with his microcurrent Dermatron device.

EAV research provided much valuable understanding of the therapeutic effects of microcurrents on the human body. Voll described the specific therapeutic characteristics of microcurrent therapy as follows[208]:

- Spasmolysis and tonification of the smooth muscles of the arterial and venous blood vessels, the large lymph vessels, and the hollow organs such as the stomach, intestines, gall bladder and urinary bladder. These effects are necessary to relieve stasis and constrictions.

- Tonification of elastic fibers, as is required in problems of lung capacity such as emphysema and some cases of asthma.

- Reduction of inflammatory processes by reducing exudative processes and accelerating cicatrisation[209]

- Reduction of incipient degenerative processes by promoting normal fluid transfer in and between the cells, as well as normal functioning of connective tissues and fascia. Voll stated that the early stages of scleroses, fibroses, cirrhoses, indurations and malignancies could be corrected with low frequency currents, yet advanced conditions would require drug or surgical treatment.

- Restoration of polarization in the nerves. Energy is required to maintain ionic equilibrium between the cell interior and interstitial fluids, and deficiency conditions can fail to make enough energy available for this vital balance. Lack of equilibrium can lead to chronic pain, stiffness and disability. Microcurrents can add the energy that may be lacking.

- Stimulus of ATP in injured muscles. When cellular ATP production is inadequate, chronic muscle tension and contraction is the result. Microcurrent therapies can significantly increase ATP levels in the cells.

In the early part of his work with electroacupuncture, Voll mainly used frequency-specific microcurrent stimulation through distal meridian points as therapy. Later, he moved his emphasis to use of potentized homeopathic substances for treatment. Voll was the originator of remedy testing. This is the practice of testing a patient with EMT to obtain baseline readings, and then placing a therapeutic substance in his electro-magnetic field and retesting. He found that the electronic test reading would significantly improve if the substance were curative.

Electronic meridian testing is now widely used in many modern systems such as the Vegatest, Computron and Best devices. A complete elaboration on the EAV system and remedy testing is beyond the scope of this book, however there are two valuable methods described below that are relevant to microcurrent electro-acupuncture. These are distal meridian point balancing and quadrant balancing treatment.

Distal Meridian Point Balancing

As mentioned above, this method kept Voll alive for several decades longer than his doctors predicted. This is similar to therapy in Ryodoraku, in that each meridian with abnormal

---

[208] R. Voll, <u>20 Years of Electroacupuncture Therapy Using Low-Frequency Current Pulses</u>., American Journal of Acupuncture, special EAV edition
[209] Normal formation of scar tissues in the healing process.

readings is individually stimulated to bring its reading into balance. In Ryodoraku either tonification and sedation or regulatory points are used, while in EAV the 5 distal points on each meridian are balanced. Either system is valuable for overall body balancing (Step One in the Four-Step protocol) and preventive medicine. In EAV system, the measurement meter has a 0 – 100 scale. "50" is considered to be the balanced, optimal average reading for meridian test points, with readings up to 65 considered acceptable.[210] Ryodoraku often uses a 0 – 160 scale, with a more complex calculation needed to arrive at the average reading for an individual.

To balance an individual meridian on a device with a 0 – 100 meter scale, follow these instructions:

1. **If the reading is below 50, the meridian is deficient and tonification is applicable.** Set the polarity of the treating electrode to negative (electron donating), frequency in the 0.6 – 10 Hz range, and intensity to the tickling level, which may require several hundred microamps. Place trigger probe on tonification, source or other relevant meridian point, and have patient hold a brass hand mass in the hand on the opposite side from the part being tested. Voll simply balanced the 5 distal test points themselves. I prefer the method described later in this chapter.

   Treat with very light pressure, alternated with brief conductivity test periods. Treat until meter reads 50 - 55, then stop. Do not overtreat. Quality microcurrent devices allow you to easily alternate between test and treat modes by simply pressing the trigger switch of the test probe.

2. **If the reading on the meridian is above 65, which is considered excess, it can be sedated as follows**: Set treating electrode to positive polarity, which reduces the charge where it is placed, frequency to 80 – 130 Hz, and intensity to minimal setting of 25 – 50 µA. This should be considerably less current than the tickling intensity specified for tonification. Place on sedation, source or other point and again, have patient hold a hand mass to complete the circuit. Use a light touch, and sedate for 10 – 60 seconds, or until reading comes down in search mode to as close to 50 as possible. Again, do not overtreat! Just use the minimum time necessary to bring down the reading.

   The above steps are used to balance individual meridians. As you will soon learn, the meridian balancing system taught in this book does not attempt to balance each meridian separately in that way, but rather balances by treating the overall pattern. In the opinion of the author, this is a superior and more holistic way to regulate the body. By determining and balancing the most critical meridian imbalances, the other, lesser imbalances are usually resolved without treating them directly.

Quadrant Measurement and Balancing

This is a valuable method to create overall energetic balance between the regions of the body. It is indicated if a patient's meridian readings don't seem to make sense, or all seem abnormally low. This may be due to poor circulation of Qi and Blood to the extremities, or overall energetic Deficiency.

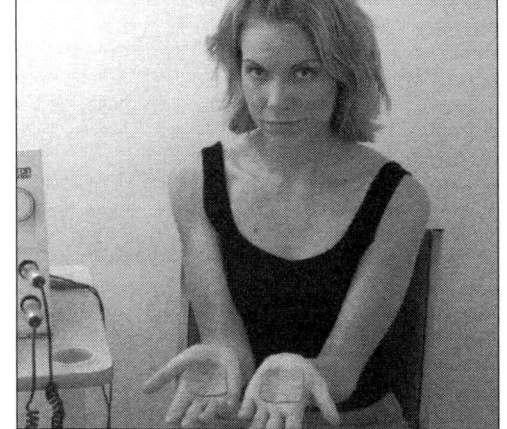

Figure 16.1: Hand-to-hand quadrant testing

---

[210] There are minor differences in the optimal reading on the meridians, yet using this average will work quite well.

Quadrant balancing can help to correct this condition. It can be used as a treatment in its own right, or used prior to EMT to provide more accurate readings.

The body is divided into four quadrants, each including one extremity and a quarter of the body trunk.

There are six kinds of quadrant measurements, each consisting of a set of hands and/or feet:

1. Hand to hand
2. Foot to foot
3. Right hand to right foot
4. Left hand to left foot
5. Right hand to left foot
6. Left hand to right foot

To take a measurement choose a treatment channel on your device using its GSR[211] measurement capabilities, and firmly touch the electrodes to one or more of the above pairs. This can be done with probe or pad electrodes. A simple way to do this is use one set of pads, with one pad on the palm of each hand, sole of feet or combination. When using probes, have the patient hold a hand mass in one hand, and pinch the tip of the trigger probe between thumb and forefinger of her other hand and note the reading. It is interesting to measure some or all of the six quadrant measurements and compare the readings. Such readings can reveal left-right imbalances, or disequilibrium between the upper and lower body.

If the GSR reading is below 50 on a 0 – 100 scale meter for any set, the energy circulation between those areas can be boosted. Leave the electrodes in place, and the following parameters may be used for 5 – 10 minutes[212]:

- 50 - 100 µA intensity, 25µA for very sensitive patients.
- 10 Hz frequency
- Biphasic polarity
- Square or Slope waveform
- 2:1 Modulation (if available)

If treating more than one pair of quadrants, the treatment time can be reduced to a total time of 10 – 20 minutes, depending on degree of deficiency. There may be some other benefits to microcurrent quadrant stimulation at 10 Hz. There is intriguing evidence that low-level current applied in this way can boost the immune system and potentially deactivate some harmful viruses and parasites[213]. Further research in this area is highly warranted.

Choice of EMT Test Points

The test points used for EMT are on or near the Jing points or the Source points. The instructions below utilize BFD points, which are slightly proximal to the Jing points. Meridians are more superficial than Organs, and so the superficial Qi at the level of the Jing points will

---

[211] Galvanic Skin Response
[212] For Acutron Mentor, use Probe #1 or uA Pad # 1 and adjust intensity up to 100 µA
[213] See work of Bob Beck and Hulva Clark, searchable through any internet search engine.

give information primarily about the status of the meridians. Thus, they are most useful as test points when myofascial pain management is the primary objective.

The Japanese Ryodoraku system primarily uses Source points for testing. These are the same as the Shu or Earth points on the Yin meridians. On Yang meridians, the Source points are not one of the Five-Element master points. Source points give more balanced information about both the meridian and the Organ. As mentioned earlier, Source points have major electrical connections into the fascial planes that house the meridians and connect directly to Organs.

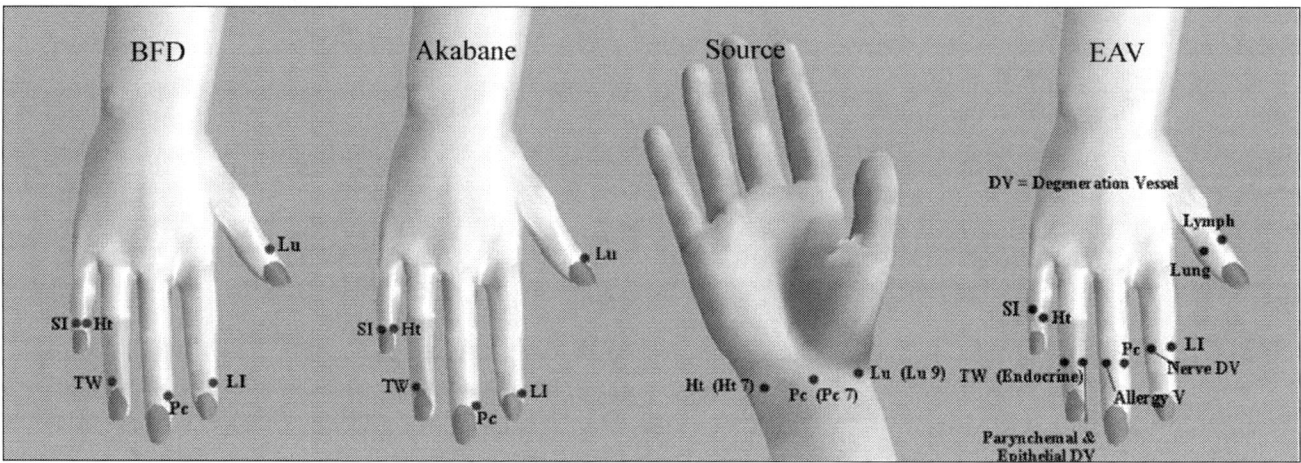

Figure 16.2: Test point systems – BFD, Akabane, Source and EAV

The Front Mu-Alarm and Back Shu points, being directly connected to the Organs rather than the meridians, primarily give information about the status of the Organs. These are not very useful for EMT, however. The choice of test points for EMT therefore depends on whether the patient is being primarily treated for myofascial pain management or internal medical disorders and deep organic pain. While both systems of test points reflect both Organ and meridian energetics, Source points are more weighted toward Organ information, while Ting and BFD points reveal more about the meridians, and hence myofascial pain conditions.

The Law of Resonance and EMT

Another way to understand meridian testing is through the principle of resonance. Voll and Nakatani both understood the effects of stimulation of acu-points through the action on the autonomic nervous and other bodily systems, in other words, through Western physiological principles. Neither man referred to "Qi" in their writings. Therefore, what is the relationship between these systems and movement of Qi though TCM? In studying literature about Qi, it is a substance that is part physical and part energetic. Ted Kaptchuk defines it as "energy on the verge of becoming matter, and matter on the verge of becoming energy."[214] This is not a one-to-one synonym for electrical energy, although it is closely associated with it. The term Qi implies a life-force with aspects of consciousness. Qi cannot be directly measured with an ohmmeter, and the domain of Qi cannot be limited to the nervous and endocrine systems. Yet, it is true that the quantity of Qi in each meridian can be ascertained by measuring skin resistance with EMT. Therefore, a resonance must exist between electrical changes on the

---

[214] From The Web That Has No Weaver, Chapter 1

skin surface and Qi movement in the body. We are *indirectly* measuring Qi through EMT. This is an important example of the Law of Resonance, the "As Above, So Below" principle. In the same way, Spirit is a substance that is even subtler than Qi. Resonance exists on many levels, as illustrated in the following diagram:

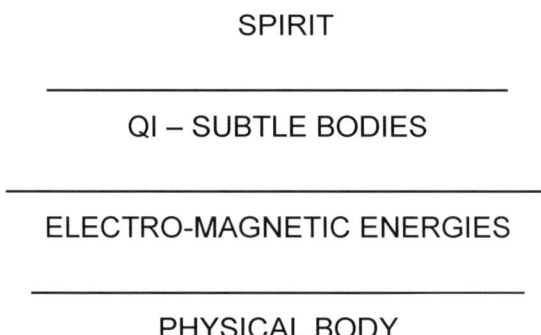

SPIRIT

QI – SUBTLE BODIES

ELECTRO-MAGNETIC ENERGIES

PHYSICAL BODY

AcuLogic™ Software

I recently produced an innovative software program that greatly simplifies EMT. As readings are taken, they immediately appear on a colorful Windows-based graph screen.[215] Once all the meridians are graphed, the user can view all the readings at once in graphical format, which can be stored in database or made into a printed report. This simplifies evaluation and treatment planning. The software also offers many additional intake, evaluation and report functions. You may contact me at the address and phone number given in the Resource section for additional information about this system.

Electronic Meridian Testing Instructions

The instructions that follow are for use with a device that has the following features:

- 0 – 100 meter scale, with a 500 k Ohm load indicating the midpoint, or approximately "50". For devices with other scales, determine which value is considered normal and healthy, and adjust instructions accordingly.

- Grounding hand mass the patient can hold in her hand not being tested to complete the circuit

- Probe tip that is about 3mm in diameter on testing probe, for testing Jing or BFD point. The low-force probe tip design is best. This is a flat tipped 3mm brass tip with a shallow circular indentation to hold water through surface tension.

- Q-tip electrodes will be too large for accurate measurements of BFD points, but may be used to test Source points. Some manufacturers have produced spring-loaded probe tips in an attempt to equalize point pressure. The reviews on these are mixed.

- A small cup of tap water or a wet sponge set up conveniently on your equipment cart.

---

[215] Users that do not have a device with RS-232 port for automatic input to the software can manually enter test readings.

If you do not have automatic recording software as mentioned above, use a chart to write the readings for each meridian, or manually enter the readings into an EMT software program through the keyboard.

Instructions for performing BFD test

BFD stands for **B**iologically **F**unctional **D**iagnostic points. BFD is one of the electro-diagnostic methods developed in Germany in an attempt to simplify the complex EAV system. While EAV specifies multiple test and treatment points in different locations on each meridian, BFD points are located on the same, easy to locate, anatomical location on each finger and toe. As mentioned above, BFD points, being near the Jing points of each meridian, register the condition of the meridian system more than the Organ. Since myofascial pain conditions are primarily meridian related, these will be more applicable.

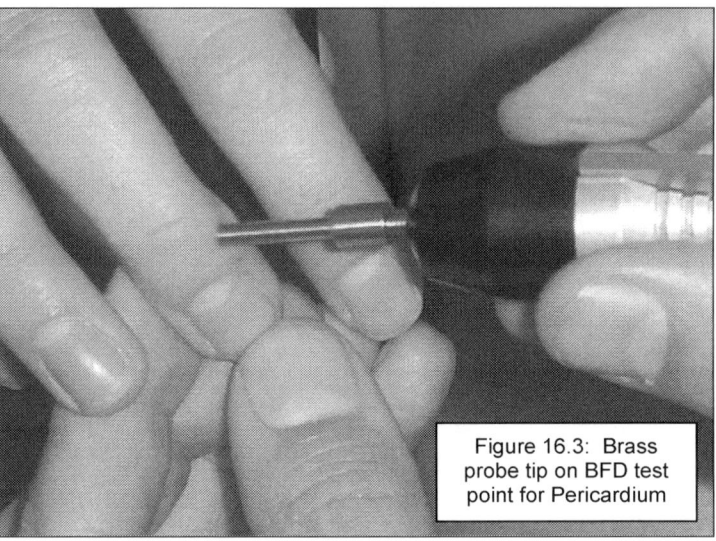

Figure 16.3: Brass probe tip on BFD test point for Pericardium

1. Guide patient into a comfortable sitting position. If she is unable to sit, testing may be performed supine.

2. Sit in front of her, with testing device on the side of your dominant hand.

3. Plug in the hand mass and its cord into the unit. Ask your patient to hold the hand mass in her hand on the side of the body not being tested. Make sure the 3 mm tip is installed on your trigger (test) probe.

4. With her palm facing down, hold the patient's finger to be tested with your free hand (the one not holding the test probe). With your testing hand, hold the trigger probe. Hold it close to the tip between your thumb and first two fingers. Experiment until you find the way of holding it that allows the most precise control.

5. Dip the probe tip into a small container of water, and shake off the excess water so only a wet film remains. It is important that it is not dripping wet. For patients with moist skin, this step is not necessary if using the brass probe tip.

6. Holding the probe in line with the finger to be tested, gently touch the probe tip to the test point with no pressure, only the weight of the probe. Hold it almost perpendicular to the finger, with a slight angling toward the hand. BFD points are found at the initial osseous angle of the distal interphalangeal joint (DIP). If the probe tip starts to ride up on the joint itself, you have gone too far. The BFD point is the same distance from the edge of the finger as the Jing point.

7. Once you are on the point, very gradually increase the pressure. When using a brass low-force tip, very little pressure is needed. The average correct amount is similar to the pressure needed to make a postal scale read less than 1 ounce. Determining the correct

pressure for accurate readings takes practice. Too much pressure will certainly yield overly high readings. Note the reading, and then move onto the next test point.

8. Dip the probe in water and shake it off before each reading if the patient's skin is dry. It will take some experimentation to learn to determine when re-wetting is necessary.

9. If you will test both sides of the body, start with patient's right hand and then move to left hand, then right foot, left foot. If just wanting a quick overall evaluation, you can just test the patient's dominant side, although this will not reveal left-right imbalances.

When first learning EMT technique, it is valuable to measure each point 2 or 3 times to make sure the readings are consistent. It is common for beginning testers to feel unsure of their results, and wonder if the readings are accurate or just artifacts. The only way to get past this stage is to follow the above instructions exactly and test a lot of people. After testing 10 – 20 people, most practitioners develop the familiarity and motor skills to become confident in their readings. This skill is well worth developing, as it makes a valuable diagnostic tool available to you for the rest of your career. You will start to understand the correct amount of pressure to apply to the test points with the probe tip once you see the difference between deficient (low) readings and normal or high readings. Truly deficient readings will read below 50 on the meter even with slightly increased pressure, while normal or high readings will read above 50 without much pressure. It is helpful to attend a hands-on training in which an experienced tester can show you the correct technique.

The following factors can cause unclear or inaccurate readings:

- Probe tip on wrong test point location.
- Probe tip at wrong angle.
- Probe tip too wet or too dry.
- Incorrect pressure on test point.
- Patient may need to be energetically cleared if readings don't make sense, or may require quadrant balancing prior to testing.

Interpreting Electronic Meridian Testing Patterns

Once you've dealt with your initial learning curve and start to perform EMT with a reasonable level of confidence, the fun and fascinating part begins. Now you can grasp the diagnostic significance of the data you have recorded.

As mentioned earlier, Ryodoraku and other related electro-diagnostic systems mainly measure and balance one meridian at a time. If the Lung is deficient, tonify it. If the Liver is excess, sedate it. Some instructors have offered meridian balancing formulas based on Five Element relationships, but this is still largely focused on balancing individual meridians. These are valid, but limited methods. Even a brief study of TCM, Ayurveda or other major traditional healing arts reveals that a majority of diagnostic and therapeutic methods are based on whole-body pattern recognition. This is the primary difference between energetic medicines and modern Western medicine. While modern medicine will diagnose a kidney disease and treat the physical organ directly to control dangerous symptoms, energetic medicine seeks to correct overall physical and energetic patterns of the body.

In the same way, it is my opinion and experience that results with EMT and its indicated treatments are superior when overall patterns are recognized and treated. The overall pattern of the readings is most useful for understanding the unique presentation of the patient. A low electronic reading on any single meridian can only lead to a proper treatment if viewed in the context of the other meridians. Because EMT is such a new and rarely used modality in the West, those practicing it have rarely had access to good information about pattern recognition through its use. The information that follows is offered to help fill this void. It comes from my own experience and observations by Charles McWilliams, as well as research by Yosio Nakatani.

Electronic meridian testing provides a reading on a 0 - 100 scale for each individual meridian test point on the fingers and toes. The results can be entered on a graph for analysis.

Understanding EMT readings

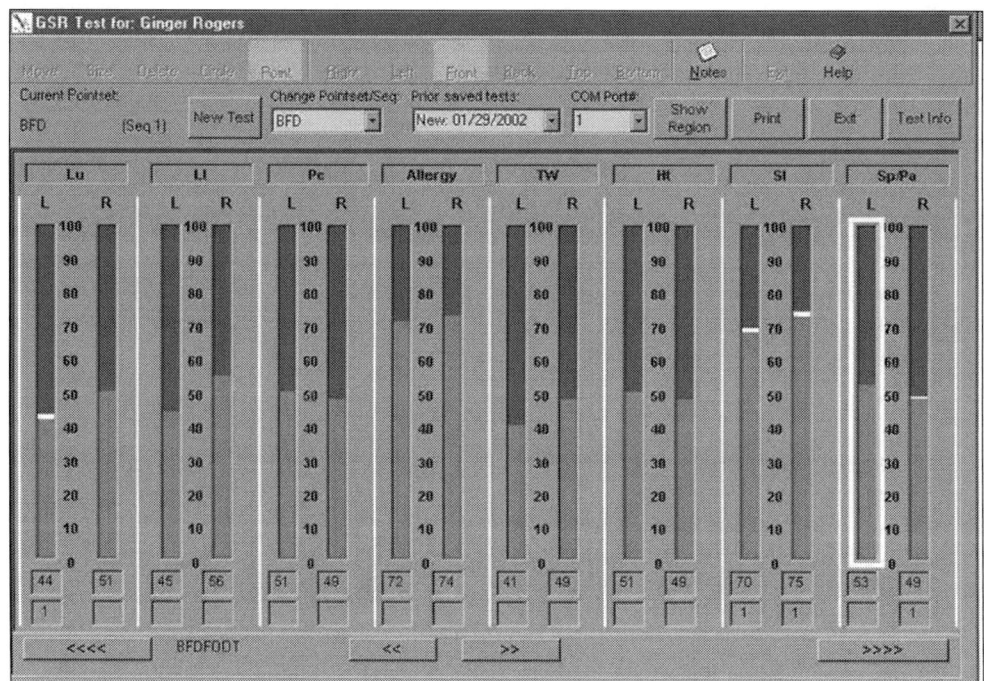

Figure 16.4: AcuLogic sample test screen

There are three main types of EMT readings:

1. *High reading (above 65% and stable)* - indicates excess energy (shi) or inflammation in the meridian or associated Organ. Can also indicate pain or toxicity in the meridian or Organ. Technically, any reading above 50 can be excess, but 50 - 65 or as much as 70[216] may show normal cycles of high energy in healthy people. *The higher the reading, the greater the excess, inflammation or toxicity.*

2. *Low reading (below 50%)* - indicates low energy (deficiency or xu) in the meridian or associated Organ. Readings from 40 - 49 may indicate a low ebb of energy in an otherwise healthy person, however any reading below 40 generally indicates significant deficiency.

---

[216] Readings of 65-70 may be normal in major cities, where intensity of stress and stimulation are more constant, especially New York City (as noted by the author).

Low readings on meridians that run through areas of chronic pain often indicate that there is a long standing blockage in the flow of Qi through that area, and opening this blockage may help to relieve the pain. In cases of deficiency with chronic pain, patients are also often depressed emotionally. A combination of meridian therapy with nutritional or herbal support can help to alleviate this condition. Low readings may also indicate an area in which the patient has shut off their feeling and life force, and so intuitive counseling to help them resolve these root issues is often essential. *The lower the reading, the more profound the deficiency or degeneration.*

It is important to mention that the numerical ranges referenced above are averages. The normal or most healthy reading can vary from person to person and from meridian to meridian. Relatively less energetic patients, including many of the elderly may have readings of 40 -50 as their norm. In these cases, such readings are not considered pathologically deficient. "Hot" constitutional persons, such as "type A" personality, may show normal readings in 55 - 65 range. One simple way to determine the normal reading is to add all of the patient's EMT readings together and then divide them by the number of readings to arrive at an average reading. This can then be considered the normal reading for that person on that day.

Experienced EMT practitioners can simply make a mental adjustment for each patient based on the readings to determine which readings are clinically significant. The most significant readings are those that stand out from most of the others. For example, if Liver reading is 20 points higher than any other meridians, this may point to a condition of hepatitis. In most cases, however, the overall pattern of meridian readings leads to a diagnosis.

3. *Unstable reading, or indicator drops* - In this case the indicator goes to a high point and then drifts down, even though you are maintaining steady probe pressure on the test point. According to EAV theory, this phenomenon indicates organic degeneration or allergic responses in the patient relative to that meridian. The following chart gives guidelines for understanding the meaning of indicator drops[217]:

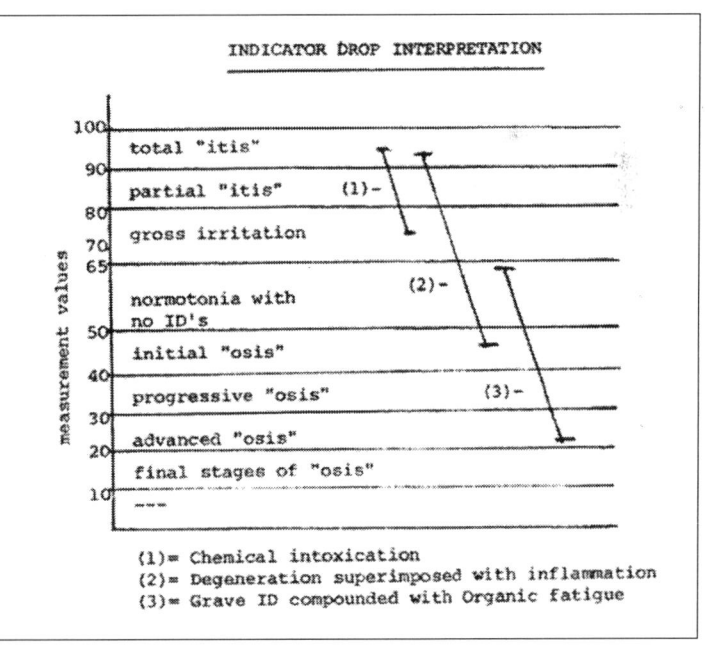

Figure 16.5: Indicator drop diagram

---

[217] Indicator drop chart from book <u>Electroacupuncture, Volume One and Two</u> courtesy Charles McWilliams, Panam Institute, Nevis

Figure 16.6: EMT Diagnostic Patterns

CONDITION	TREATMENT PRINCIPLE / RELEVANT ACU-POINTS	COMMENTS
1) Most hand points high and steady; most feet points normal; may signify an acute cold, flu, fever, or reaction to toxics in an otherwise healthy person; may also signify an acute, short-term allergic reaction	Clear the surface, sedate Heat (if indicated only) Disperse LI 4, Lu 7, LI 11, St 44, TW 5, Du 14, GB 20, UB 12 SI 3 (+) and UB 62 (-)	Surface clearing herbs, sweating may be indicated for cold and flu; detoxification and fasting may be indicated for individuals who are not acutely sick.
2) Most hand points high and steady, most feet points also high: Major inflammatory process in the body, generally a very sick individual in a crisis. "Hot" condition according to Eight Principles diagnosis.	Sedate Heat or Fire: Disperse Lv 2, GB 40, K1, Du 13, Du 14, LI 4, LI 11, St 43, St 44, also local acu-points in area of inflammation, TW 5 (-) and GB 41 (+) Nourish Yin (when indicated): Tonify K 3, Sp 6, Pc 6 (-) and Sp 4 (+) or K 6 (-) and LU 7 (+)	This is the kind of patient likely to need Western medical diagnosis or treatment for acute infections. Chinese heat clearing herbs may be indicated.
3) Most hand points high with indicator drops (I.D.'s): Allergic response or toxic load in body, possibly lymphatic stasis. Check test point on Allergy vessel (ulnar side of middle finger) for confirmation. <u>If feet readings are normal</u>, allergy is in superficial parts of body, <u>if feet points low or with I.D.'s</u>, allergy is overlaid over significant bodily weakness and possible organ degeneration.	Support Normal Qi: St 36, LI 11, Sp 6, Ren 6, focus on individualized support Subdue Fire: See 2), above	For such conditions, Chinese herbal therapies are indicated, and/or homeopathic remedies. Electrodermal screening[218] is useful for determining and clearing specific allergic sensitivities.
4) Most feet points low, especially Kidney, Spleen-Pancreas, Liver: Significant deficiency of Qi in deep internal Organs. These patients almost always have chronic health problems and frequently present fatigue, allergy, autoimmune disorders, or degenerative disease. If patient has come with main complaint of pain, the practitioner must make some judgments about treating the Root or Branch of their complaint. In this case, the Root would be the organic insufficiencies, the Branch the symptom of pain. <u>The Four-Step protocol is ideal for such patients.</u>	Tonify affected Organs, Qi and Blood, balance Qi, address herbal or nutritional deficiencies. Tonify affected Organs, Qi and Blood, balance Qi, address herbal or nutritional deficiencies. Tonify Qi with St 36, Ren 4, Ren 6, Ren 12, tonification points for individual affected Organs, K 6 (-) and Lu 7 (+) and/or Pc 6 (-) and Sp 4 (+). Polarity may need to be reversed. Moxibustion is very useful.	Herbal and nutritional support is essential for these patients. Gentle Qi Gong and self-empowerment work will help deal with their Root issues in many cases.

---

[218] Electrodermal screening is the increasingly popular practice of using an EMT device to test for allergies, infections, toxicity or disease by exposing the patient's energy field to samples of vibrational substances. Nosodes are samples of homeopathically potentized disease organisms or tissues, sarcodes are potentized samples of normal organ and tissue, and both are used in testing along with allergens, nutritional and healing remedies and much more. Some ED devices sample disharmonious bodily energies, harmonize them and inject them back into the body for healing purposes, and some create energetic medicines that can be orally administered. No claims for effectiveness of such devices are made by the author.

5) **Most feet points low, most hand points high**: Some aspect of auto-immune disease or Yin deficiency, in which the body's hormonal control is faulty, and the internal metabolic heat (Fire) of the body is not being balanced by its cooling and moistening functions. This creates fatigue, nervousness, and annoying heat symptoms, especially in the upper body such as low fever, hot face, hands and feet, headaches, stiff shoulders, mental and emotional upset and confusion, insomnia, and in extreme cases, stroke, tachycardia and mental illness. This pattern may be seen with RA, lupus, MS, and in some cancers.	Tonify Yin, balance endocrine function, cool Heat Tonify Yin: K 3, Sp 6, <u>K 6 (-) and Lu 7 (+) and/or Pc 6 (-) and Sp 4 (+)</u> Polarity may need to be reversed. Tonification of affected meridians and Organs. Manaka's Cross Syndrome: <u>with Pc 6 (-) and Sp 4 (+) R side, TW 5(-) and GB 41(+), left side</u>	See 4 above
6) **Most hand and foot points low and/or dropping- Kidney test point almost always low**: Severe constitutional deficiency and fatigue, Kidney Yang deficiency. Patient is usually weak, cold, either overweight or emaciated, with weak pulse, pale tongue, and presenting any of a host of medical problems, including kidney disease, congestive heart disease, mental illness, cancer or HIV	Support normal Qi, tonify Yang, address nutritional deficiencies Support normal Qi: St 36, LI 4, Sp 6, Pc 6, Ren 6, UB 13, 20, 23, moxa applicable Tonify Kidney Yang: Ren 4, Du 4, UB 23, K 7, K 3, <u>K 6 (-) and Lu 7 (+)</u>, Du 20	See comments, #4
7) **Meridians of Fire low or dropping (Pericardium, Triple Warmer, Small Intestine, Heart), Liver low or high**: Middle age burnout syndrome, frequently encountered in health practitioners, especially acupuncturists!, around age of 35 - 50, mid-life crisis, emotional broken heart after divorce, separation, or sexual disappointments. This pattern often shows in people who are "breaking down" prior to a new stage of spiritual awakening, so take hope!	Pray, meditate, win the lottery, fall in love, tonify Fire, balance Kidneys and Heart <u>Pc 6 (-) and Sp 4 (+)</u>, Lv 3, Sp 6, K 3, Du 4, Du 14, Ren 17, Ren 4, Du 4	Physician, heal thyself.
8) **Spleen-Pancreas and/or Stomach meridians low, Triple Warmer, Small Intestine, Large Intestine may also be low or dropping: Spleen/Pancreas low**. Patient presents with digestive problems, appetite disorders, weak pulse, often flabby, overweight or emaciated, may have fluid imbalances.	Tonify Spleen Qi, straighten out diet, move out of Houston or Washington D.C. St 36, LI 11, Sp 2, Sp 3, Sp 9, UB 20, UB 21, Ren 12, Lv 13, Ren 6 (moxa useful).	Often a sequela of the Great American Diet and sedentary lifestyle. A comprehensive program of nutritional improvement, herbs, exercise, deep breathing, acupuncture and addressing emotional/spiritual issues.

Common EMT Patterns

The table above contains some common EMT patterns, with suggestions of how to use this information to arrive at a Chinese medical diagnostic pattern. Suggested acu-points are listed to address each pattern, including a pair of Extraordinary Vessel Master points that may be applicable. The + and - shows the most likely polarity of probes to use on each point[219]. It is not necessary or recommended to treat all the listed points; point selection must be based on individual assessments and experience of the practitioner.

The suggested treatments should be confirmed for applicability with each individual patient, including the indicated polarities. This can be done through checking key imbalance EMT readings after treatment, or by using kinesiology, pulse diagnosis or changes in pressure sensitive points. This will ensure that readings are balancing. Some adjunctive therapies are also listed, a few of which are offered from a light-hearted perspective.

Chapter 11 offers more specific methods to choose and confirm treatment points. The therapies here are offered as a starting point. To review, the term "points high" refers to readings that are abnormally high, usually above 65, while "points low" are those below 45.

More EMT patterns from Nakatani

The following patterns, some of which overlap with those presented above, were discovered through experiments on 4,446 volunteers in Japan by Yosio Nakatani and his colleagues[220] (see next page).

---

[219] Choose Probe preset #2 on Acutron Mentor, trigger probe on - points and counterprobe on + points, treat 12 - 30 seconds per point combo)
[220] As tabulated in Ryodoraku Textbook by Hirohisa Oda, Naniwasha Publishing Inc.

Figure 16.7: Nakatani EMT patterns

Common Symptomatic Presentation

All hand meridians high, all foot meridians low	Problems of peripheral circulation
All hand meridians low, all foot meridians high	Mental disorders
Stiff shoulder, rush of blood to the head, hemorrhoids, asthma	
Lung high, Liver low	Prolapsed anus
Lung and Large Intestine high	Facial spasms, trigeminal neuralgia
Lung and Pericardium high, Large Intestine low	Stiff shoulders
Stiff shoulders, decreased muscle strength and abnormality of upper limbs	
Pericardium high, Lung low	Upper limb neuralgia
Pericardium high, Liver, Gall Bladder and Stomach low	vertigo (low blood pressure)
Heart high	Bloated stomach, constipation
Heart high, Spleen low	Abdominal evacuation
Small Intestine high	Bloated stomach
Small Intestine and Urinary Bladder high	Headache
Triple Warmer high	Bladder dysfunction
Large Intestine high	Frequent urination
Large Intestine, Urinary Bladder high	Stiff neck
Large Intestine high, Kidney low	Coldness in low back and legs
Large Intestine high, Gall Bladder low	Blurred vision
Coldness in lower back and legs, knee problems, stomach disease, purulent lung disease	
Spleen and Liver high or Spleen high and Liver low	Stomach disorders
Spleen and Urinary Bladder high	Nape of neck stiffness
Liver high	Hepatitis
Liver high and Kidney low	Disorders of sexual organs
Liver and Stomach low	Depression
Kidney low	Weak constitution, sciatica
Kidney and Urinary Bladder low	Nocturia (bed wetting)
Urinary Bladder low	Lumbago
Gall Bladder low	Feelings of heaviness in the limbs, eye disorders

This information was gathered in a similar way to the determination of Voll's "new" meridians and points in Germany. This was through testing meridians in patients with known medically diagnosed conditions. When similar meridian patterns showed up over and over in a number of patients with the same disease, the correlation were drawn. A well-trained acupuncturist can see many obvious correlations in the above list, such as weak Kidney reading associated with deficient constitution and high readings in Small Intestine and Bladder leading to headaches. Many of the associations are not so obvious, however, such as Heart high with constipation. It would be a mistake to take this list as "gospel truth", as this data requires additional research and confirmation. I certainly encourage you to check these associations out for yourself, which is quite easy to do once you are practicing EMT. I can imagine how this information can be used as a valuable screening tool for emergency medical practitioners and medical statisticians and researchers.

Nakatani observed that when patient's symptoms and associated abnormal meridian readings match the above chart, their disorders are relatively easy to cure. If the symptoms and readings do not follow the chart, it will be much more difficult to cure the patient.

Abnormal readings in Triple Warmer and Gall Bladder are considered the most significant for detecting cancer. Pericardium and Heart dysfunction gives clues about the progression of the disease, while Liver and Kidney readings reveal degree of resistance to cancer. Dr. Kobayashi of Tokyo developed a scoring system for these readings to determine a patients susceptibility to cancer, the so-called "cancer constitution" or the presence of existing cancer.[221]

Conclusion

Electronic meridian testing is a very valuable diagnostic tool. It is easy to perform, reproducible, and lends itself to well to modern computer-based testing and documentation. EMT can help empower patients by allowing them to see the condition of their meridians for themselves, and to witness improvement (hopefully) in their readings as therapy progresses. The German and Japanese researchers who pioneered EMT expended thousands of hours of diligent research charting the information presented in this chapter, and much more. EMT provides an excellent bridge between traditional energy medicines such as acupuncture with modern empirical scientific research and diagnosis.

It is highly recommended that you compare the readings of EMT with other, known diagnostic methods such as pulse and abdominal diagnosis, as well as western medical lab test results. When, as Nakatani discovered, the different methods correlate, it is easy to use this method with confidence. Chapter 11 offers specific instructions for using EMT and Alarm Point kinesiology readings to erect an accurate energetic evaluation of a patient.

---

[221] For more information, see <u>Ryodoraku Textbook</u> by Hirohisa Oda, Naniwasha Publishing Inc..

Chapter 17

POLAR MERIDIAN PAIRS AND GASTROCNEMIUS DIAGNOSIS

Introduction

Polar meridians are pairs of meridian/Organ[222] systems that are each at peak energy at opposite times during the daily circadian rhythm of the body. This daily rhythm of the meridians is described through a diagram often called the Chinese clock, which is divided into 12 two-hour segments. During each segment, one function is at its peak flow of energy, while another is at its lowest level. An example of a polar meridian pair is Spleen-Triple Warmer. Spleen is at its peak energy during the period of 9 – 11 AM, while Triple Warmer is at its peak energy between 9 – 11 PM. Each function is at its lowest energy during the peak of the other. The Chinese clock is often depicted as the diagram below:

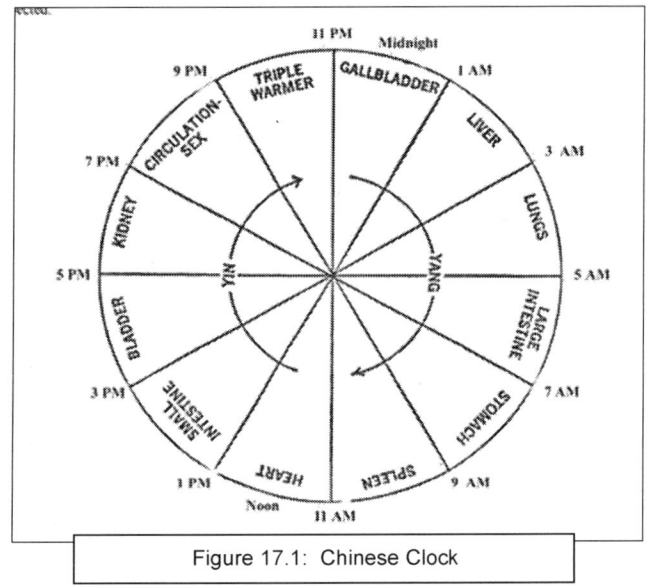

Figure 17.1: Chinese Clock

---

[222] Although both Organ and meridian function are included on the Chinese clock, I will use the simple word "meridian" to describe both functions in this explanation.

The polar meridian pairs are as follows, followed by their peak energy times:

A. Spleen (9 AM – 11 AM)	Triple Warmer (9 PM – 11 PM)
B. Kidney (5 PM – 7 PM)	Large Intestine (5 AM – 7 AM)
C. Liver (1 AM – 3 AM)	Small Intestine (1 PM – 3 PM)
D. Stomach (7 AM – 9 AM)	Pericardium (7 PM – 9 PM)
E. Urinary Bladder (3 PM – 5 PM)	Lung (3 AM – 5 AM)
F. Gall Bladder (11 PM – 1 AM)	Heart (11 AM – 1 PM)

The need for polar meridian treatment is indicated by abdominal and gastrocnemius evaluations utilizing palpation and/or O ring kinesiology. Treatment is administered by stimulating combinations of tonification and sedation points[223] of the selected meridians with specific polarities. Thus, two meridians are chosen, one of which is at its peak energy and the other at its lowest energy. Due to their polar relationship, treatment of these meridian pairs tends to have a deep root level balancing effect. This is the level at which Step One treatments are directed.

Chapter 8 on the Great Loops details some of the meridian relationships that may be utilized for pain management and energy balancing therapies. Polar meridian pairs are one of the most clinically useful relationships. Please review the Manaka Meridian Balancing chart in Chapter 11. The upper part of the chart is for treatment of Extraordinary vessels. The lower part is for treatment of polar meridian pairs. Manaka recommended his students to mainly work with Extraordinary Vessels when first learning this system, as they are indicated in more cases, and to draw from polar meridian pairs if Extraordinary Vessel treatment was not an effective counter-bias.[224]

Micro-systems and the Gastrocnemius

Micro-systems are regions of the body that contain a map of points that correspond to the body as a whole. The most well known are the micro-systems of the ear, hand, face, sole of the foot and iris of the eye. Each of these regions can be used to either diagnose or treat disorders of the entire body, or both. There are many other such systems used for diagnosis and treatment. In reality, every cell of our body is a micro-system that contains genetic information that corresponds to our entire body, and some day may be used to clone entire new beings in our likeness. (May wisdom be used!)

The gastrocnemius muscles of the legs are another micro-system that contains zones that correspond to the entire meridian system. Manaka described a system of palpation points on

---

[223] Also called Mother and Son points in Five Element acupuncture
[224] For explanation of biases, see Chapters Three and Ten

these muscles that correspond to the polar meridian pairs[225]. Gastrocnemius palpation is a simple method that is useful for determining polar meridian pair imbalances. It is presented here in this book after the explanations of O Ring kinesiology and EMT because it is another important diagnostic system used for the Four-Step protocol.

Palpation Points Location and Method

For the rest of this chapter we will refer to the polar pairs by their A – F letter designators:

A. Spleen/Triple Warmer

B. Kidney/Large Intestine

C. Liver/Small Intestine

D. Stomach/Pericardium

E. Bladder/Lung

F. Gall Bladder/Heart

A., B., and C. are about three-finger widths medial to the midline of the back of the leg (Urinary Bladder meridian), while D., E., and F. are about the same width lateral. A., B., and C. are therefore on the medial, yin aspect of the calf while D., E. and F. are on the lateral, yang aspect. B. and E. are found at the widest level of the calf. A. and D. are about two finger widths above B. and E., while C. and F. are about two finger widths below. These measurements must be adjusted depending on the size of the patient's legs.

To palpate these points, the patient can either lay prone on a treatment table with the back of the legs upward, or lay on his back while placing the bottoms of his feet on the table to bend the knees at a 90 degree angle. Palpate with a steady, gentle pressure, comparing the right and left sides at each level – A. and D., B. and E., C. and F. The points will often be found along tense bands of muscle. Once the tenderest point is noted, palpate the same points on the other leg to compare. In most cases one of the palpation points will be most sore, and will be clearly more reactive on one leg than the other. The most tender point and leg should be noted. If Step One meridian balancing procedures calls for treatment of polar meridian pairs,[226] stimulate all the treatment points on the side of the body <u>opposite</u> to the most sore gastrocnemius palpation point. This will usually also be homolateral to the most reactive side of the abdomen.

After a successful treatment, the sore point on the gastrocnemius corresponding to the meridians treated should be noticeably more relaxed and less sore. During Step Two treatment of yang meridians, the gastrocnemius palpation points themselves can be treated if still markedly sore, although back-shu points along the spine are used in the majority of cases.

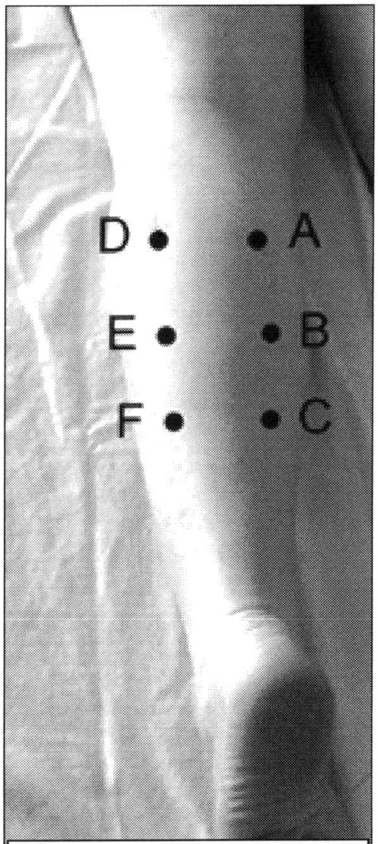

Figure 17.1: Gastroc points

---

[225] This micro-system first observed by Osama Honda of Osaka, Japan
[226] Explained in detail in Chapter Eleven

Treatment points

For treatment of polar meridian pair imbalances, Manaka prescribed simultaneous treatment of the tonification and sedation points on each meridian of the pair, using specific polarities. These treatment points are listed in the Manaka Meridian Balancing Method chart in Chapter 11.

The meaning of tonification and sedation points can be understood through reference to the Law of Five Elements. The tonification point is the point on a principal meridian that corresponds to the "mother" of its Elemental quality. This point will draw extra Qi into the meridian from the mother Organ/meridian. For example, Lu 9 is the Earth point of the Lung meridian, and will draw Qi into the Lungs from the Spleen and Stomach (Earth element). A sedation point is the point that corresponds to the "son" Organ/meridian. This point will draw Qi away from the meridian being treated to the son. It is not customary in TCM to treat tonification and sedation points together, yet this is what Manaka found to be most effective for balancing polar meridian pairs. This practice is consistent with the whole concept of polar pairs, as we are treating functions with opposite energy peaks simultaneously.

The prescribed polarities require some discussion. As mentioned earlier in this text, negative electrical polarity is electron donating, and so adds energy and is locally tonifying. The positive polarity is electron receptive, and so reduces energy and is locally sedating. I use the word "locally" to emphasize that other, systemic, effects are likely. Manaka taught, and I have verified, that a negative, tonifying agent must be placed on the sedation point of the treated meridian, and that a positive, sedating agent must be placed on the tonification point, for effective treatment of polar meridian pairs. At first look this may appear to be a contradiction, yet upon some reflection it makes sense. There are many levels of energy movement within our bodies. Superficial energy moving in one direction may induce deeper energy to move in the opposite direction. To illustrate this point, I can offer a memory from my childhood. On hot summer days when it felt good to cool a room in our New Jersey home, my dad would often open a window and place a fan blowing outward. I remember asking him why he aimed it outside instead of blowing the cool air in. He replied that blowing the air out the window was creating a negative pressure on the air in the room, which was drawing the cool air in through the other window. It worked! I believe this is a good analogy for the value of seemingly paradoxical stimulation of tonification and sedation points. This effect, in combination with the simultaneous stimulation of polar meridians with opposite energy conditions, is powerful and effective.

Section V

TREATMENT FORMULARIES

Treatment Formulary Section I

TREATMENT FORMULARY

BY BODY AREA

This section is divided according to sections of the body. Specific points and protocols are described, with diagrams of the body on the facing page. Information provided for each body area includes the following:

Common Trigger Points (TP's)

Common trigger points are given that are often key in releasing myofascial tension in the affected area. For each area, I reference charts and page numbers from Travell & Simons Trigger Point Flip Charts.[227] It is recommended that you obtain this or another source book for complete diagrams of trigger points. Some diagrams of some common trigger points from the Flip Charts are reproduced here for your convenience.[228] On the diagrams in the Flip Chart, the painful areas are shown in solid red and secondary pain areas in stippled red. Common trigger points are marked with "X". Refer to the indicated charts, and determine which ones most closely reflect your patient's pain pattern. Palpate the TP's shown on those charts. If the TP's (X's) are tight, painful, ropy or otherwise unusual, and radiate pain, treat them with needles, moxa or microcurrent probes. In most cases the TP's overlap with named acu-points. Trigger points often respond rapidly to microcurrent treatment. Please see Chapter 7 for details on the Acute probe technique which is valuable for this purpose.

Indicated Local and Distal Acu-Points

For each body area, local and distal acu-points are given that can be used in the style of sotai by stimulating them while the patient is stretching, mobilizing or exercising the painful or restricted body area. The local points suggested are those found to be tender or constricted upon palpation, which may or may not be in classic acupuncture point locations. The distal points given may be treated on the same, or opposite side, to the area of complaint. I suggest

---

[227] Williams and Wilkins, 1996, order at (800) 638-0672 in the US, (410) 528-4223 other countries, fax (410) 528-8550
[228] By permission of the publisher

palpating the indicated distal points on the patient's right and left extremities, and treating those that are most tender. When in doubt, treat the distal points on the opposite side, as this practice has a better record of effectiveness. An excellent way to treat these points is to set up your microcurrent device for polarized probe treatment, and place the + probe on the local painful area and the – probe on indicated distal point(s), usually on the opposite side. This is an application of microcurrent Great Loops technique as explained in Chapter 8.

For example, in the Shoulder section below, distal points St 38 and Sp 9a are listed. You could place the + probe on a focal point of pain in the shoulder, and the – probe on those distal points and treat. Alternatively, you could place acupuncture needles in the distal points, and microcurrent interferential pads to surround the shoulder, and then manipulate the needles to obtain Qi sensation while the pads are applying microcurrents. For sciatica pain, you can place a + electrode on affected lower back nerve roots, and the – probe on distal points on the opposite hand. Richard Tan's Ling Ku combination is excellent for this purpose[229].

I have not included Extraordinary Vessel Master points, such as SI 3 and UB 62, TW 5 and GB 41 or P 6 and Sp 4 that may be useful for these conditions. The adjustment of this energetic level is best dealt with separately in Step One treatments. This is done, as explained in Chapter 11, by choosing the indicated Master points, treating with indicated microcurrent polarity, and then confirming efficacy after treatment. I suggest performing such global body balancing prior to the described treatments.

The symbol → placed between acu-point names indicates a treatment using two probe electrodes to connect the two points. If it is in the Local Acu-Points section, biphasic current is used and it doesn't matter in which sequence the probes are placed on the points. In the Local-Distal Acu-Points listings, the + probe will generally be placed on the acu-point to the left of the → symbol, and the – probe on the one to the right. This will not <u>always</u> be accurate, so monitor your patients carefully and switch polarity if necessary.

Treatment Methods & Protocols

For each disease, pain or pathology category, the preferred method(s) of treatment are listed along with tips and commentary on each method, as appropriate. In many cases, the Trigger Point, Acu-Point, and Kinetic Electro-therapy steps of treatment overlap with each other, but are presented separately here for clarity.

Chapter 7 contains microcurrent probe methods that are valuable for releasing trigger points – specifically the Dermatome and Distal and Acute techniques. There are three main methods to release TP's with microcurrent:

1. Use Acute probe technique to connect local TP's in the affected area, or to simply pinch the TP between the probe tips from several angles. Treatment time 15 – 30 seconds per set of points.

2. Use Dermatome and Distal polarized probe treatment to connect TP with distal meridian point, using + on TP and – on distal point. Treatment time 15 – 30 seconds per set of points. Use 10 – 40 Hz.

3. Use microcurrent polarized pads for same applications as 2., but use with simultaneous stretching and exercise. Microcurrent ice treatment may be used in this way for acute, hot TP's.

---

[229] See page 221 in this Section

Specific instructions and protocols particular to the body region are described, including probe, pad and kinetic electro-therapy treatments. Refer to main portion of the book for specific device parameters, including the device settings and treatment times.

Most Step Three treatments involve stimulation of acu-points with movement. I am summarizing all of these techniques under the term kinetic electro-acupuncture (KEA). You can determine appropriate treatment methods either through trial and error, or through kinesiology. To test the effectiveness of any electrotherapy treatment with kinesiology, first clear the body[230], then place the first probe or pad set-up, give one second of stimulation and test the indicator muscle. Then try the alternative placement, stimulate for one second, and retest. The placement that makes the indicator muscle stronger will probably be the more effective treatment.

---

[230] See Chapter Twelve for instructions for kinesiology

HEAD REGION

TRIGGER POINTS / ACU-POINTS	TREATMENT METHODS
TP's: Chart 1, pp. 2-3 **Acu-points - Local** Areas of pain or tenderness. Major points include: Taiyang, Yintang, eye orbit, GB channel (temples), trigeminal nerve pathways of face, GV 20 and Sishencong, GB 19, GB 20 (occiput). **Acu-points - Distal (by region)** + probe at points on painful head region, - probe at distal point *Frontal* (for pain in Yangming Zone): LI 4, St 44, St 36, Lv 2, Lv 3 if eye area pain *Temporal* (for pain in Shaoyang Zone): TW 5, GB 41 (treat most tender side), Lv 3, GB 40 *Occipital* (for pain in Taiyang Zone): SI 3, UB 60 or 62, K 3, Du 4, Du 14 *Vertex:* Lv,2, Lv 3, P 5 or P 6, K 1 **Acu-points - Distal (by TCM diagnosis)** *Wind-Cold:* Lu 7, LI 4, LI 11 (moxibustion applicable) *Wind-Heat:* TW 5, SI 3, LI 4, Lu 7 *Hyperactive Liver Yang:* Lv 2, Lv 3, K 1, P 6, K 3 *Congealed Blood:* LI 11, Sp 10 *Blood Vacuity:* Sp 3, St 36, LI 11, UB 20 *Spleen Vacuity:* St 36, Sp 2, Ren 6, UB 20 *Kidney Yin Vacuity:* K 3, Sp 6, Ren 4 *Spleen Dampness:* Sp 6, Sp 9, St 36, UB 20, Ren 6 *Stagnant Food:* Ren 12, St 25, St 44, LI 4 *Migraine prevention:* St 36, GB 20, Sp 6, Lv 3, LI 4 **Acu-points - Ear** Forehead, occiput, brain, Shenmen, sympathetic, subcortex, cervical vertebrae, valium	**Local-Distal Polarized Probe Treatment:** Polarized microcurrent probe treatment is very effective for many types of headaches, and works more quickly than needle acupuncture in many cases. **NOTE**: Local biphasic treatment with both probes on the head can be quite effective, also, but may be more likely to aggravate sensitive patients. Use with care. Please also see Treatment Formulary - Section III for EAV headache treatment parameters. *Acute headache:* Polarity: + probe at painful head region, - probe at distal point Intensity: 50 – 75 μA Frequency: 80 Hz (acute/replete); 0.6 Hz (chronic) NOTE: also can use kinesiology to test for other resonant frequencies Time: 12-20 sec/pt then re-test If improved or same, treat additional local-distal point combination *Chronic / concurrent disease:* When treating patients who have chronic headaches or concurrent health imbalances and diseases, it is vital to first give Step One & Step Two assessment and treatment for Root level, and then follow with symptomatic treatment. Release of TP's indicated in Travell and Simon's charts for head pain is often essential for effective headache treatment. This can be done with probe stimulation, needling or electro-massage. Check for nutritional imbalances and/or medical conditions that may be causing headaches **Electro-massage / 4-pad Microcurrent Interferential Pad Treatment for Tension / Migraine Headache:** TP release with probe, needle acupuncture and/or electro-massage. Place 1 pad of each channel on tight shoulder region, other pad on therapists hands. Wet head, neck, trapezius area. Start current and massage tight, painful areas and TP's. Combine with needle or microcurrent probe stimulation of distal points. Treat first with probes or retain needles with period manipulation during massage *Polarity:* biphasic

Head Region Trigger Points

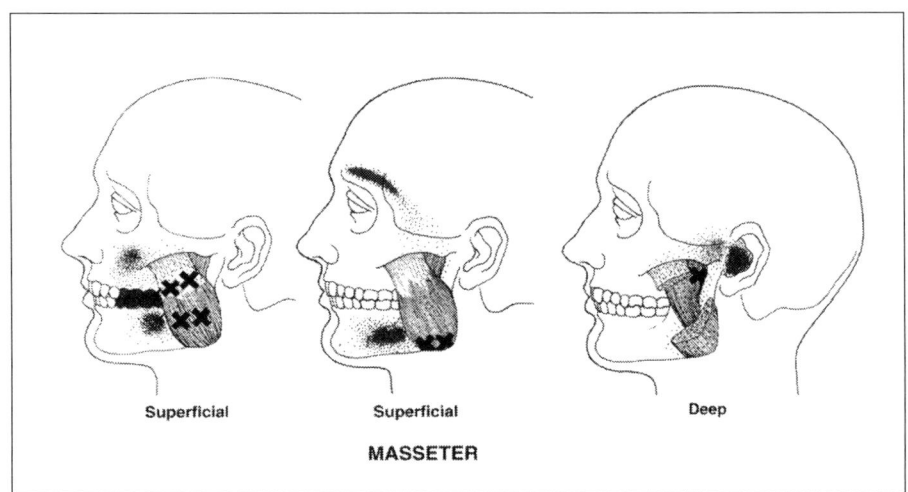

Distal Acu-Points

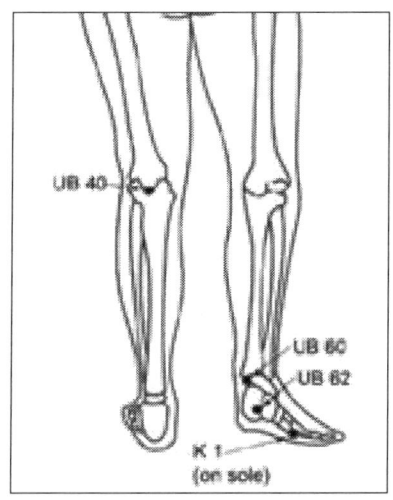
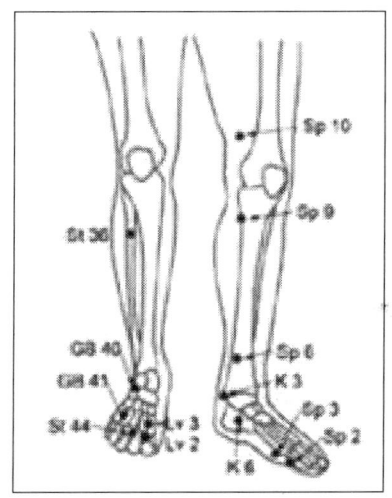

Local Acu-Points

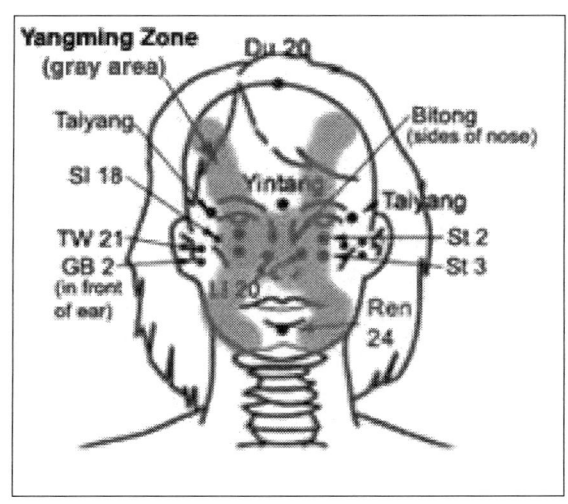
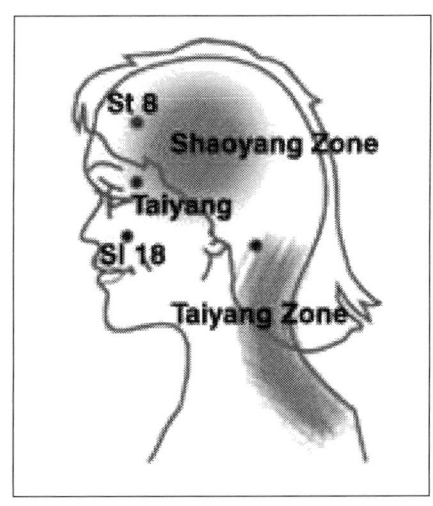

HEAD REGION, CONTINUED

Acu-points for Sinus Headache: St 2, St 3, LI 20, SI 18, Bitong (bilaterally); can also use probe or needle on Yintang, GB 20, LI 4, St 44	**Local-Distal Biphasic Probe Treatment for Sinus Headache:** Sinus-related pain responds very well to microcurrent probe stimulation. Using the Intensity and Frequency parameters below brings about excellent pain relief and sinus drainage. Relief is immediate to several hours post-treatment. *Intensity:* mild stinging sensation (with caution) *Frequency:* 80 Hz
Acu-points for TMJ St 3, 4, 5, 6, 7, SI 18, TW 17, TW 21, GB 2, GB 20, LI 4, St 44; Ear: TMJ point	**TMJ Electrode Treatment for TMJ pain:** Use TMJ electrode treatment for dysfunction of jaw joint and supportive tissues responsible for headache; also treat TP's in masseter, pterygoid and other facial muscles. SCM muscle can cause jaw pain and recalcitrant headaches. Treatment sandwiches affected tissues between probe tips and releases TP's very quickly *Polarity:* biphasic *Intensity:* 25 – 75 µA (depending on patient's sensitivity) *Frequency:* 0.3 Hz *Note:* treat bilaterally, even if pain is unilateral or can create more imbalance *Steps:* Attach TMJ extension electrode to counterprobe, insert Q-tip, place 3" segment of plastic straw over shaft. Wet Q-tip. Ask patient to hold TMJ electrode inside mouth at site of pain. Using trigger probe, search and treat acu-points on face.

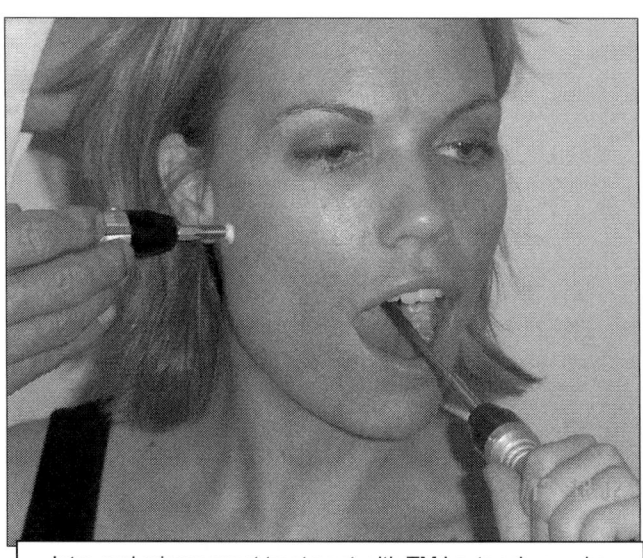

Intra-oral microcurrent treatment with TMJ extension probe

HEAD REGION DISTAL ACU-POINTS, CONT'D

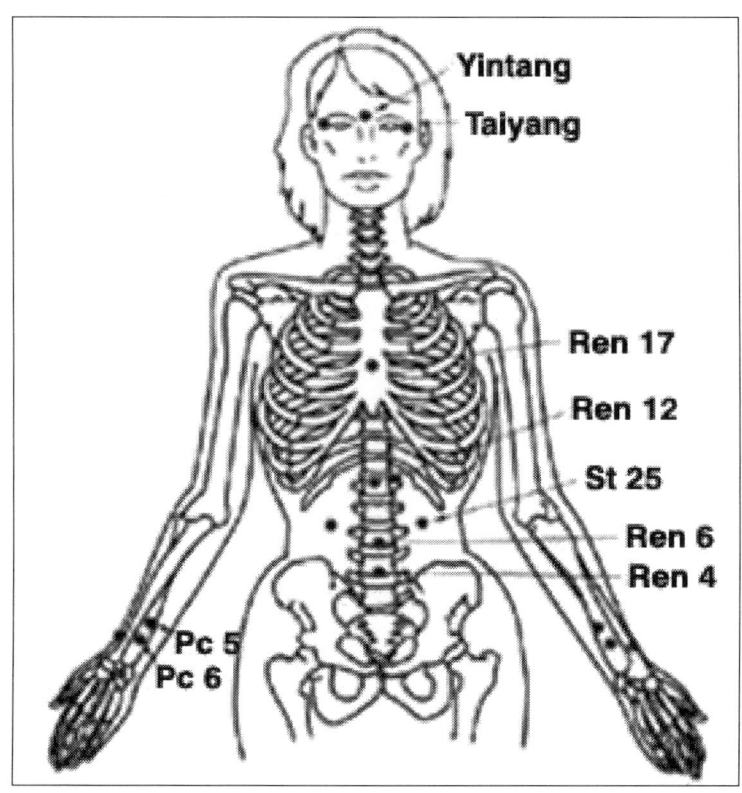

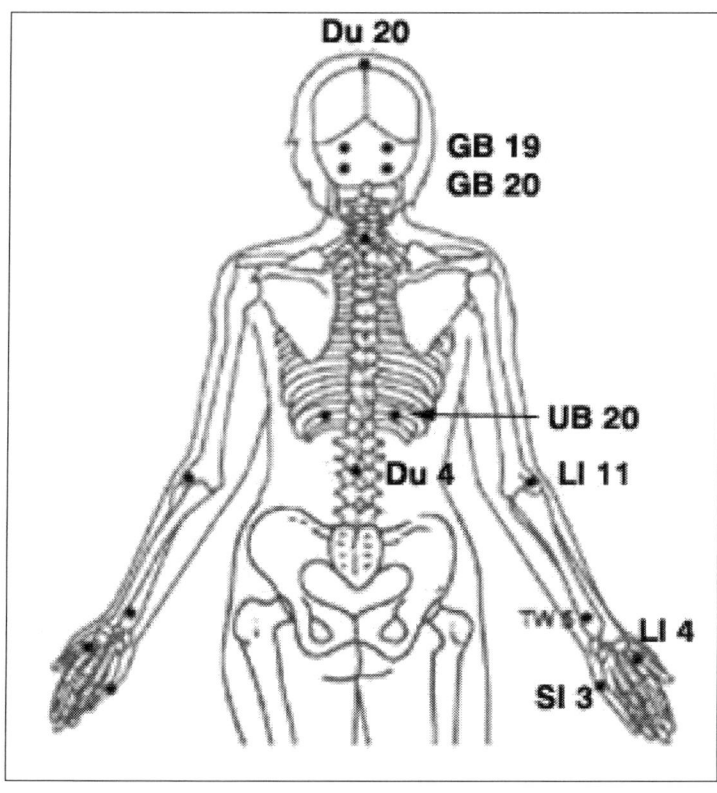

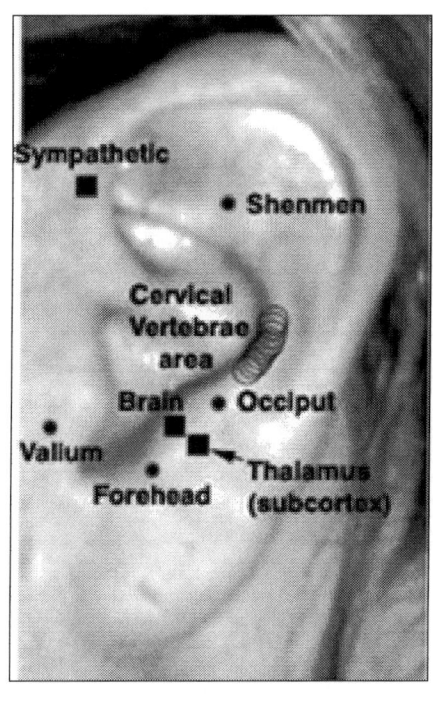

NECK REGION

Trigger Points / Acu-Points	Treatment Protocol & Methods
TP's: Chart 1, pp. 1-3	
Acu-points - Local GB 20, UB 10, and neck nerve root points	**Local Biphasic Probe Treatment for General Neck Release:** Brief biphasic bilateral probe treatment of distal hand points while patient is moving her neck, frequently increases range of motion to significant degree. *Acutron Mentor:* Probe preset #1 *Intensity:* 75 µA *Frequency:* 10 Hz *Time:* 12 seconds per point *Steps:* ask patient to sit up in a chair with her hands palm down on her knees to facilitate stimulating these points. Ask her to practice rotation, side flexion, and forward and backward flexion while the hand points are being stimulated
Acu-points - Distal Hand Points *Release rotation of neck, relax facet joint irritation:* Luozhen, So Jing Dian, SI 3 (have strong effect of releasing restricted ROM of neck)	**Local Biphasic Probe Bilateral Nerve Root Stimulation** *For overall neck and shoulder pain and some headaches, to adjust sympathetic nervous system:* Start at GB 20 and UB 10 and work down the back of the neck in approximately 1" intervals. At each level, use the searching function of your device to select the highest conductivity acu-points and treat them. Palpate along top of trapezius muscle from the acromion to the neck. Place one probe on the sorest, tightest point, with the other probe search for the highest conductivity point along neck nerve roots (C1 to C7) approx.1 " lateral to midline. Treat while patient rotates head away from probes. Repeat on other side.
Acu-points - Local/Distal *Whiplash, acute stiff neck:* Ah shi points of lateral neck (+)→ GB 39 (-) Extraordinary Vessels *Neck rotation problems and torticollis associated with trapezius pain and nervous system / psychological issues:* GB 21, ah shi (+)→ Ht 4 (-) *Recalcitrant trapezius tension and knots:* GB 21 (+)→ GB 41 (-) **Microcurrent IF Pads:** *Whiplash:* GB 20 (+)→ Levator Scapulae TP's/ SI 14 / SI 15 (-)	**Local Polarized Probe Treatment:** **Whiplash, Acute Stiff Neck and Neck Rotational Problems:** See Chapter 7 for device parameters. Such injuries tend to traumatize the smaller and more delicate muscles such as the scalenes and sterno-cleido-mastoid. Origin-insertion probe work is very valuable for treating and adjusting the tone of these muscles. For this application, increase the tone of muscles that have become weakened and slackened, and decrease tone of muscles that feel overly tense. Manaka's Extraordinary Vessel whiplash protocol can be very effective (see Treatment Formulary Section II - Whiplash).

Neck Region Trigger Points

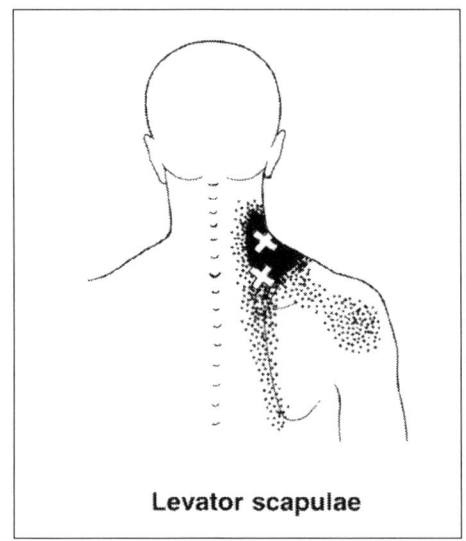

Levator scapulae

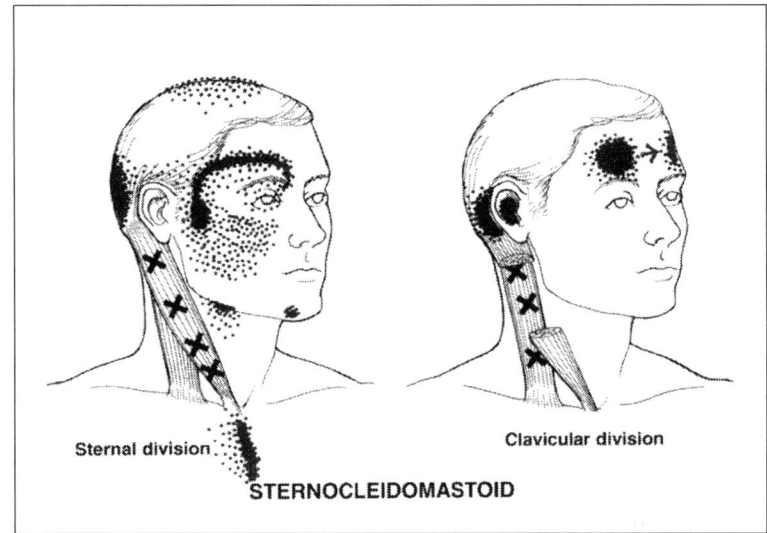

Sternal division · Clavicular division
STERNOCLEIDOMASTOID

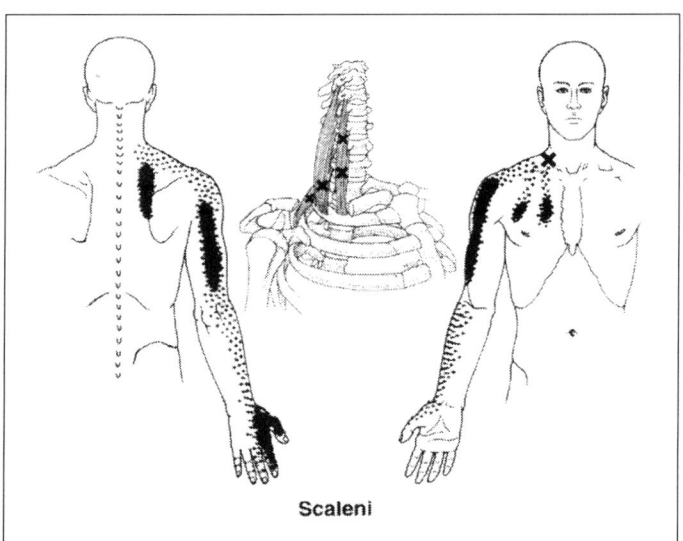

Scaleni

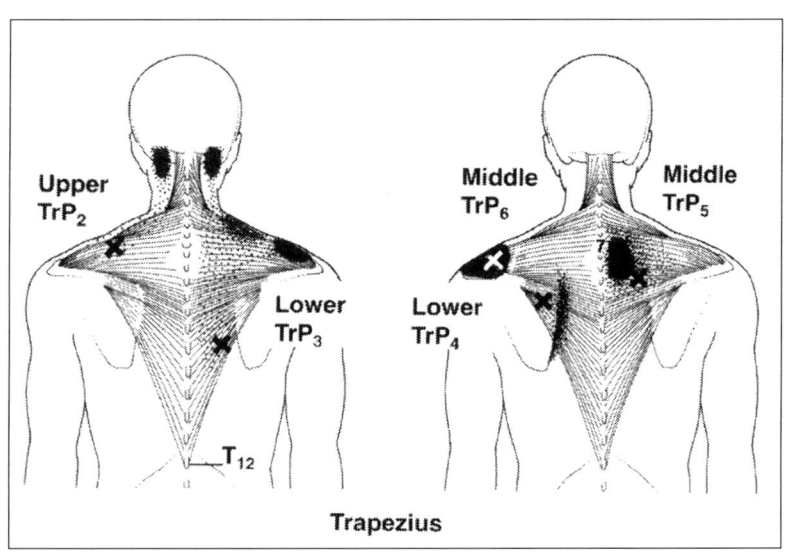

Upper TrP$_2$ · Lower TrP$_3$ · Middle TrP$_6$ · Middle TrP$_5$ · Lower TrP$_4$ · T$_{12}$

Trapezius

NECK REGION, CONTINUED

	Trapezius Tension and Knots: Place (+) probe on tight area on trapezius and the (-) probe on distal GB channel unilaterally, digging into both points with a bit of pressure if possible. Deep releasing breaths on the part of the patient enhances the effect. **Polarized microcurrent interferential pads for Whiplash** Use Acutron Mentor I.F. Pad Preset #3.

Other Treatment Techniques:

Sotai-Type Neck Treatment *for Rotational Problems:*
Determine which direction of neck movement is most restricted, and choose a tight adjacent acu-point that is related to the constriction. Stimulate it while the patient moves his head toward the unrestricted side, while exhaling. When he reaches the maximum point of arc, use your hand to place some resistance against his movement while he holds his breath for a few seconds. Then, remove stimulation and tell him to relax completely and breathe deeply. Recheck ROM and if there is not a clear improvement, choose a different treatment point or different movement pattern and try again. Use caution with patients having degenerative disk disorders of the neck.
Degenerative Cervical Disks:
When disk degeneration leads to neck pain and stiffness, some practitioners have found neck traction with simultaneous microcurrent interferential pad stimulation through the affected area very valuable. Before using this method, it is essential that any pronounced tilt of the head and neck to one side be corrected first. This can be accomplished through combinations of extraordinary vessel treatment, origin-insertion balancing of the muscles of the neck (see Chapter 7), chiropractic manipulation, or myofascial release methods.

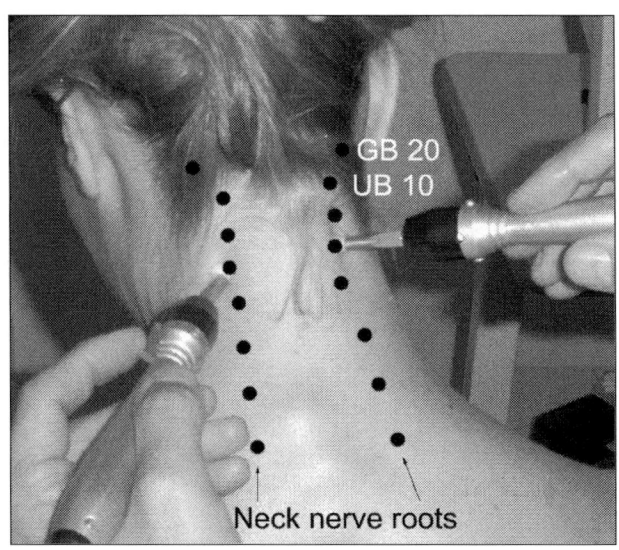

TREATMENT FORMULARY I: BY BODY AREA 239

NECK REGION DISTAL ACU-POINTS

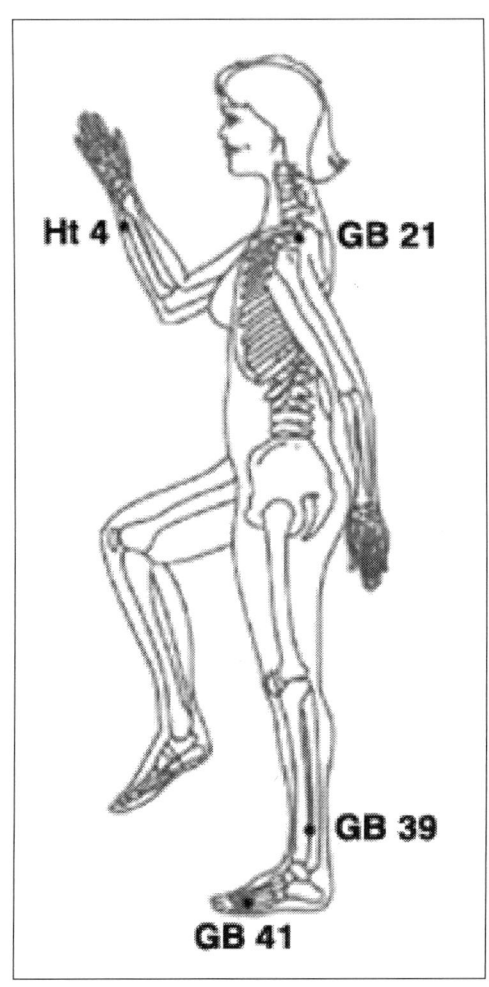

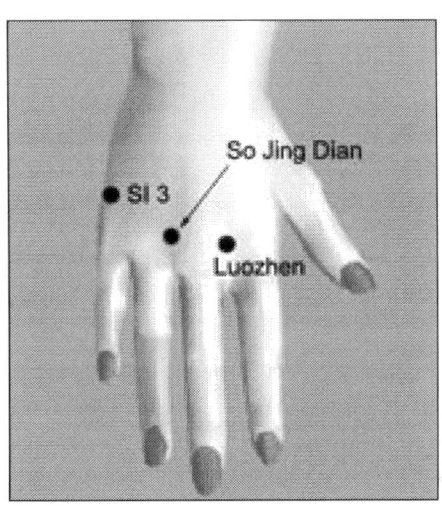

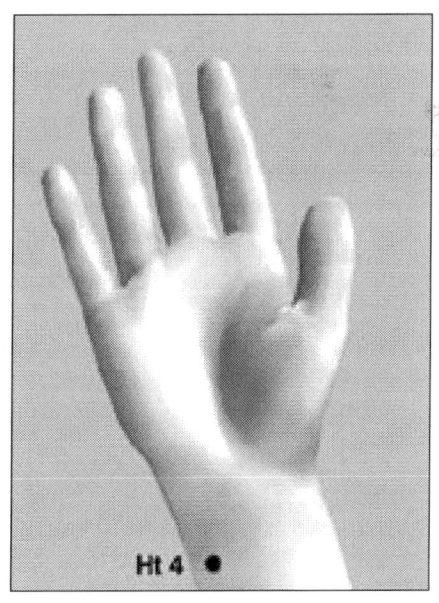

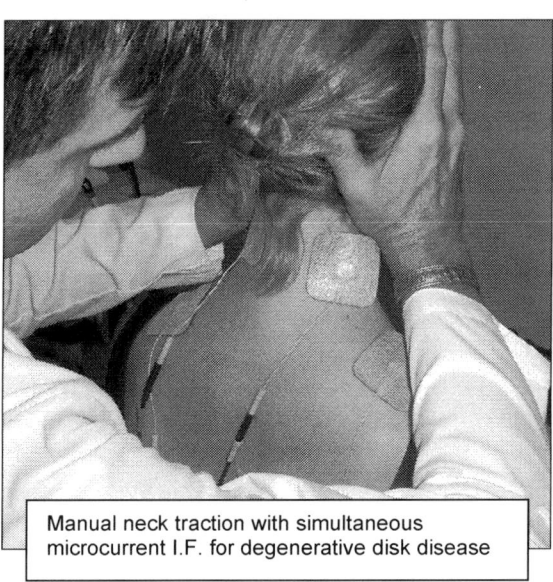

Manual neck traction with simultaneous microcurrent I.F. for degenerative disk disease

SHOULDER REGION

TRIGGER POINTS / ACU-POINTS	TREATMENT METHODS AND PROTOCOLS
TP's: Chart 2, pp. 4-9	TP release in specific muscles of the rotator cuff is especially important for effective treatment of the complex shoulder joint. Shoulder treatment through specific muscles may be performed as follows:
Levator Scapula: Elevates the scapula and rotates the scapula downwards. Elevates and retracts the scapula with the trapezius. This muscle is a common cause of acute torticollis and posterior shoulder and neck pain. When TP's are active, pain may radiate up into the neck/occiput or down into scapula. Pain usually predominates on one side. **Acu-points - Distal** *Neck rotation limitation:* TP (+)→ SI 3 (-) (good overall distal point for this muscle) *Neck flexion/extension:* TP (+) → UB 60/ 62 (-) *Acute Torticolis & Whiplash:* TP (+)→GB 39 (-) **I.F. Pads:** GB 20 (+) SI 14/SI 15 (-)	**Local-Distal Polarized Probe treatment** TP (+) → distal point on same or related meridian (-) **Microcurrent I.F. pads (Acutron I.F. #3) treatment** GB 20 (+) → levator scapula SI 14 / SI 15 area (-)
Supraspinatus: Abducts humerus at the shoulder joint, stabilizes the glenohumeral joint. When TP's are active can cause deep pain in the deltoid region that may radiate down the arm toward acu-point LI 11, mimicking symptoms of "tennis elbow". Arm may be difficult to raise above head. **Acu-points - Local:** Jianneling, LI 16, SI 10, SI 15 **Acu-points - Distal:** SI 3	**Local-Distal Polarized Probe treatment** (TP +, distal point -) **Local Biphasic Treatment ("Circling the Dragon")** **Polarized Pad Treatment** Polarized microamp pads run from local TP's (+) to distal SI points (-) with simultaneous stretching
Infraspinatus: Stabilizes the humeral head in the glenoid fossa, and facilitates lateral rotation of the humerus at the shoulder. Active TP's in infraspinatus also present with deep pain in the shoulder join, aggravated by reaching hand behind back such as to hook a bra. Pain may be localized or may radiate down the arm, approximately along the Lung channel. May aggravate or mimic carpal tunnel syndrome.	**Treatment principles and points are the same as for Supraspinatus, except for location of local TP's.**

SHOULDER REGION TRIGGER POINTS

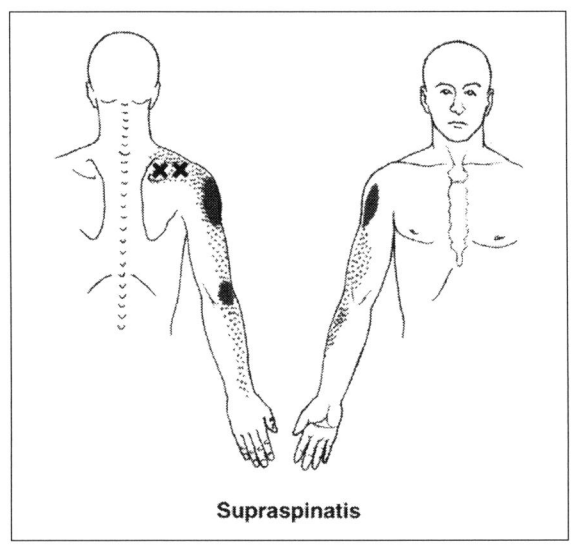
Supraspinatus

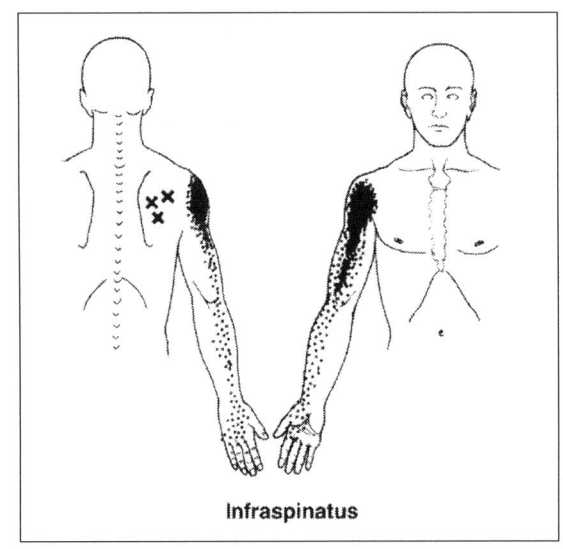
Infraspinatus

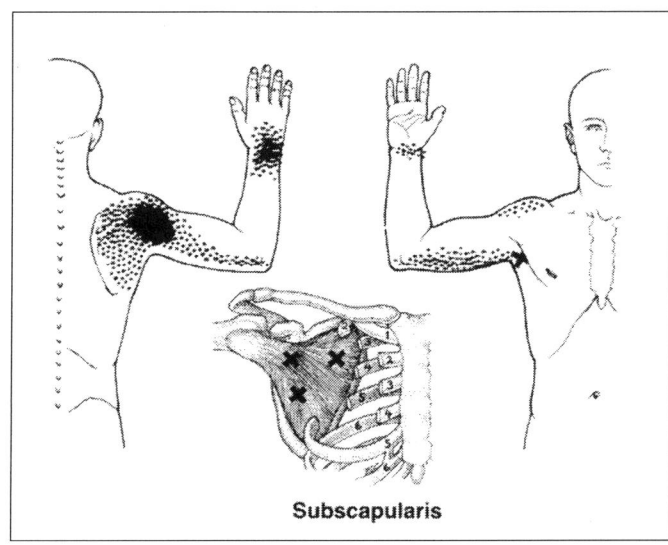
Subscapularis

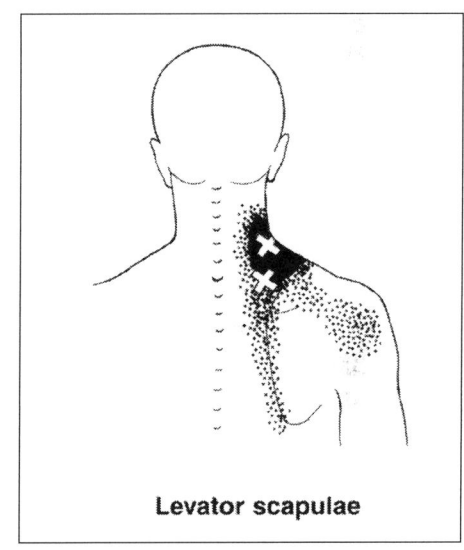
Levator scapulae

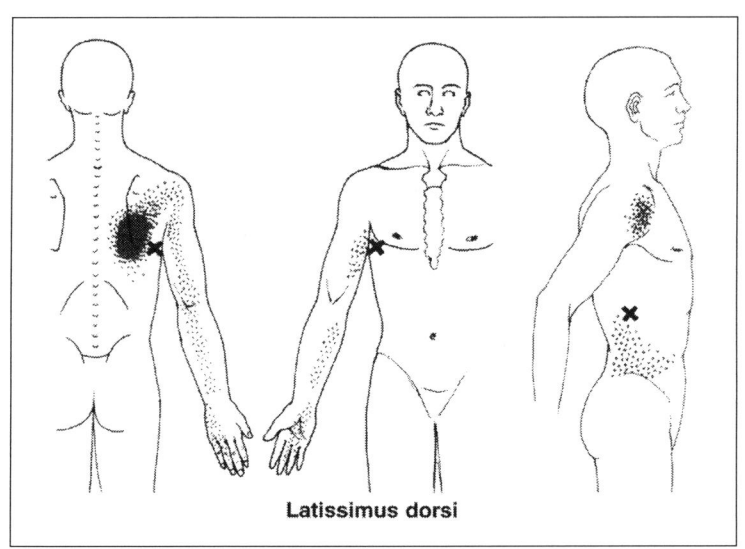
Latissimus dorsi

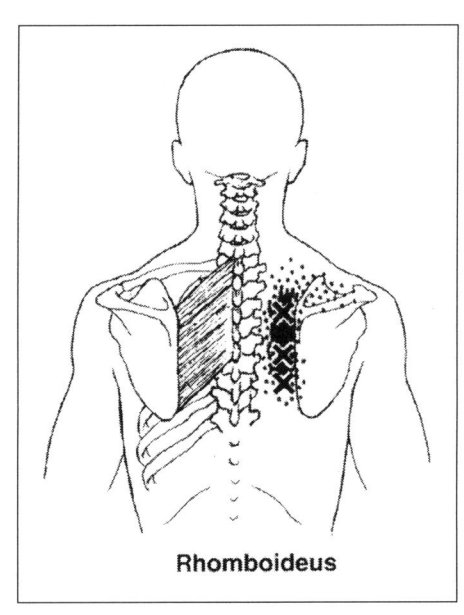
Rhomboideus

SHOULDER REGION, CONTINUED

TRIGGER POINTS / ACU-POINTS	TREATMENT METHODS AND PROTOCOLS
Subscapularis: Stabilizes the gleno-humeral joint and effects medial rotation of the humerus at the shoulder. Often associated with "Frozen shoulder" syndrome, which may be caused by build-up of adhesions and tightening of the tissues surrounding the gleno-humeral joint. **TP's in axillary region** **Acu-points - Distal:** ST 38, GB 34, SP 9a (opposite quadrant of body) **Acu-points - Local:** Ah shi points along medial border of scapula	**Local Biphasic Treatment ("Circling the Dragon")** Connect axillary TP's with tender areas along medial border of scapula **Local-Distal Polarized Probe treatment** **Electro-massage / 4-pad Microcurrent Interferential Pad Treatment:** Place 1 pad of each channel on neck or below clavicle and other pads on therapists hands. Wet neck area. Use to gradually release adhesions using cross-fiber friction massage techniques *Intensity:* 200-600 µA **Local Polarized Probe / Distal Needle Treatment** Alternatively, use acupuncture needles on distal leg points and periodically manipulate while applying microcurrent therapies to shoulder. May be enhanced by briefly using polarized probes to connect shoulder TP's with distal needles.
Rhomboid Major and Minor: Retracts and elevates the scapula, helps to rotate the scapula downwards. These muscles may become painful due to poor posture or uneven muscle development, with pectoralis developed much more than upper back muscles. Pain is felt between shoulder blades and ropy, tight bands may be palpated under medial border of scapulae. Area may become hypersensitive when energy stagnation of Lungs has gone on for a long time, or patient is holding unresolved grief. **TP's in scapula region** **Acu-points - Distal:** Chung Tze, Chung Hsien **Acu-points - Local:** Hua-To points along thoracic spinal nerve roots Ah shi points along medial border of scapula	**Local-Distal Polarized Probe treatment** Painful area (+)→ distal hand points (-) **Local Biphasic Treatment ("Circling the Dragon")** Place one probe along thoracic spinal nerve roots and other along medial border or scapula, or alternatively both probes stimulating pairs of paints along medial border of scapula **Microcurrent Pads treatment (Acutron µA Pad Preset #5)** Place pads in an "x" pattern to stimulate entire region between scapulae. *Waveform:* sloped *Intensity:* 25 - 50 µA *Frequency:* low Hz **Microcurrent I.F. pads treatment** Stimulate entire region of rhomboids and trapezius with simultaneous stretching/exercise for sports injuries and rehabilitation **NOTE:** Do not pass any current across thoracic spine with patients with diagnosed or suspected cardiac disease or with a pacemaker. Probe treatments may be used with caution for such patients under medical supervision.

TREATMENT FORMULARY I: BY BODY AREA 243

SHOULDER REGION ACU-POINTS

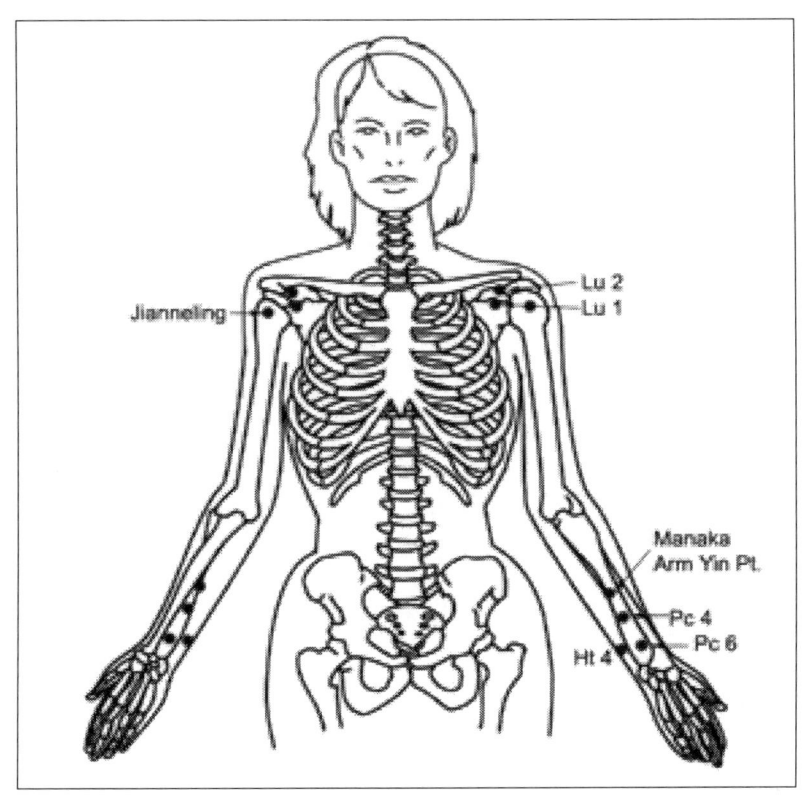
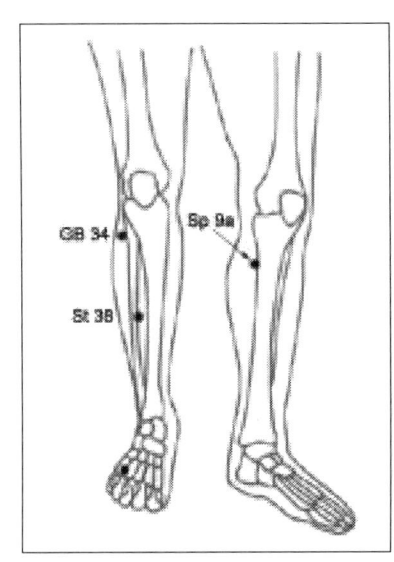
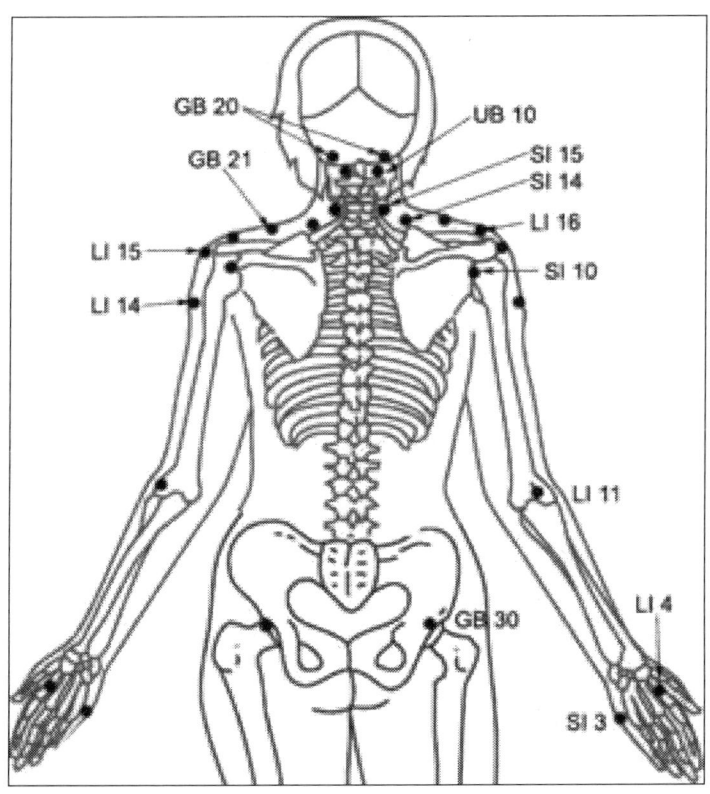
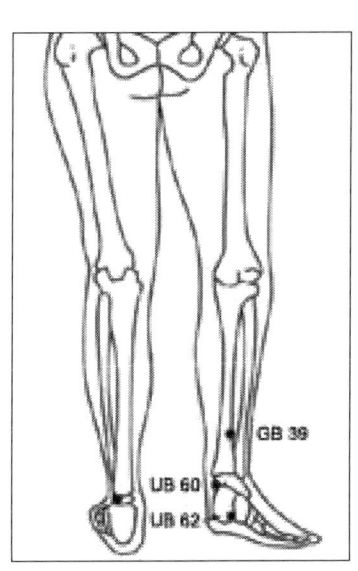

SHOULDER REGION, continued

TRIGGER POINTS / ACU-POINTS /	TREATMENT METHODS AND PROTOCOLS
Generalized Shoulder Pain **Acu-points - Local point combinations** LI 15 → LI 4, LI 15 → LI11, SI 10 → Lu 1 or Lu 2, LI 16 → LI 14, UB 10 → LI 11, C5-6 nerve roots → LI 15, SI 10 →Jianneling **Acu-points - Local-Distal Point combinations** *Frozen Shoulder:* Shoulder ah shi → contrateral St 38, GB 34, Sp 9a (palpate for most sensitive point 1-2 cun below Sp 9) *Trapezius area of whole shoulder painful:* Mostly GB channel: GB 21 (ah shi location), → GB 30 or GB 41 (most tender side) or Ht 4 area *Frontal shoulder pain and pectoral area:* Jianneling (ah shi location on anterior shoulder)→ St 41 or Sp 9a, choose leg with most tender points. Use distal PC meridain points for pectoral area P 4 - 6, or Manaka arm yin point between P3 and 4)[231] *Shoulder abduction problems* Use Large Intestine or Triple Warmer channel. *Difficulty touching the opposite shoulder by reaching across chest* Use Lung or Triple Warmer channel **Acu-points - Ear** Shoulder, shoulder joint, upper arm, thoracic vertebrae, zero, shenmen, adrenal, triple warmer	**Local-Distal Polarized Probe treatment** Using probes, connect the tightest point on the shoulder with appropriate distal points while patient repeatedly mobilizes her shoulder, trying to extend the range of motion. In spirit of sotai, it is sometimes helpful to stimulate and mobilize the opposite (healthy) shoulder when local treatment fails. Local ah shi (+), distal (-) in most cases **Myofascial Release Technique** Using Ear shoulder point, mobilize shoulder, or treat distal acup-points on opposite side and mobilize shoulder. **Electro-massage with Simultaneous Movement for Restricted Shoulder** This technique sometimes has great success. The advantage of this method is that you can feel the changes in the tissues with your fingers as treatment is administered, and can adapt your bodywork technique to follow the patient's response. **Adhesive capsulitis** Use cross-fiber friction electro-massage technique, gradually working out restricted areas. Negative polarity current has tissue softening properties, so for this condition use polarized I.F. treatment so that your massaging hand has two (-) pads on them, while two (+) pads are at least 6' away, placed so that the pathway of current passes through the tight areas. (I.F. #3) **Distal needling or microcurrent probe** of lower extremity points is also valuable while exercising the shoulder through its range of motion. **Trigger Point Release** may be necessary in the following muscles: Levator scapulae, upper trapezius, rhomboids, posterior seratus, pectoralis major, latissimus dorsi and quadratus lumborum. Origin/Insertion (O/I) technique is also applicable for specific muscles. See trigger points information above for specifics.

Jina's magic shoulder formula (using pads) - 10, 10, 10
1. Milliamp: 10 minutes turned up to strong tingling at 30 Hz (Acutron mA preset #1, modify Hz)
2. High microamp: 10 minutes 300 µA 30 Hz (Acutron uA preset #1, modify Hz and intensity)
3. Low microamp: 10 minutes 50 µA 0.3 Hz (same preset as above, modify Hz and intensity again)

---

[231] Between P 3 and P 4, palpate for most sensitive point

TREATMENT FORMULARY I: BY BODY AREA   245

SHOULDER REGION – AURICULAR PTS/ MICROCURRENT TECHNIQUES

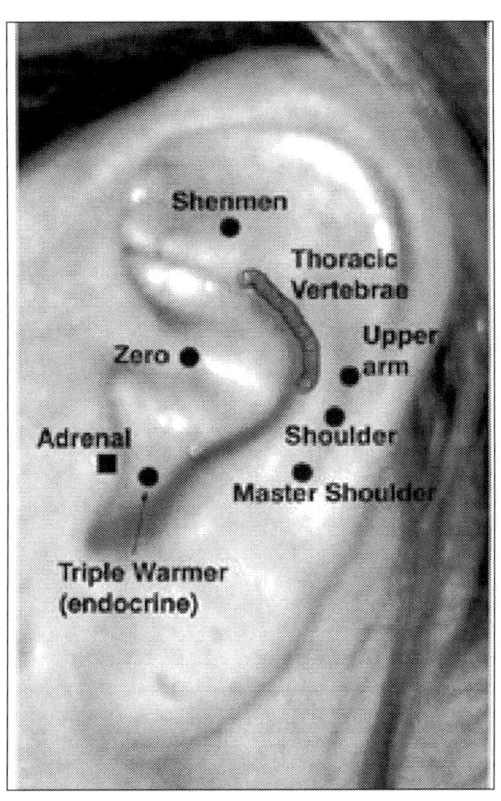

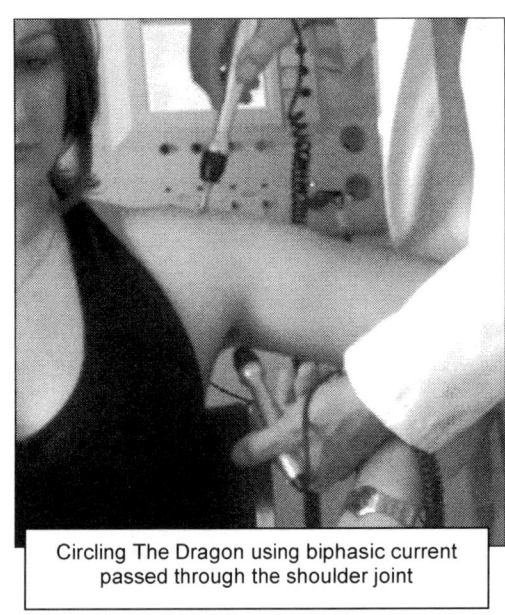

Circling The Dragon using biphasic current passed through the shoulder joint

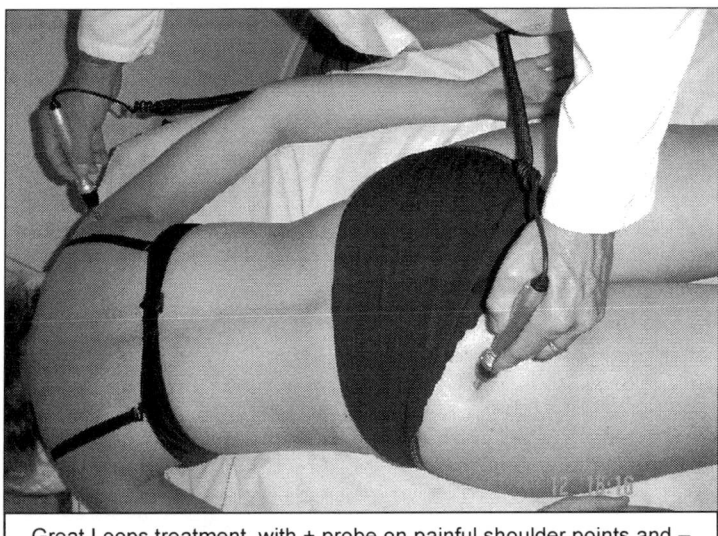

Great Loops treatment, with + probe on painful shoulder points and – probe on tender points on opposite hip

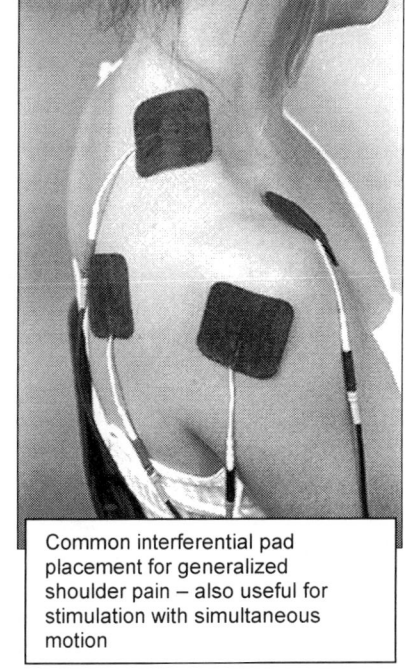

Common interferential pad placement for generalized shoulder pain – also useful for stimulation with simultaneous motion

ELBOW AREA

TRIGGER POINTS / ACU-POINTS	TREATMENT PROTOCOL & METHODS
TP's: Chart 2, pp. 8-9 **Acu-points - Local point combinations** LI 11 → H 3, P3 → TW 11, P3 → P7, P3 → Ling Ku, LI 11 → LI 4 or LI 5 C5-8 nerve roots → ah shi points of elbow *Arthritic pain, add:* H 4, SI 4, TW 3, TW 5 when tender **Acu-points - Local/Distal combinations** (+) Local ah shi, (-) distal Local ah shi → opposite GB 33/GB 34, Sp 9/ Sp 9a, or tender leg St point(s) 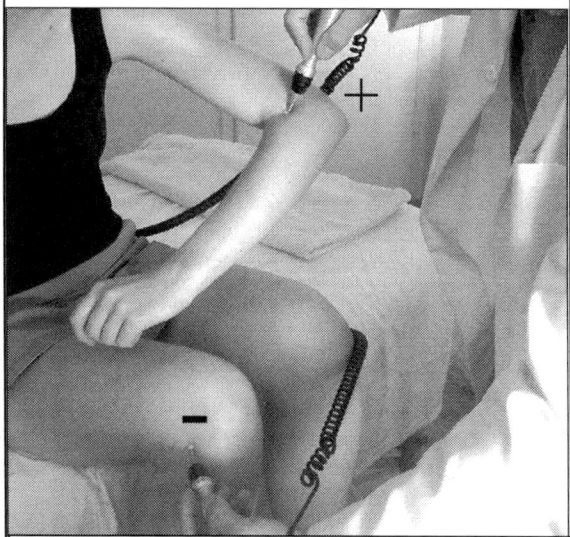 Great Loops treatment from painful elbow region to tender point on opposite knee	**Local, Biphasic "Circling The Dragon" Stimulation Using Dual Probes:** Choose point combinations that pass microcurrent through the affected area, and search and treat each set in 6-second increments until the conductivity meter reaches its maximum. Then move onto the next set of two points and repeat. It is best to use palpation to choose the most significant points to treat, then use GSR meter guidance to zero in on the exact points to stimulate. **Proximal - Local Point Treatment** Place (+) probe on proximal C5-C8 nerve roots, on area of lateral neck or other proximal affected area around shoulders or pectoral girdle, and (-) probe on painful local points on elbow. Treat each set of points until conductivity meter peaks. **Local - Distal Point Treatment** Place (+) probe on local painful points on elbow and (-) probe on distal points on opposite knee area. Select distal points that are tender to palpation and have meridian relationships to affected elbow area (see Chapter 8) **Polarized Interferential Microcurrent Pad Treatment** For longer-standing cases, polarized interferential microcurrent pad placements should be used after completing probe work (2-3 minutes). Using Acutron I.F. preset #3, use "Dermatome Interferential" placement shown on previous page. Use both sets of pads and set them up in a crossing pattern. Once pads are in place and treatment current has been turned on, instruct the patient to gently move the elbow through its range of motion. Watch for areas of pain and restriction, and work with these areas through additional probe work, needling, or electro-massage.

TREATMENT FORMULARY I: BY BODY AREA 247

ELBOW REGION ACU-POINTS

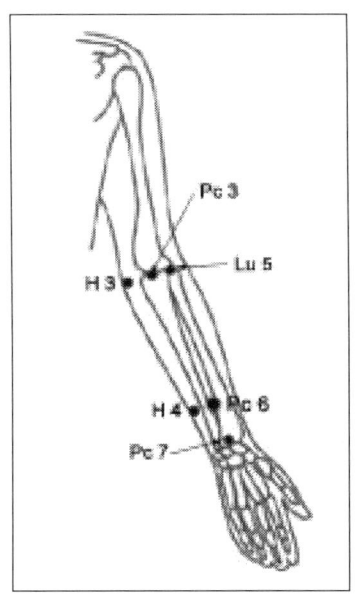

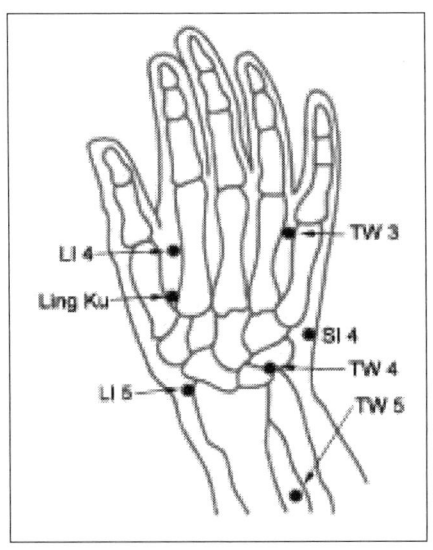

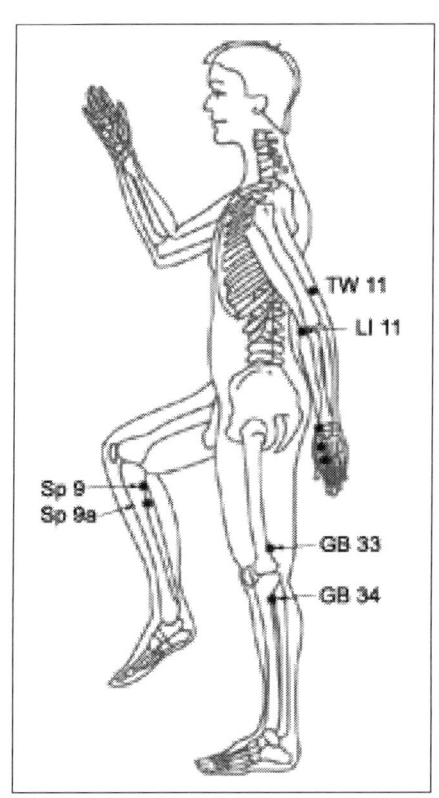

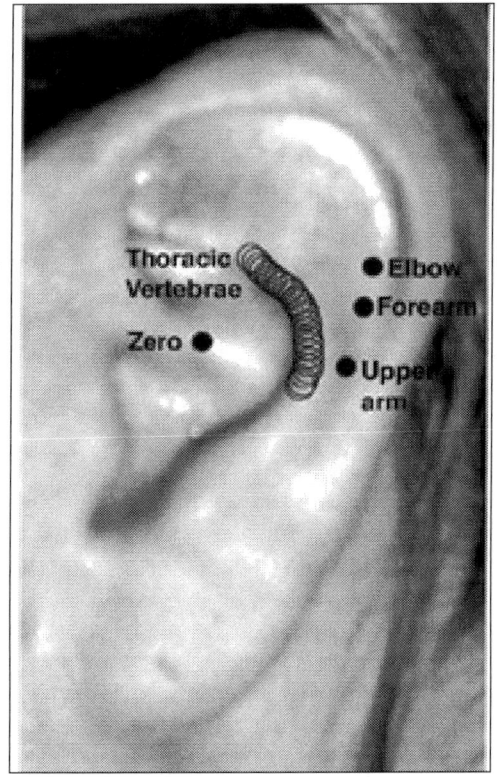

FOREARMS, WRISTS AND HANDS

TRIGGER POINTS / ACU-POINTS	TREATMENT PROTOCOL & METHODS
TP's: Chart 3, pp. 10-11 for forearm and hand pain Chart 2, pp. 4-9 for proximal TP's that can refer pain to the arms and hands. **Local Point Combinations:** LI 10 → LI 4 or LI 5 P 3 → P 7 P 6 → TW 5 (often treated with one needle through technique) LI 11 → Baxie points (between knuckles) TW 4 → Baxie points Lu 10 → L1 4 LI 4 → SI 3 or SI 4 C6-C8 nerve roots of neck (+) → local ah shi points (-) **Local - Distal Point Combinations:** Local ah shi points → opposite St 41, Lv 4 or other tender ankle points Wrists: St 41, Lv 4 or other tender ankle points on opposite side, P 3 on same side, tender proximal points along affected arm channels, for proximal stimulation.	**Local, Biphasic "Circling The Dragon" Stimulation Using Dual Probes** **Polarized "Great Loops" Probe Treatment** Connect local points of pain to reactive distal points (see facing page) (use following local, biphasic treatment above) **Polarized Interferential Microcurrent Pad Treatment** etic electro therapy is very useful. Probe treatment can followed by pad treatments connecting spinal nerve roots h local regions. The affected joint can be gently exercised ile stimulation is applied. **Carpal Tunnel Syndrome:** Start with polarized probe treatment along local dermatomes or through Great Loops technique, connecting to opposite quadrant of body. Can be followed with polarized interferential microcurrent (I.F. #3). For channel A, place (+) pad over C6-C8 nerve roots of the neck, and (-) pad over the heel of the hand. For channel B, place two pads on the ulnar and radial sides of the wrist, respectively, so as to sandwich the affected area between them.

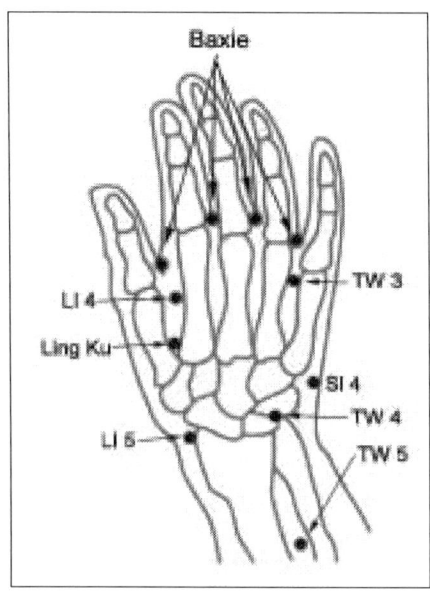

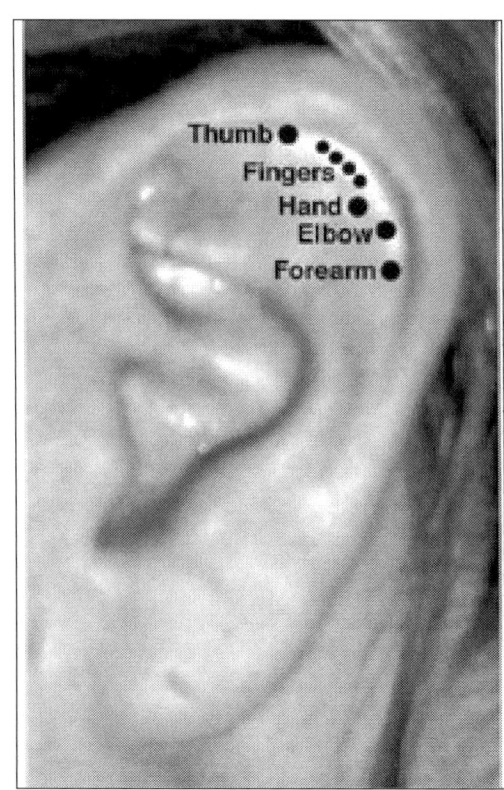

FOREARM, WRISTS AND HANDS REGION

Trigger Points

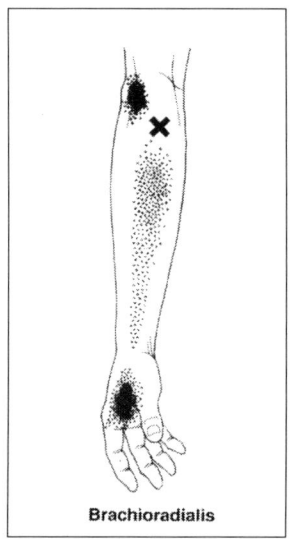
Brachioradialis

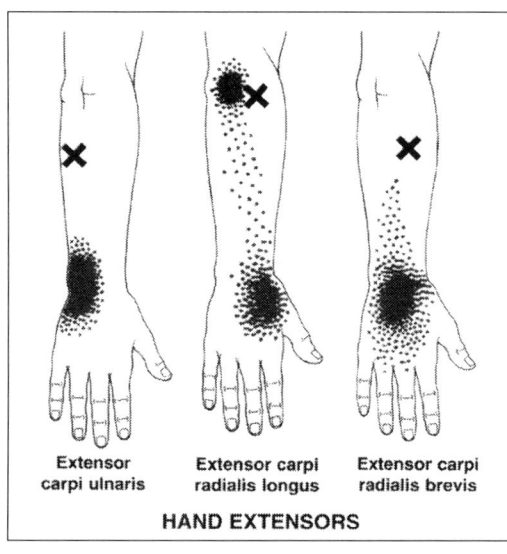
Extensor carpi ulnaris | Extensor carpi radialis longus | Extensor carpi radialis brevis
HAND EXTENSORS

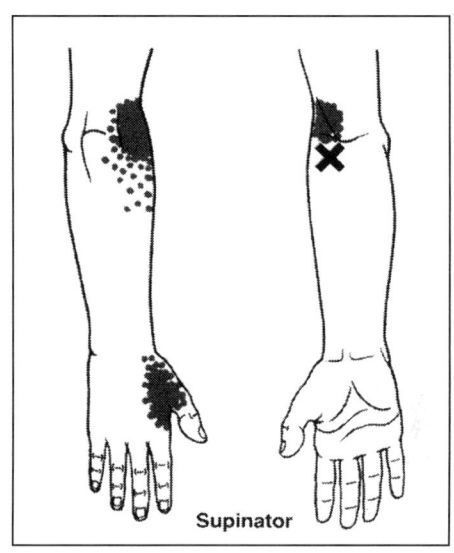
Supinator

Acu-Points

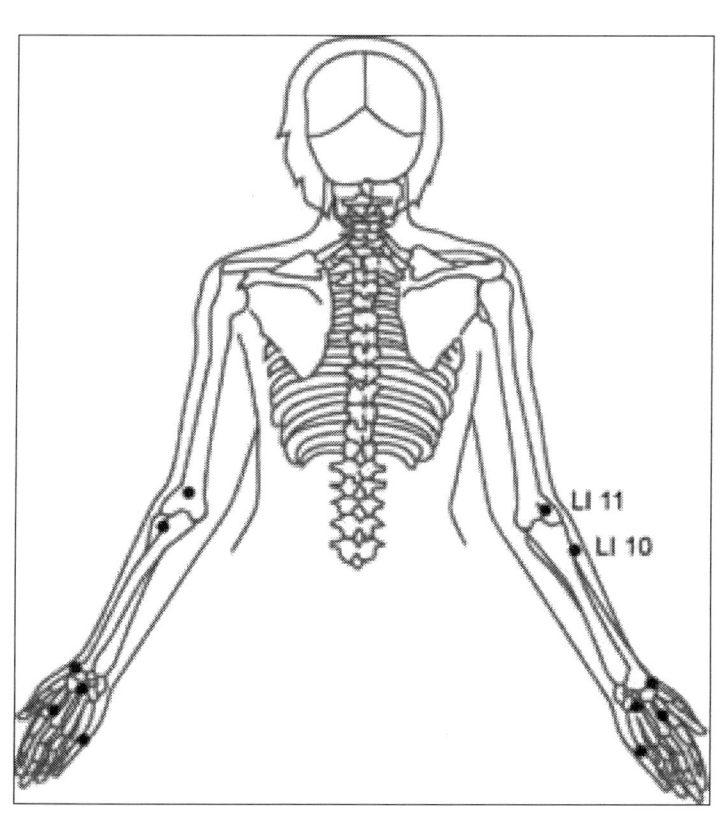
LI 11
LI 10

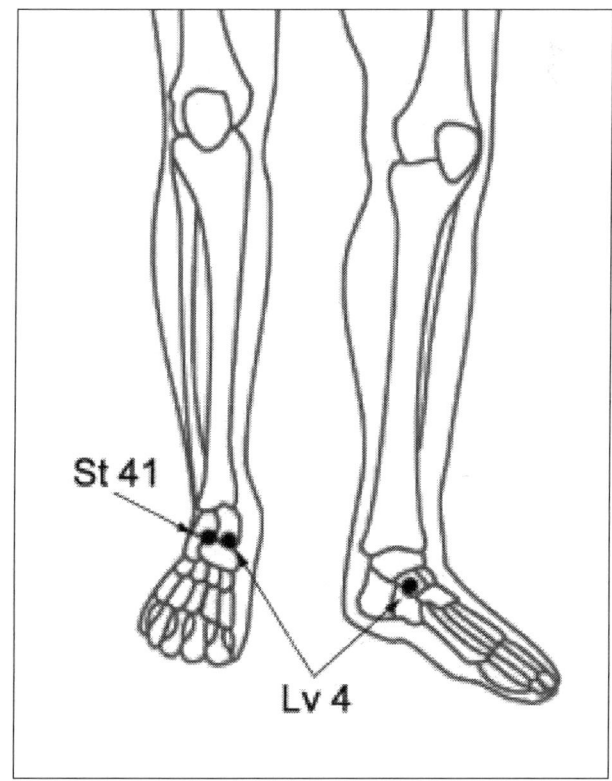
St 41
Lv 4

ABDOMINAL AREA

TRIGGER POINTS / ACU-POINTS	TREATMENT PROTOCOL & METHODS
TP's: Chart 4, pp. 13-14 **Acu-point - Local Combinations:** Microcurrent Mu-Shu techniques: Alarm points (+) →Back-Shu points (-) St 25 bilaterally Circle Dragon around umbilicus Sacral foramen (Liao points) → tender abdominal points Treat other points directly, especially those that refer pain elsewhere Consider Ren 3, Ren 4, Ren 6, Ren 9, Ren 12, St 30 and the Kidney channel **Acu-point - Local/Distal Combinations:** Proximal (+), Distal (-) Ren 6 or Ren 12 → St 36 St 25 → St 36 TW 15 → GB 34 Abdominal ah shi → Sp 6 or Sp 4 Genital area → Lv 6 or 8 Ren 12 → P 6 P 6 → St 36 (check polarity with kinesiology since both points are distal) **IMPORTANT NOTE:** Abdominal cross-currents are contra-indicated in the case of cancer of the abdominal organs, active bleeding, or during pregnancy.	**Important Caution:** In cases of pain in the abdomen, it is vital to first give or refer the patient for a thorough medical examination to check for disease of the internal organs that may require emergency intervention, such as appendicitis, colon cancer or stomach ulcers. Once these are ruled out or dealt with, acupuncture treatment can proceed. **Step One and Two Root Treatments:** Step One Balancing of Extraordinary Vessels and Step Two treatment of Back Shu points are indicated prior to direct treatment of abdominal pain, and such Root treatment may go a long way toward clearing it. **Dispersion of TP's in Abdominal Area** Dispersion of TP's can have far-reaching beneficial effects. In many cases. These TP's can cause dysfunction of the internal organs through retardation of the free flow of Qi and Blood. This can eventually lead to Blood stasis, which can degenerate into tumors and severe organ disease. Dispersion of abdominal TP's to prevent and treat organ dysfunction is frequently overlooked treatment of great significance. Japanese acupuncture methods focus on this much more than is commonly practiced in TCM and other styles. **Local-Distal Polarized Probe treatment** painful abdominal points (+)→ distal points (-) It is often beneficial to use distal points on the same or related channels as the local point. For example, you can create circuits between St 25 and St 36, or TW 15 and P 6 (Yin-Yang couple relationship) **Electro-massage / 4-pad Microcurrent Interferential Pad Treatment:** Place 1 pad of each channel on lower back, choosing tender or tight point, and place the other two pads on the backs of therapist's hands, so that when the patient is touched the current pathways will crisscross from right to left and vice-versa. Palpate for constricted areas, nodules, ropy regions and weak, collapsed areas, and use appropriate manual massage methods to release or support these. Polarity therapy method has been utilized to release abdominal TP's with success. This involves holding the resistant abdominal point with one hand, and a reactive distal point down the leg or on the low back with the other hand. The patient then holds their breath until the therapist feels an equal pulsing through the two points, after which the patient releases the breath.

TREATMENT FORMULARY I: BY BODY AREA 251

ABDOMINAL REGION ACU-POINTS

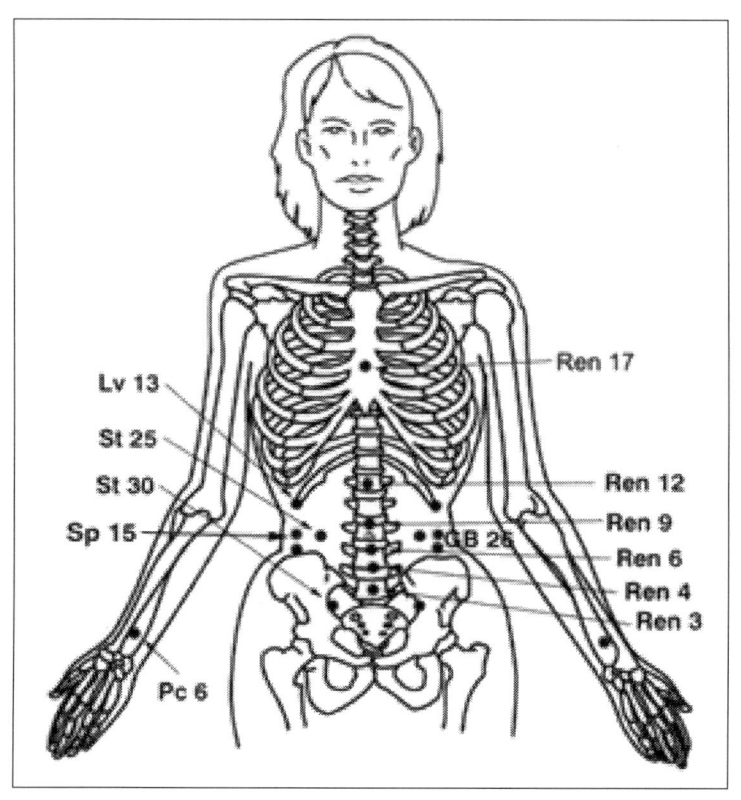

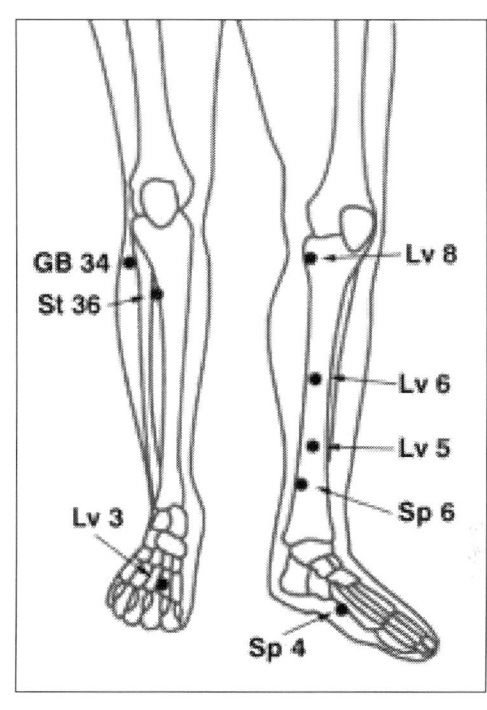

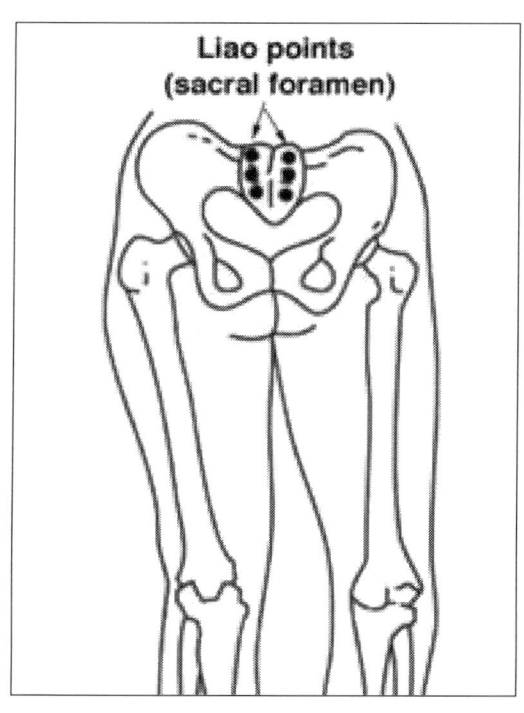

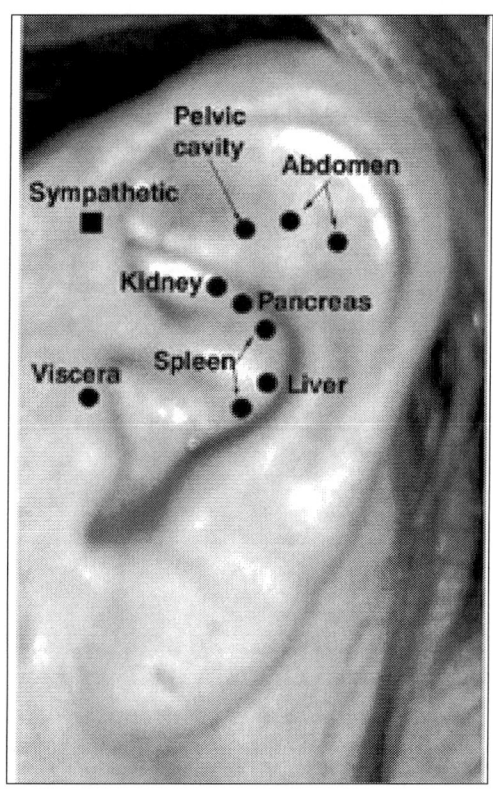

Low Back

Trigger Points / Acu-Points	Treatment Protocol & Methods
TP's: Chart 4, pp. 12-14 **Acu-point - Local Combinations:** UB 22 or UB 23 → UB 25 GB 25 bilaterally *Any painful spinal section:* Bilateral ah shi or Back Shu points Anterior-posterior treatment - Abdominal TP's (+), painful back points (-) Bilateral treatment of sacral foramen and sacro-iliac joint TP's **Acu-point - Local/Distal Combinations:** Proximal (+), Distal (-) UB 23 → UB 40 Back ah shi points → UB 58, UB 58 1/2[232] or UB 61-62 area (choose tender spot) UB 23 → K 2 or K 3 GB 26 → GB 40 Ah shi points → "Ling Ku combination"[233] of hand on opposite side to back pain, GB 26, UB 2 on face for acute disorders (needle or (-) probe) *Whole back release:* UB 10 (+) → UB 40 (-), SI 3 (+) → UB 62 (-) **Acu-points - Ear** Lumbo-sacral, thoracic vertebrae, buttocks, sciatica, lumbago, zero, shenmen	**Local-Distal Polarized Probe treatment** Back ah shi (+), distal point (-); Use kinesiology to confirm polarities, and reverse if indicated. To release the whole dorsal region, use UB 10(+) → UB 40 (-) To open dorsal region, use points SI 3 (+) → UB 62 (-) **Local Biphasic Treatment ("Circling the Dragon")** Connect ah shi points and to create cross-hatching stimulation pattern over painful areas. **Polarized Pad Treatment** Polarized microamp pads run from local TP's (+) to distal S-I points (-) with simultaneous mobilization. **4-pad Interferential Pad Treatment:** Interferential therapies can be very effective for acute back pain. The I.F. combination therapy, which provide a few minutes of intense classic IF followed by gentle microcurrent IF, is one of the most popular I.F. treatments for this purpose (I.F. #5). Adding simultaneous microcurrent or needle stimulation to distal points such as Ling Ku, Zong Bai, UB 40 or 58 can enhance results **Sotai** is excellent for relaxing tight back muscles. See the example given in Chapter 13, plus further techniques given in the books <u>Chasing the Dragon's Tail</u> and <u>Hara Diagnosis</u>.[234] **Electro-massage / 4-pad Microcurrent Interferential Pad Treatment:** Place 1 pad of each channel on rectus abdominus muscles of the abdomen with the patient lying prone on the treatment table. Place the other two pads, one from each channel, on the backs of therapists hands. The therapist positions his hand over the patient's right low back (same channel as the pad on his <u>left</u> abdomen and vice-versa). This forms a crossing pattern of the two current pathways throughout the abdominal/lower back area. After wetting the low back area and turning on the current, palpate and massage all the tight and restricted areas of the low back.

---

[232] UB 58 1/2 is a special Japanese point on the lateral gastrocnemius muscle below UB 58 that is found by palpation
[233] This consists of the extra points Ling Ku, Da Bai, and Zong Bail as described by Dr. Richard Tan in his book "*12 and 12 in Acupuncture*"
[234] By Matsumoto and Birch, Paradigm Publications, 1988

Low Back Region
Trigger Points/Head Acu-Points

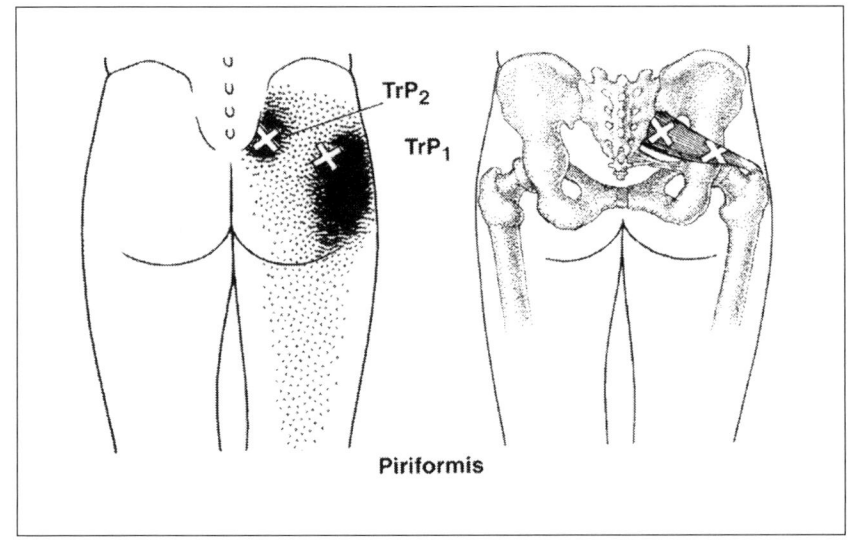

Piriformis

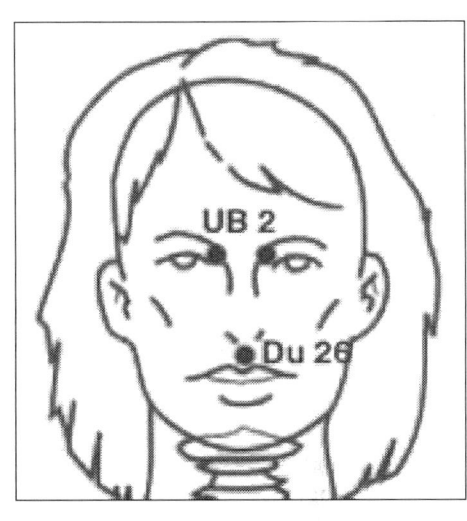

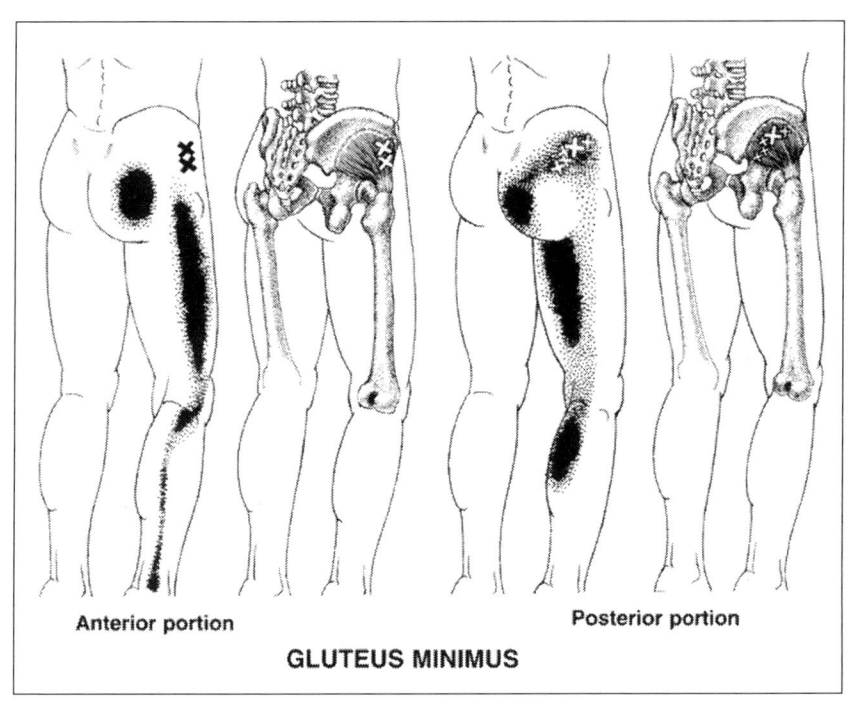

GLUTEUS MINIMUS — Anterior portion / Posterior portion

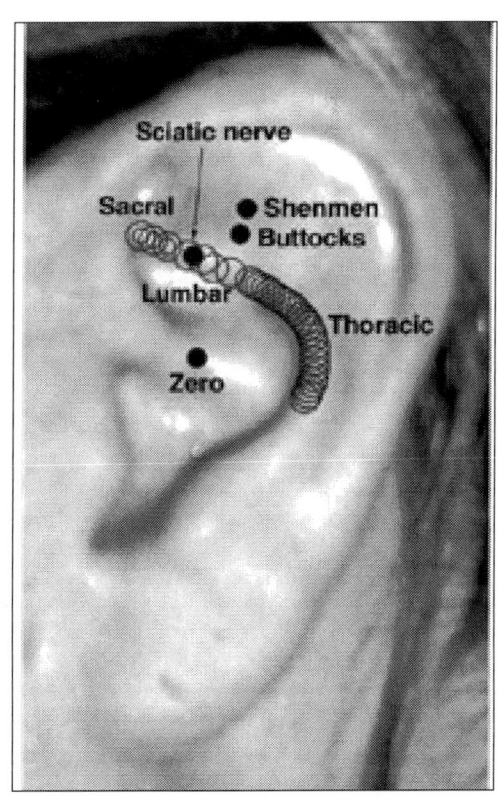

LOW BACK, CONTINUED

TRIGGER POINTS / ACU-POINTS	TREATMENT PROTOCOL & METHODS
	Some simple sotai moves can be added into this approach, such as raising the leg off the table that is looser, and holding and lowering it as explained above while stimulating a significant TP on the back or leg. **Hatha Yoga** Another useful approach for patients that are in the rehabilitative stage of treatment is to perform simple hatha yoga postures and movements with simultaneous microcurrent stimulation. Yoga is one of the finest ways to prevent musculoskeletal disorders, and to heal them once they have occurred. The addition of microcurrent with the postures can help make a stiff patient's muscles and ligaments more flexible and plastic to facilitate neuromuscular re-education. The Cobra yoga pose to be particularly helpful for many kinds of disk disorders, and the addition of simultaneous microcurrent interferential or probe treatments can help adjust the disk's support muscles. This pose is not appropriate for all disk patients. Check x-rays or MRI's with a qualified chiropractor or D.O. when this is in question. **Kinetic Electro-acupuncture** The KEA principle can apply to any indicated yoga posture. I particularly recommend the system of 18 postures taught by M. Govindan.[235] In his book and video, he clearly explains the health benefits for each posture, many of which address the whole range of myofascial disorders. Any of these postures can be enhanced with probe stimulation of TP's or with microcurrent interferential treatment.
Piriformis Syndrome: A frequent cause of low back pain is hypertonia of the piriformis muscle of the buttocks. This is a deep muscle that can compress the sciatic nerve, causing symptoms of sciatica	**Local Biphasic Treatment ("Circling the Dragon")** Apply deep pressure over origin and insertion of piriformis muscle. The patient lies on side with painful side up and leg bent to open muscle area. **Local-Distal Polarized Probe treatment** w back ah shi , or UB 32, GB 30 or lateral border of crum(+), distal point UB 57, UB 58, or UB 59, ichever is more tender (-) **Polarized Microcurrent Pad treatment:** Use same locations as above and instruct patient to stretch buttocks while current is flowing.

---

[235] *Babaji's Kriya Hatha Yoga Publications*, tel (450) 297-0258, fax (450) 297-3957

Low Back Region Acu-Points

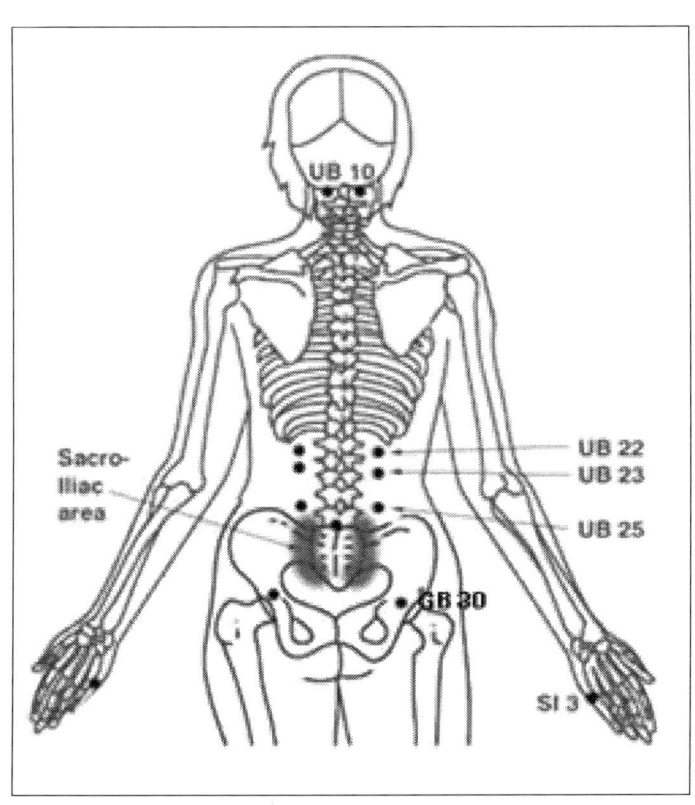

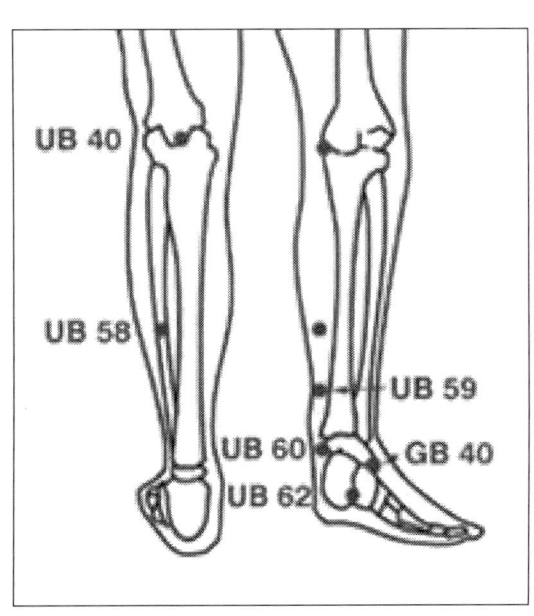

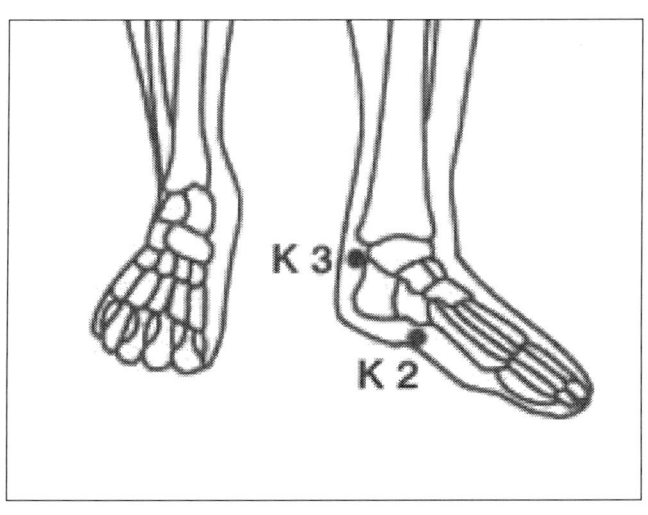

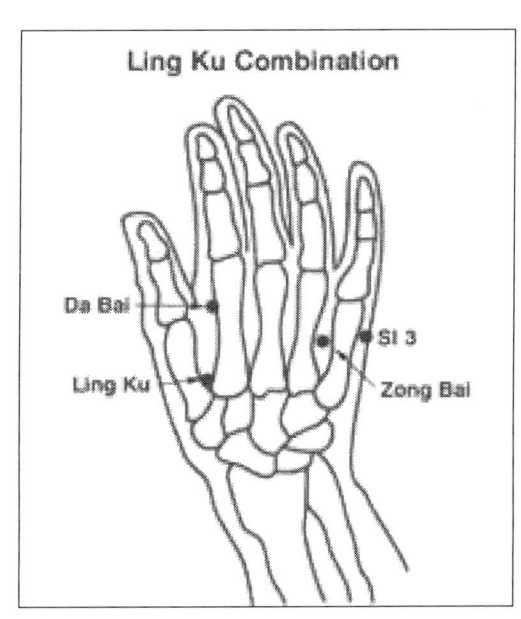

HIP AND KNEES

TRIGGER POINTS / ACU-POINTS	TREATMENT PROTOCOL & METHODS
TP's: Charts 5 and 6, pp. 15-19 *Hips* **Acu-point - Local Combinations:** GB 30 → Lv 11 area of inguinal region GB 30 → GB 31 GB 26 → GB 29 UB 54 → St 31 Huan Zong (center of buttocks) → GB 29 **Acu-point - Local/Distal Combinations:** Proximal (+), Distal (−) GB 30 → GB 34, GB 39, GB 40 or other tender distal points on GB channel Ah shi hip points → LI 15 or TW 14 / TW 15 Ah shi hip points → opp. Lu 2a[236] GB 30 → opposite side H 7 & and/or P 6 for elderly; these wrist points can also be needled while applying kinetic pad therapy to hips *Knees* **Acu-point - Local Combinations:** Eye of knee - ST 35 and medial Xiyan → UB 40 Heding (above patella) → eyes of knee Lv 8 area → GB 34 *Lateral knee injury:* GB 33 → GB 34 *Medial knee injury:* Sp 10 → Sp 9 **Acu-point - Local/Distal Combinations:** Proximal (+), Distal (−) Medial knee ah shi point → opposite P 6 Medial knee point → ipsilateral SP 6 or K 7 K 10 → opposite Lu 5 GB 33 or GB 34 → GB 40 Lateral knee ah shi points → opposite LI 11 **Internally-caused hip and knee pain** This type of pain can stem from disorders of the Kidneys, Liver, Gall Bladder, or Blood. It is very common among elderly patients to have progressive pain in these areas, mostly due to internal Organ degeneration and decline of Qi and Blood. This may present as deficiency of Yang Qi to warm and irrigate these vital joints or Yin deficiency with Heat signs.	Pain in the region of hips and knees can be due to external or internal causes. Trauma is the major external cause of pain, followed by invasion of pathogenic environmental factors such as cold, heat, wind and dampness. Such disorders can respond well to needle or microcurrent electro-acupuncture. **Polarized Great Loops Treatment** Local acu-point (+), distal acu-point (−) in most cases Connect painful local points to some of the acu-points listed, usually on the opposite side of the body, will often significantly reduce pain and improve pain-free range of motion. **4-pad Interferential Microcurrent Pad Treatment:** Rehabilitation is furthered through microcurrent interferential pad placements around the affected area with simultaneous exercise. For example, apply current while patient is using exercise bicycle or continuous passive motion (CPM) device. **Internally-caused Hip and Knee Pain:** Step One and Step Two Balancing **Step Three Treatment:** **Biphasic Probe Treatment with Motion:** Following Step One and Two, ask the patient to lay down in supine posture, raising his legs to make a bicycling motion in the air, and to continue this during probe and I.F. pad stimulation (2-3 minutes). It is also appropriate for you to move the patient's legs for him if he is unable to do so. **4-pad Interferential Microcurrent Pad Treatment** If you have a device with the capacity to set up two sets of interferential, you can treat the right and left hips and knees at the same time. Choose polarized treatment by placing the pads to create intersecting circuits connecting the hips and knees. Using channels A and B for the left hip and knee, place Channel A (red/+) over left sacro-iliac joint, Channel A (black/−) just below patella on same side[237]. Place Channel B (+) in the inguinal crease of the same side and Channel B (−) pad on back of knee, over UB 40.

[236] Palpate the area lateral to LU 2 on the anterior shoulder, and choose most tender and reactive point to indicate LU 2a location.
[237] Acutron Mentor preset IF #3

Hips and Knees Region Acu-Points

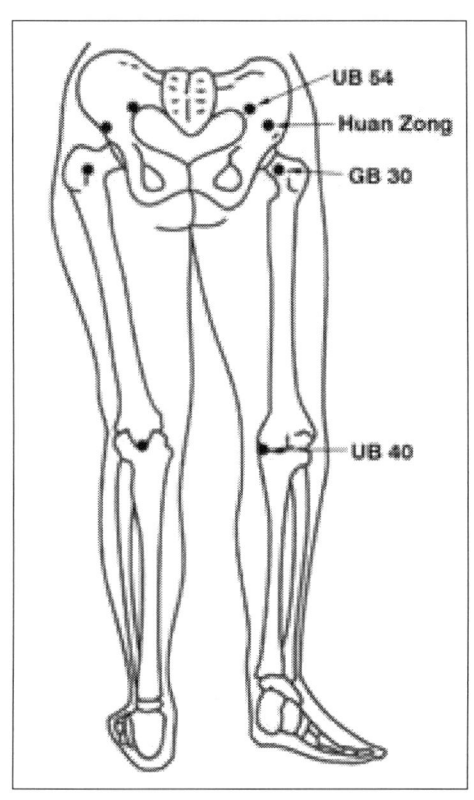

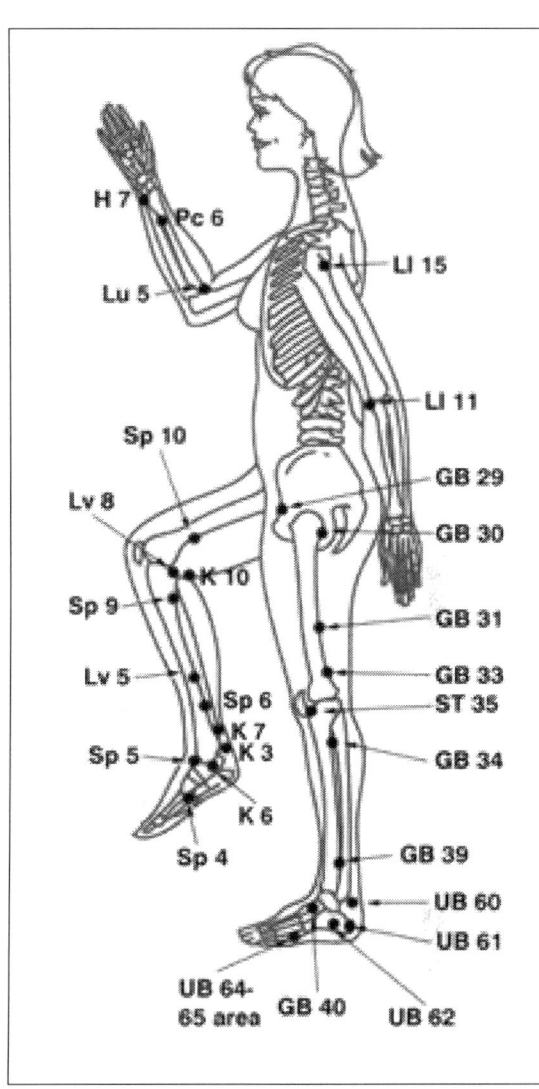

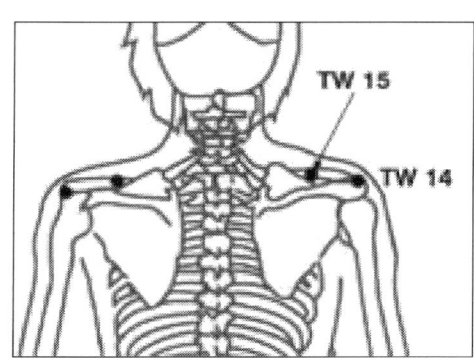

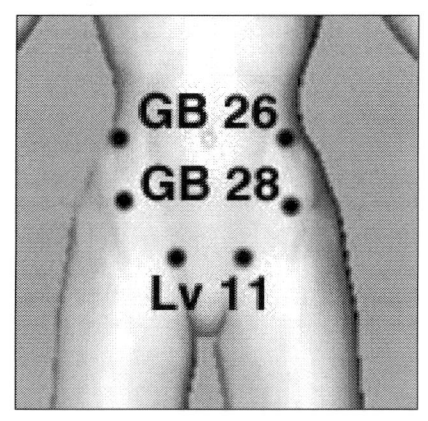

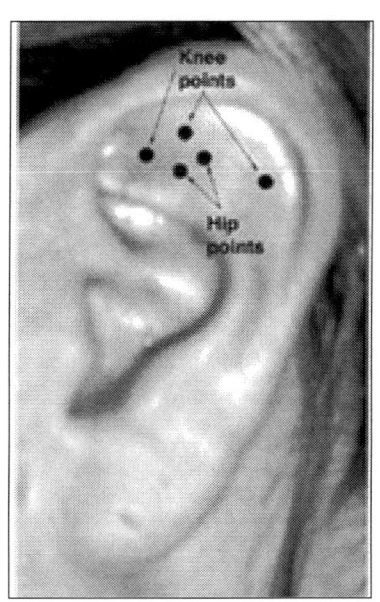

LEGS, ANKLES AND FEET

TRIGGER POINTS / ACU-POINTS	TREATMENT PROTOCOL & METHODS
TP's: Chart 7, pp. 20 - 22 *Ankles* **Acu-point - Local Combinations:** K 3 → St 41 K 6 → UB 61 or UB 62 Sp 5 → GB 40 Lv 4 → UB 60 K 7 → K 1 **Acu-point Local-Distal Point Combinations:** Ah shi ankle point (+) → opp. LI 5 (-) Ah shi ankle point (+) → opp. Lu 2a (-) Tender proximal points along affected leg channels (+) → local ah shi Sacro-iliac joint (+) → local ah shi points (-) *Numbness of Leg and Feet (including peripheral neuropathy):* **Acu-point - Local Combinations:** K 1 → Lv 3 St 41 → Shangbaxie [238] points of foot Sp 4 → UB 64-65 GB 41 → ah shi points on soles of foot GB 40 → GB 41 GB 40 → K 2 **Acu-point Local-Distal Point Combinations:** Du 2 → sacral foramen GB 30 → GB 31 GB 34 → GB 40 Sp 9 → Sp 6 St 36 → Sp 6 GB 34 → GB 39 Lv 5 → K 2 Manaka leg 3 Yin point[239] → ah shi loc. of K 6 *Spasm of gastrocnemius muscle:* UB 56, UB 57 *Pain in sole of foot:* K 1	The following three techniques may be used in sequence: **Local Biphasic ("Circling the Dragon") Dual Probe Stimulation** Choose local point combinations. Search and treat each set in 6-second increments until the conductivity meter reaches its maximum. Choose the next set of two points and repeat. It is best to palpate the points and choose those that are most tender and reactive to treat. Then use GSR meter guidance to zero in on the exact points to stimulate. Check to see how much pain relief and increased ROM has resulted from this step, and then follow with local-distal point treatment. **Local-Distal Polarized Probe treatment** Most painful lower leg or foot point (+), distal point (-), using the following principles: 1. (+) probe on proximal nerve root, usually around S-I joint area or other proximal affected area; (-) probe on painful local point 2. (+) probe on local painful points; (-) probe on distal points on opposite quadrant of body according to the principles of the Great Loops (see list of distal points) It is best to try both approaches for extremity joint pain, as one of the other will work most effectively. Once you are familiar with these probe techniques, they should require no more than 2-3 minutes. Then use following technique for longer-standing cases. **Polarized Interferential Microcurrent Pad Treatment** Place (+) pads more proximal and (-) pads around the area of pain or injury. Use both sets of pads and set them up in a crossing pattern. Once pads are in place and treatment current has been turned on, instruct the patient to gently move the ankle and foot through its range of motion. Watch for areas of pain and restriction, and work with these areas through additional probe work, needling, or electro-acupuncture.

---

[238] Located in web spaces between toes
[239] Palpate above Sp 10 for most tender point)

Legs, Ankles and Feet Trigger Points/Techniques

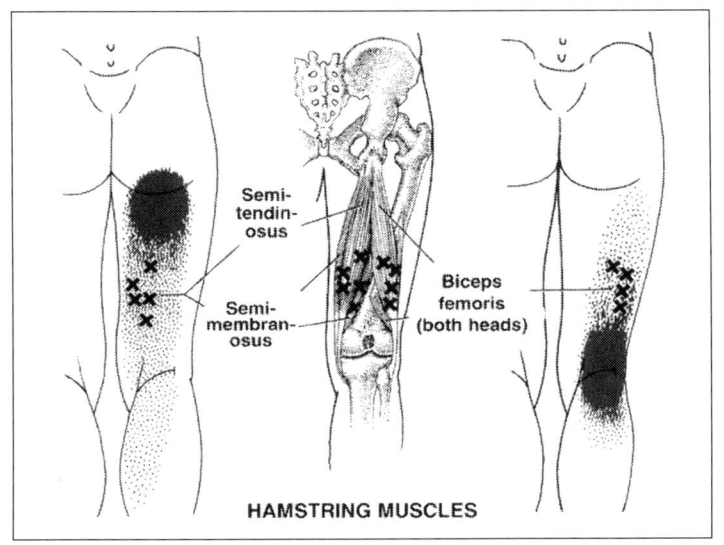

HAMSTRING MUSCLES

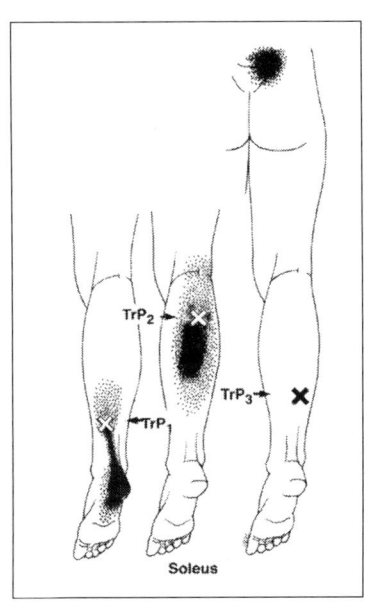

Soleus

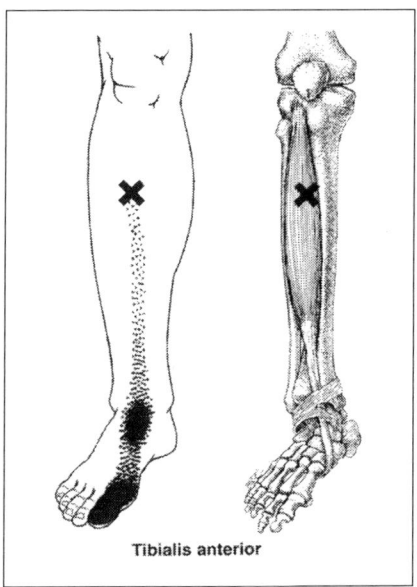

Tibialis anterior

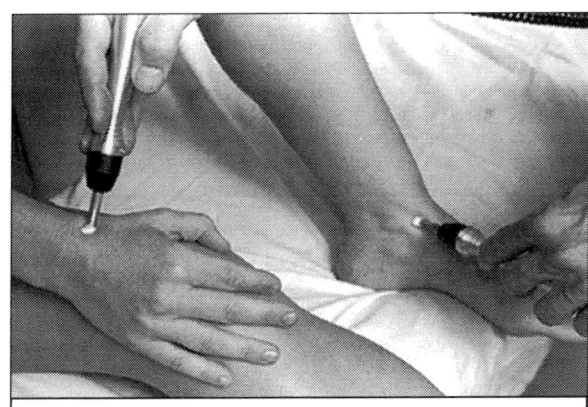

Great Loops treatment for ankle pain, with + probe on painful ankle and − probe on opposite tender wrist point

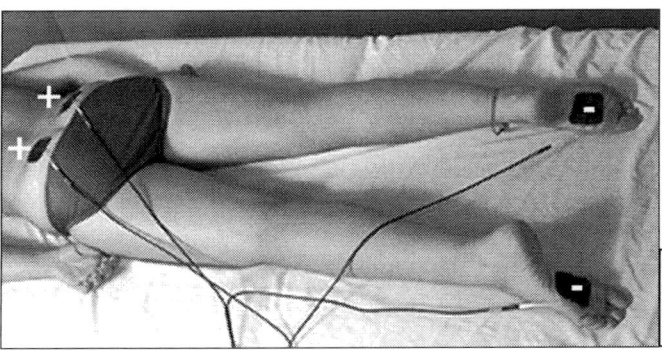

Polarized 4-pad treatment for peripheral neuropathy or circulatory disorders of the legs, with + pads proximal and − pads distal

LEGS, ANKLES AND FEET, CONTINUED

TRIGGER POINTS / ACU-POINTS	TREATMENT PROTOCOL & METHODS
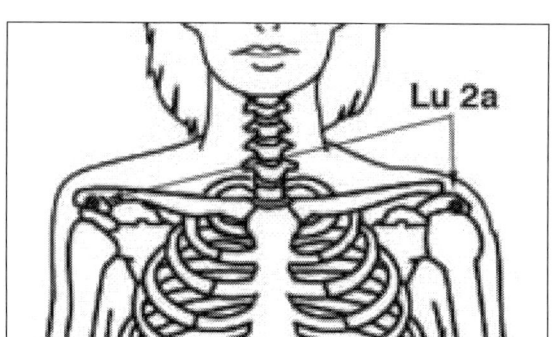 **Pain in heel:** **Acu-points - Local** UB 61, Lv 3, K 8, K 7, K 3, K 5, K 6, extra point at bottom of heel - combine freely with biphasic probes to pass currents through heel area **Acu-point Local-Distal Point Combinations:** UB 57 → ah shi heel point Ah shi heel points → Mu Guan and Gu Guan on heel of hand[240] Sacro-iliac joint → ah shi heel points (Use kinesiology to confirm proper polarity, as this can be variable with these points) K 1 → ah shi heel point (needle electro-acupuncture may be applicable here)[241]	**Combination Probe and Pad Treatment for Specific Muscles or Joints.** Athletic hamstring injuries respond well to Origin/Insertion probe treatments or electro-massage. For calf spasm and pain use probes to connect acu-point UB 57, which is slightly above center of midline of gastrocnemius muscles on back of leg to proximal distal UB points. Use interferential placements for knee and ankle injuries. **Flooding Technique for Paresthesias and Leg Circulation Problems:** Place one large pad over S-I joint and other pad of that channel on sole of foot. *Polarity:* Biphasic *Intensity:* tickling sensation *Frequency:* 0.6 Hz *Time:* 10 minutes For numbness, peripheral neuropathies and nerve conduction problems, use dermatome treatments with (+) over sacral nerve roots and (-) over furthest area of numbness of tingling sensations **Combination Needle and Microcurrent Probe Technique for Plantar Fascitis and other Heel Pain** Use probes from heel to under toes. Move them together gradually while flexing and extending. Heel pain often requires a combination of acupuncture needling with microcurrent stimulation for best results. Try needling the Kidney channel points listed, with stimulation directed toward the heel, followed by probe and/or interferential microcurrent treatment. Plantar fascitis often responds will to dermatome interferential of lower extremities

---

[240] Described in Dr. Tan's book 12 and 12 in Acupuncture
[241] Devitt, Michael, Electroacupuncture for Plantar Fascitis, Acupuncture Today, December 2001

LEGS, ANKLES AND FEET ACU-POINTS

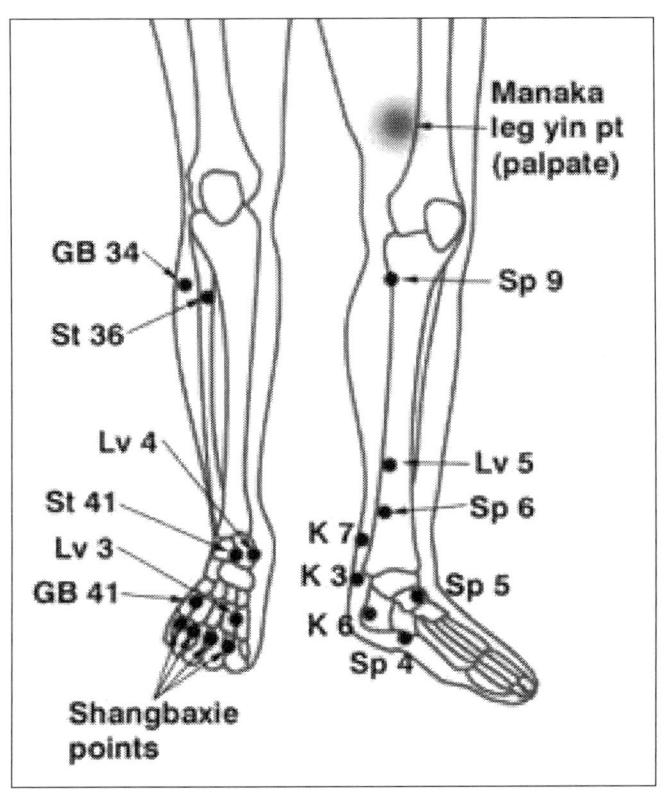
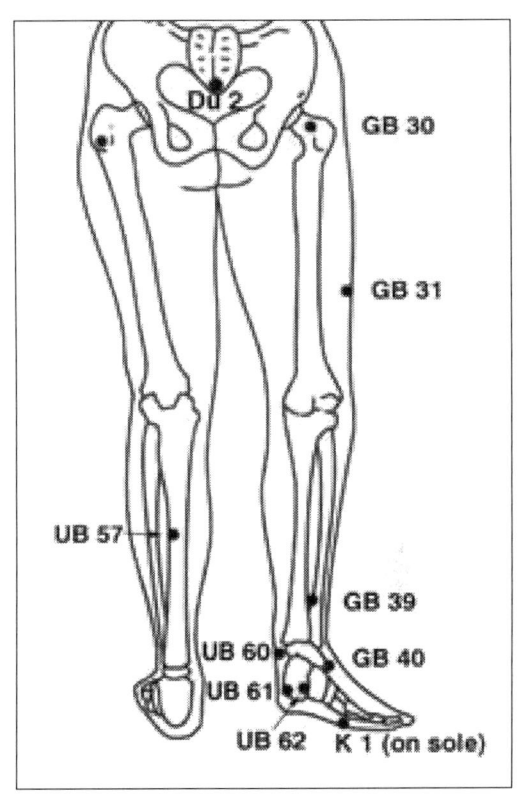
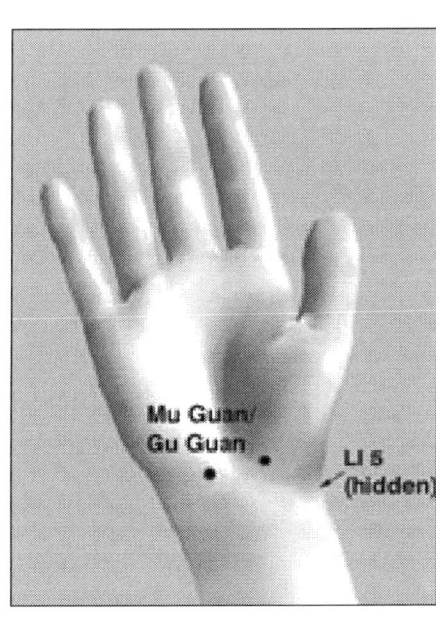
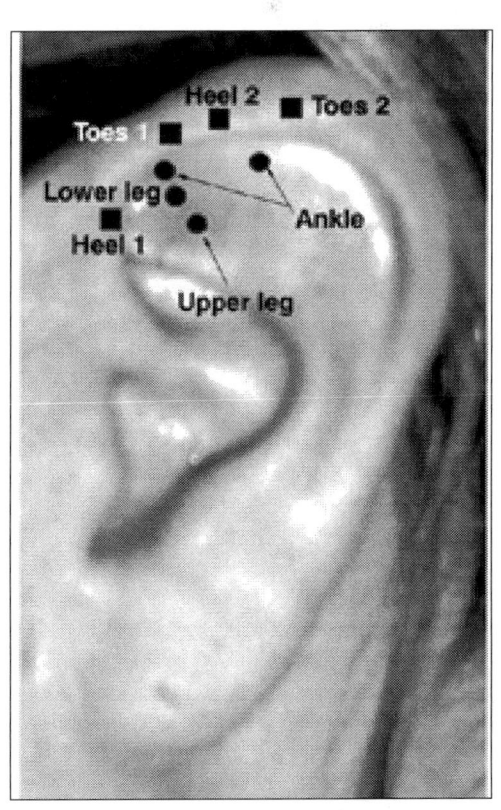

Treatment Formulary Section II

OTHER SPECIFIC CONDITIONS

Many of the conditions listed in this section are associated with internal Organ imbalance. For this reason, it is recommended to first give Step One evaluation and treatment (see Chapter 11) to augment results. Such global energy balancing will improve the effectiveness and carry-over of results. When Step One treatments are of particular importance for a condition dealt with in this Chapter, such treatments will be specifically discussed.

Differential diagnosis is essential for accurate, safe and effective treatment. Space in this book does not permit a thorough elaboration of differential diagnosis for all the conditions listed. Acu-points, protocols and techniques are offered as resource guidelines only, to be used as part of an individual patient assessment and treatment plan.

ACNE

Acne is associated with areas of energetic stagnation coupled with toxins in the Blood often induced by inappropriate diet. In many cases, microcurrent probe treatment can help disperse the lesions simply by placing the probe tips on either side for 40 – 60 seconds each. This must be coupled with dietary adjustments and/or blood-clearing herbal treatment.

Adjunctive Treatments: Increase amount of fresh fruits, vegetable and fibre in diet, decrease fats. Raw vegetable juices are supportive. Vitamins A, B complex, B6, C and zinc valuable. Facial applications of calendula, witch hazel and bentonite masks help to clean pores.

ALLERGIES

TREATMENT METHODS	ACU-POINTS
Step One Treatment: Meridian/Organ balancing is particularly important for treatment of allergies, especially with children. Many children have asthma associated with allergic response to foods, vaccinations and environmental substances. Use Step One treatment with some of the ear points listed, and remove offending foods, or clean up the child's air by removing dust-carrying toys and clutter and using a room air filter. Far fewer children would require medical inhalers if this regimen were followed. **Local Polarized Treatment:** *Acutron Mentor:* Probe preset #2 Treat ear acu-points first, then local face acu-points **Local-Distal Polarized Probe Treatment:** *Acutron Mentor:* Probe preset #2 Local face acu-points (+), distal points (-)	**Acu-points - Local** GV 23, GB 13, St 3 **Acu-points - Distal** + probe at local head region, - probe at distal point St 3, Lv 3 or other indicated points **ACU-POINTS - EAR** antihistamine, endocrine, adrenal, sympathetic, kidney, hay fever, Lung, wonderful and Shenmen

Adjunctive Treatments: In most cases, it will also be important to determine what specific substances the patient is reacting to, and ask him to avoid contact with them for a month or more. During this period of desensitization, the above mentioned microcurrent treatments will be of great value in resetting the body's abnormal responses to the allergen. After the initial month of abstinence, offending foods may gradually be re-introduced, while checking for reactions.

The following regimens may be supportive of an allergy-clearing program: Digestive enzymes to reduce undigested food from reaching the intestines and supplementing with vitamins A, B complex, C, zinc, magnesium and fish liver oil. Ingestion of ginger, garlic, cayenne and black pepper stimulates secretion of IgA antibodies, which stimulate complete digestion.

TREATMENT FORMULARY II: OTHER SPECIFIC CONDITIONS 265

ALLERGIES

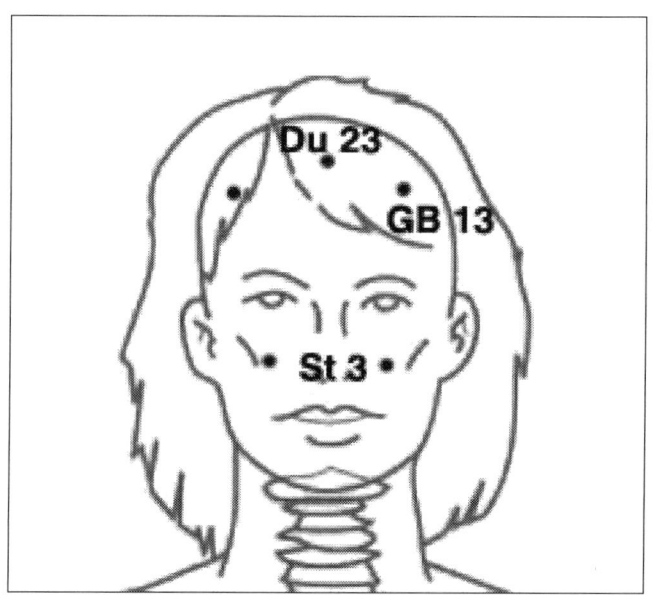
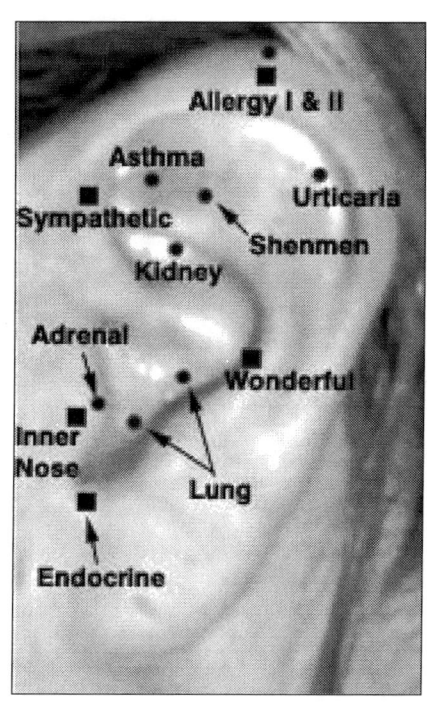

ARTHRITIS

There are two types of arthritis – osteo and rheumatoid. Osteoarthritis is a degenerative disease of the large weight-bearing joints, and is common to most elderly people to some degree. Rheumatoid arthritis is an auto-immune disease that strikes all ages, and is often associated with allergic responses. Allergies should be addressed and cleared as much as possible in any therapeutic program for this condition. Arthritic symptoms are often associated with diseases such as SLE (Systemic Lupus Erythematosus), neuropathy, Lyme's disease, Parkinson's, phlebitis, fibromyalgia and many others. While the Four-Step protocol may help alleviate any of these conditions, an accurate medical diagnosis is essential if symptoms do not resolve after a course of 10 or more treatments.

TREATMENT METHODS	ACU-POINTS
Step One Treatment Apply Extraordinary Vessel treatment bilaterally; confirm polarity with kinesiology Often used: Lu 7 (+) K 6 (-) (bilateral) **Local Biphasic Treatment:** Follow with painful or inflamed local area points and ear points as appropriate, using RA anti-inflammatory points for added effect	**Acu-points - Local** between knuckles and toes, circling the dragon around affected joints, major points of affected regions, treat along meridians that run through affected joints *RA Anti-inflammatory:* TW 5, TW 6, LI 14, LI 11, LI 15, Du 14, UB 11, UB 58 *Osteoarthritis:* BL 23, Sp 5, TW 4, TW 15, K 6 **Acu-points - Ear** Kidney, endocrine, adrenal, Shenmen, Subcortex

Adjunctive Treatments: Diet rich in fresh fruits, vegetables, and cold-water fish beneficial. Drastically reduce intake of fatty animal proteins, dairy, eggs and margarine. Many RA patients react negatively to nightshade vegetables such as potatoes, eggplant, tomatoes and tobacco. Drink lots of pure water, and consider supplementation with cod liver oil, large doses of Vitamin C and anti-inflammatory and anti-oxidant substances such as zinc, copper, selenium, manganese, pantothenic acid, methionine, SOD, proteolytic enzymes, sulfur and L-phenylalanine. Trace minerals should be supplemented, preferably in liquid form. Royal jelly, bee pollen and evening primrose oil have all been found to be effective for treatment of RA. There are several Chinese herbal formulas that are effective.

Other valuable supplements for arthritis:

OMEGA-3 ACIDS (suppresses inflammation of joints): EPA (Kyolic EPA a good product, contains garlic and EPA- 500 mg 2X day) DHA GLA
GLUCOSAMINE SULFATE: 500 mg 3X/day- helps maintain integrity of joints
CHONDROITIN- helps hydrate cartilage
BORON- Helps keep calcium in the bones
NIACINAMINE: 5-- mg 3X/day, for joint inflammation
CAPSAICIN: Extract of cayenne pepper, used topically to leach substance P from inflamed joints, relieving pain.
DEVIL'S CLAW: A very powerful herbal antioxidant and anti-inflammatory. In some research studies it has been shown to be as powerful as cortisone. Very useful for RA.
DHEA: A synthesized adrenal hormone, DHEA levels naturally decline in the body after age 25. Each individual should have their levels checked before administering. Helpful for lupus.

ARTHRITIS

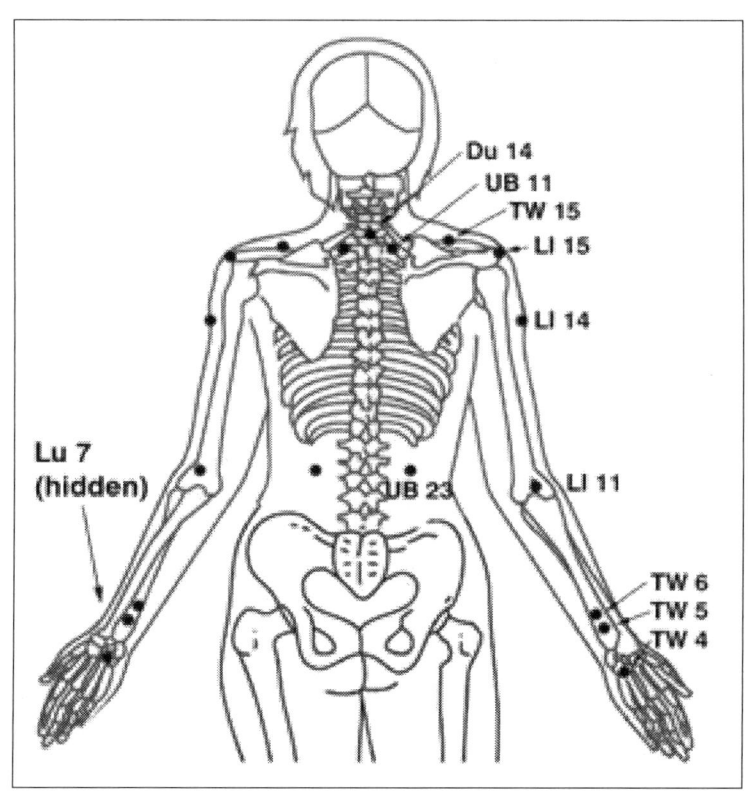
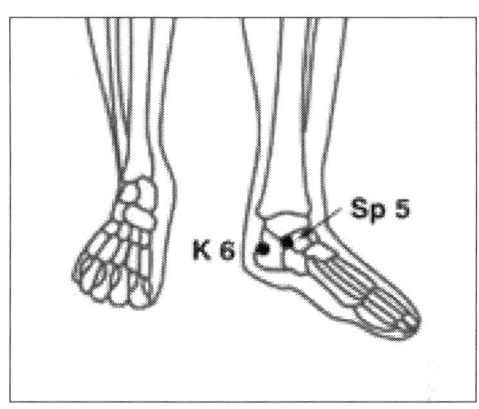
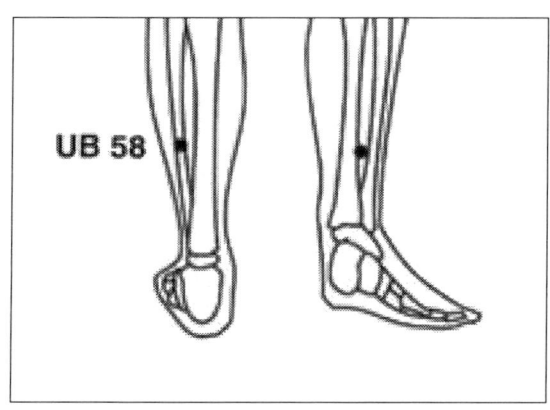
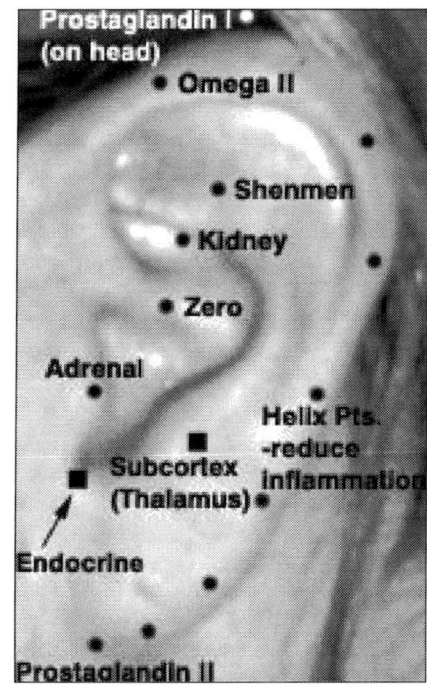

ASTHMA

Asthma is due to either External or Internal causes. External causes include unresolved colds and flu (Wind-Cold or Wind-Heat), and are associated with strong respiration, aching of the chest and back, and a full and slippery pulse. Internal causes are Root imbalance in the Kidneys, Liver or Lungs. Such patients have a weaker presentation with rapid but shallow breathing, cold limbs, sweating, and a weak and superficial pulse. It may be important to address unresolved emotional issues and allergies for long-term relief. Step One treatment is very important here.

TREATMENT METHODS	ACU-POINTS
Microcurrent Mu-Shu Treatment for External Origin Acute Attacks: See Chapter 7 for Step Two - Mu-Shu treatment. Use this method only under medical supervision if the patient also has cardiac disease. **Local Biphasic Probe Treatment:** External origin: sedate acu-points listed Internal origin: tonify acu-points listed; treat ear points Either external or internal origin: disperse ah shi points (see column 1); strongly for externally caused asthma, gently and briefly for internal origin.	**Acu-points - Local** *External Origin:* UB 12, UB 13, Lu 1, Dingchuan, and Lu 5; St 40 if Phlegm is present Acute attacks - Males: Ren 22, St 12 Acute attacks - Females: Ren 22, UB 12, GB 21 *Internal Origin:* Lu 1, K 27, UB 43, UB 23, Ren 22, Ren 4, K 3 **Ear acu-points:** Shenmen, lung, adrenal, asthma, sympathetic *Either External or Internal:* Ah shi: K 23, K 24, Du 12, St 18, Ren 12, Dingchuan, UB 11 and points along Lu channel.

Adjunctive Treatments: Test for and control food and environmental allergies, consider causes of excessive stress and try to alleviate. Core healing of emotional issues can help in many cases. Properly selected Chinese herbal formulas have been successful in relieving symptoms of asthma.

ADDICTION RELEASE

TREATMENT METHODS	ACU-POINTS
Auricular Treatment Auricular treatment is the most effective treatment for addictions. To treat the listed points, have patient hold brass hand mass of microcurrent unit, use trigger probe to stimulate ear points in sequence. It is best to use a special auricular probe tip no larger than 2 mm in diameter for precision point localization and treatment. *Acutron Mentor:* Microamp Pad preset #2; modify Hz to 00 *Polarity:* negative on ear points *Frequency:* 80 Hz *Intensity:* 25-50 µA *Duration:* 30-40 seconds for microcurrent treatment only, or touch probe tip needles in points for same amount of time.	**Acu-points - Ear** *Drug Addiction:* Lung 1, Lung 2, Zero point, Shen Men, Subcortex, Endocrine, Liver, Kidney, Master Sensorial *Alcoholism:* Drunk point, thirst, Liver, Zero, Shen Men, Endocrine, Valium point, Brain *Smoking:* Lung 1 and 2, Mouth, Zero, Shen Men, Adrenal, Master Sensorial.

Addiction Release Adjunctive Treatments: Proper diet that supports steady blood sugar metabolism is essential, eating proteins at every meal. Clear allergies and avoid simple carbohydrates (sugars) and caffeine in diet. Consider adrenal support such as Vitamin C, pantothenic acid and adrenal extracts. All vitamins and minerals should be supplemented as needed to rebuild health. Address core issues through therapy if possible. **Note- diagrams for Addiction Release acu-points are on second following page.**

ASTHMA

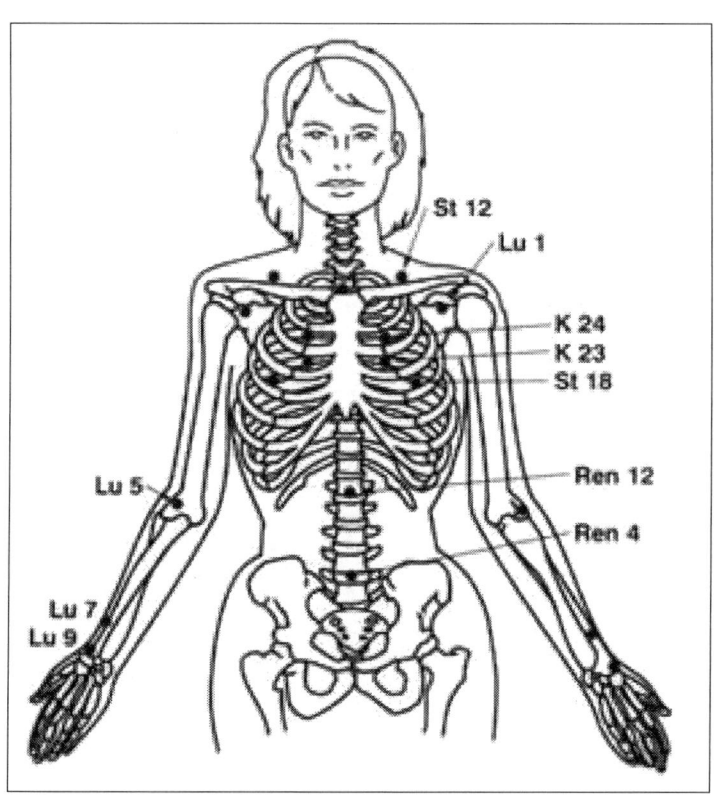
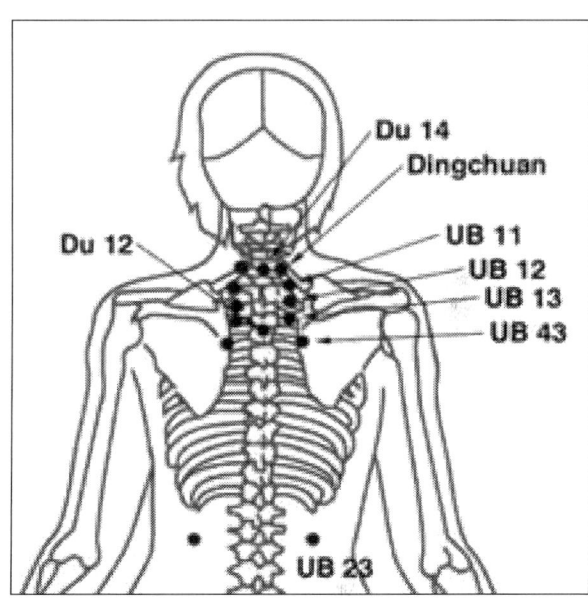
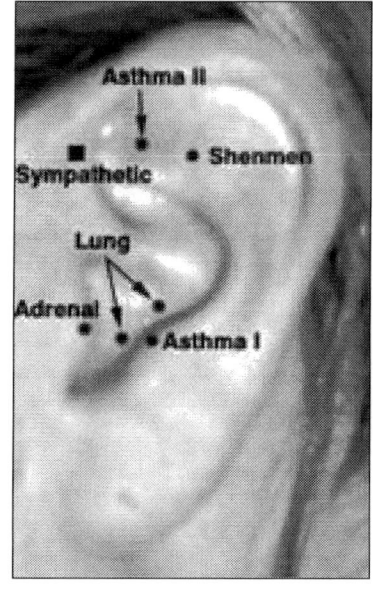
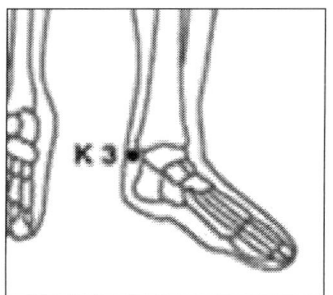

ACCELERATION OF WOUND HEALING

The most well documented effects of microcurrent stimulation in research have been its enhancement of tissue healing. Research has shown that its mechanism of action is due to increase of ATP, proliferation of amino acids for cell repair, and opening of calcium channels in the cell membranes. Microcurrent treatment is divided into three phases: acute pain treatment, chronic pain treatment, and "healing mode." Healing mode consists of very low-level micro-stimulation at very low frequencies that stimulate ion transfer through cell membranes to enhance repair activities. It is recommended to follow most acute and chronic treatments with healing mode, or to use healing mode exclusively for patients with severe and reactive pain syndromes, non-union fractures, or other non-healing wounds. The following protocol was originally developed for pressure sore treatment in nursing homes (decubitis ulcers).

TREATMENT METHODS	GENERAL PROCEDURE
Septic or mushy wounds: *Microcurrent:* Use Acutron Mentor Microamp Pad preset #2 or below parameters; modify Hz to 00 *Polarity:* negative over target area for tissue softening and/or anti-sepsis. *Frequency:* 0.3 - 0.6 Hz, or use 00 Hz (direct current), *Intensity:* 10 - 50 µA *Waveform:* slope *Duration:* l0 minutes to several hours depending on condition. **Firm, granulating wounds:** *Acutron Mentor:* Milliamp Pad preset #2; modify Hz to 100, or below parameters for other HVPG devices *Polarity:* positive over target area *Frequency:* 100 Hz *Intensity:* just below threshold of sensation *Duration:* 15-45 minutes Observe patient carefully for any uncomfortable reactions to current. In several research studies, the two above protocols have been alternated every few days to promote maximum healing. Microcurrent pad treatment is also valuable in accelerating healing of fractured bones. Place pads of an output channel above and below casting (cut distal holes in cast if necessary), or wrap small fractures of the fingers or toes with pads.	*Open wound treatment:* Attach the electrode over the wound via alligator clip adapter to a piece of metal foil cut to the size of the wound. This is then taped down over sterile, saline-soaked gauze packed directly into the open wound. The other electrode of the opposite polarity can be a TENS pad placed on an anatomically opposite aspect of the affected area. For example, for an open wound of the inner aspect of the gastocnemius muscle, the opposite electrode can be placed on the lateral aspect of the muscle. If placing electrode longitudinally along a limb, always place the – electrode distal and the + electrode proximal. Treatment parameters depend on condition of wound.

ADDICTION RELEASE EAR POINTS

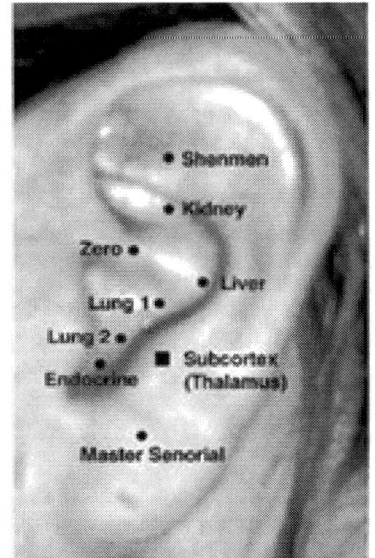

Points to release drug addiction

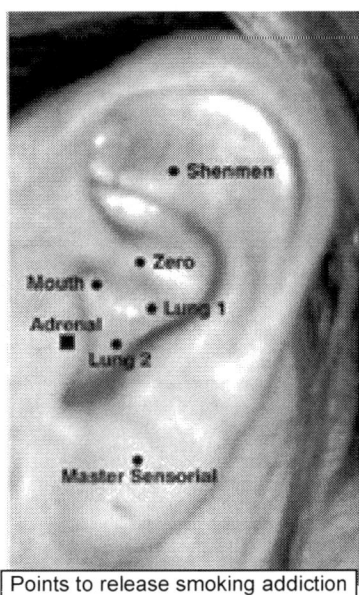

Points to release smoking addiction

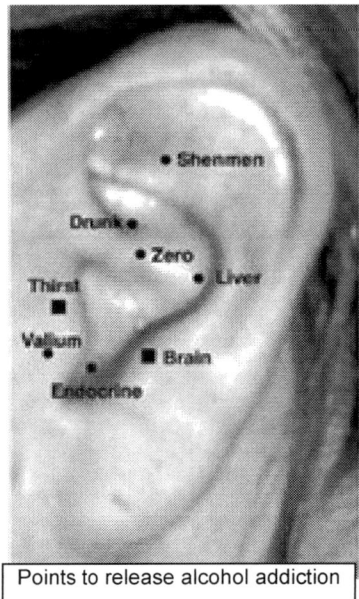

Points to release alcohol addiction

ACCELERATION OF WOUND HEALING

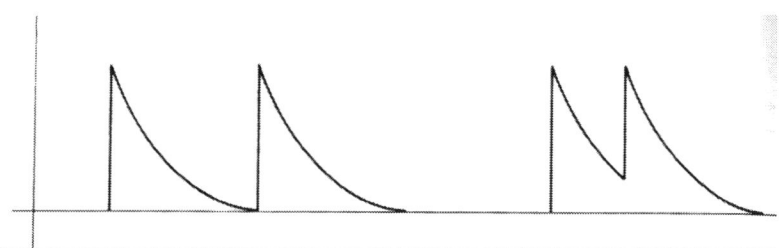

Twin peak waveform commonly used in high-volt pulsed galvanic stimulators (HVPG). These have been successfully used for wound healing acceleration

Back/Vertebral Disk Injuries

Treatment Methods
Milli-micro Combination Treatment Start treatment with milliamp interferential for first 5 – 10 minutes, follow with low frequency microcurrent for 10 – 15 minutes. Treatment principle is to enhance balanced support of disk area by surrounding muscles and nerves. *Acutron Mentor:*   I.F. preset #5 *Polarity:*   Biphasic *Frequency:*   Milliamp – high Hz, Microamp, low Hz *Intensity:* Milliamp – to comfortable tolerance, Microamp -75 – 100 µA Place X pattern of pads around affected disk region. Place set of microcurrent pads on back of knees. Also try anterior-posterior IF pad placement with microcurrent only. Once patient can begin to exercise, have him do abdominal muscle strengthening exercises with simultaneous microcurrent IF, and gradual use of Cobra pose as explained in *Treat Your Own Back* by Robin Mackenzie. This should only be used after an orthopedic examination to confirm its appropriateness. Microcurrent IF can be used with flexion-distraction treatment tables with frequent good results. This technique is an excellent adjunct to skilled chiropractic or acupuncture treatments. SEE ALSO: TREATMENT FORMULARY, SECTION I – BACK REGION

Bell's Palsy

Treatment Methods	Acu-Points
Local Biphasic Probe Treatment: Use probes on facial point and distal points. EAV frequencies 8.2 and 9.3 can be applicable for flaccid paralysis associated with this condition and Lyme's disease. Microcurrent facial rejuvenation protocol has been successful in treating this condition.	Acu-points - Local St 2, 3, 4, 5, 6, 7, Shangchengjiang (mental foramen), LI 20, SI 18, GB 20, Yuyao, Ren 24, TW 17. Acu-points - Distal LI 4, Du 20, GB 41 Acu-points - Ear Face, cheeks, forehead, subcortex, zero, Shenmen

Brachial Neuralgia, "Pinched Nerve Syndrome"

Treatment Methods
4 Pad Polarized Interferential Treatment: Pass current through brachial plexus and neck. Place + electrodes on C 3 - 6 area, and use – electrode to trace the pathway of radiation. In chronic cases use very low current and frequent treatments. 3.9 Hz may be used for neuralgia. See also Thoracic Outlet Syndrome.

TREATMENT FORMULARY II: OTHER SPECIFIC CONDITIONS 273

BACK/VERTEBRAL DISK INJURIES

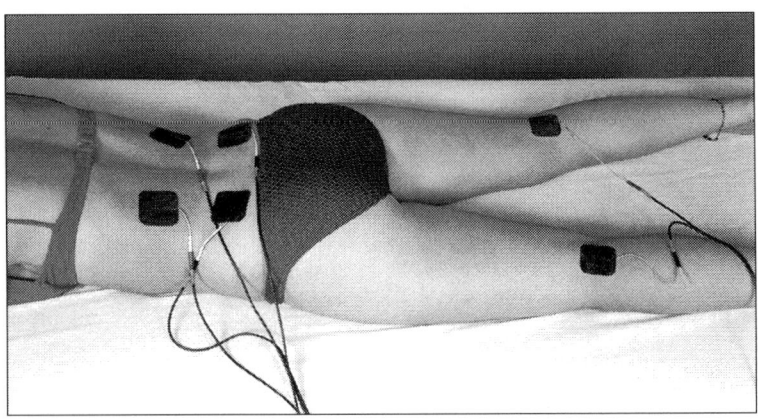

Milliamp-microamp interferential over inflamed disk area, with single set of biphasic microcurrent pads over UB 40 points on backs of knees

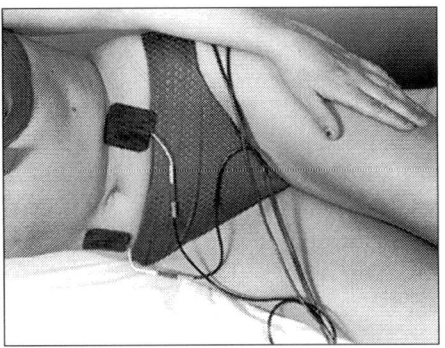

Interferential anterior-posterior placements, with each set of pads crossing midline from front to back

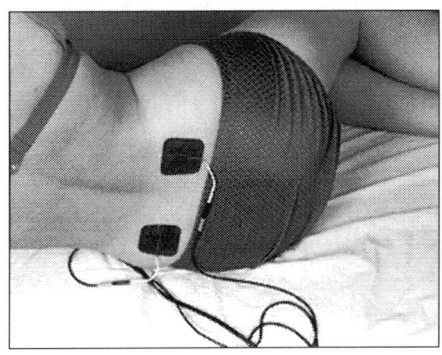

BELLS PALSY

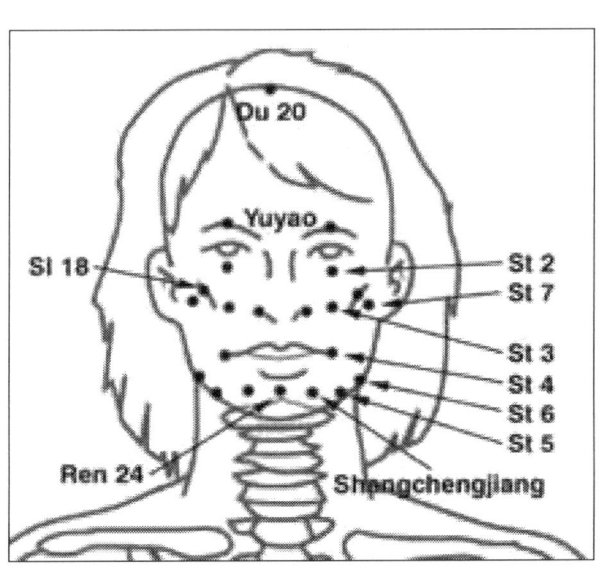

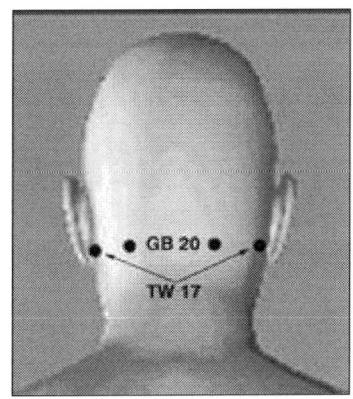

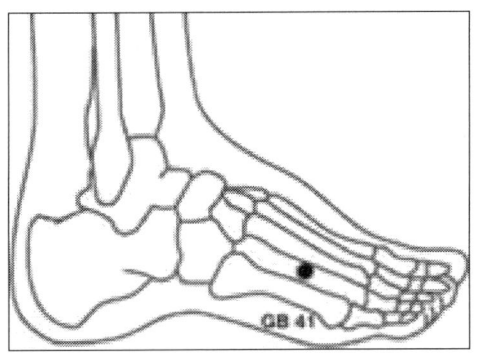

CANCER PAIN

Acupuncture and microcurrent therapies have been demonstrated effective for relieving cancer pain in many cases. Due to effects on the endocrine, immune and nervous system, acupuncture and microcurrent can also be a support in helping some patients recover from cancer. The pioneering work of Bjorn Nordenstrom[242] has demonstrated that polarized microcurrents, through electrode wires implanted directly into some kinds of tumors, can have profound pain relieving effects. In some cases, such treatment can also cause regression of the cancer itself. Improper use of this technique, however, can potentially cause the cancer to grow and spread, so it should not be attempted without further research, except in the terminally ill. Nordenstrom's work demonstrated that cancerous tumors possess different electrical qualities than healthy tissues, and are exquisitely sensitive to external electric energy. This could account for why some communities of people living close to electrical power lines and switching stations have demonstrated high cancer rates.[243]

TREATMENT METHODS	ACU-POINTS

1. It is contraindicated to place pad electrodes over known or suspected cancerous areas of the body due to the possibility that improper use of polarity may energize the growth of the cancer. Brief probe therapies are safe in most cases, however, due to the very limited amount and duration of current employed.
2. Cancer is often associated with energetic stagnation. Local and distal point stimulation is helpful to reduce stagnation, thereby relieving pain. Meridian stretching with simultaneous polarized microcurrent probe therapy can be even more valuable than passive stimulation. Place + probe on a proximal meridian point and − probe on distal point, and place body part in position to create maximum stretch along specific meridian pathway(s).
  1. Having the patient practice simple Qi Gong exercises to bring energy and blood circulation to the affected area prior to stimulation will enhance the results of therapy. Many cancer patients have low vitality, and require energizing the treatment for best response. This can be done through focused breath and visualization of energy flowing to the area. There are excellent CD's available on Medical Qigong exercises that are very beneficial for cancer patients.[244]
  2. Microsystem points of the ear, hand and foot are valuable in cancer pain treatment. You can use the auricular micro-macro technique or needles with brief application of microcurrent probes to periodically energize them.[245]
  3. Polarized treatment along extremities and across the body through the Great Loops is applicable.
	Acu-points - Local and Distal
	Local and distal points for cancer pain may be selected according to affected body part[246]:
	
	Brain and throat cancer:
	St 8, St 9, LI 7, Du 4, Du 14, Du 17
	
	Lung cancer:
	Lu 1, Lu 7, Lu 8, P 6
	
	Breast cancer:
	SI 1, Ht 7, LI 16, Lv 14, Sp 21
	
	Stomach, pancreas, esophageal and duodenal cancer: St 36, Sp 4, Lv 13, UB 20, UB 21, P 6
	
	Liver cancer:
	Lv 3, Lv 9, Lv 14
	
	Ovary, uterus and urinary bladder cancer:
	UB 59, UB 65, St 39, K 5-6 area
	
	General cancer pain points:
	LI 4, GB 38

---

[242] For more information about Nordenstrom's work see site: http://www.ursus.se/publications.htm
[243] See book <u>Cross Currents</u> by Robert Becker, Tarcher 1990 for specifics on electropollution and cancer
[244] Author's recommendation: CD set <u>Medical Qigong</u> by Donna McDermott, Center for Excellence (602) 943-4222
[245] See Chapter 14 for details on this technique.
[246] A portion of this point information was derived from the article <u>Acupuncture and Cancer Pain</u> by Magnolia Goh, Pacific College Journal, Summer 2001

From the perspective of subtle energy anatomy, cancer can be considered a physical manifestation of etheric energy cysts in the body. Among other causes, toxic substances and deeply held emotional issues[247] can create stagnation, resulting in these energy cysts. The power of the mind to reverse cancer has been well demonstrated by many doctors and healers.[248] One perspective of energetic healing is that many diseases arise from unlearned life lessons and spiritual passages. From this viewpoint, it is essential for cancer patients to "take charge" of their healing process, powerfully affirming love of life, self-love, spiritual connectedness and self-responsibility. It is also important in many cases for such patients to clear any unfinished emotional business with family members or other close relationships and to evaluate environmental stresses such as electromagnetic pollution, geopathic stress[249] and improper diet.

Adjunctive Treatments: There are many nutritive and cleansing regimens that have been credited with helping to drive cancer into remission. These include raw vegetable juice fasting, macrobiotic diets, extensive use of vitamins, minerals and anti-oxidants, brown algin-containing seaweeds, garlic, trace minerals, copper, selenium and many other substances. There are numerous alternative approaches for treating cancer with impressive track records that may be researched through organizations such as Cancer Control Society (Los Angeles, CA, 213-663-7801), Int'l Assoc. for Cancer Victors (Playa del Rey, CA, 310-822-5032) and People Against Cancer (Otho, IA, 515-972-4444).

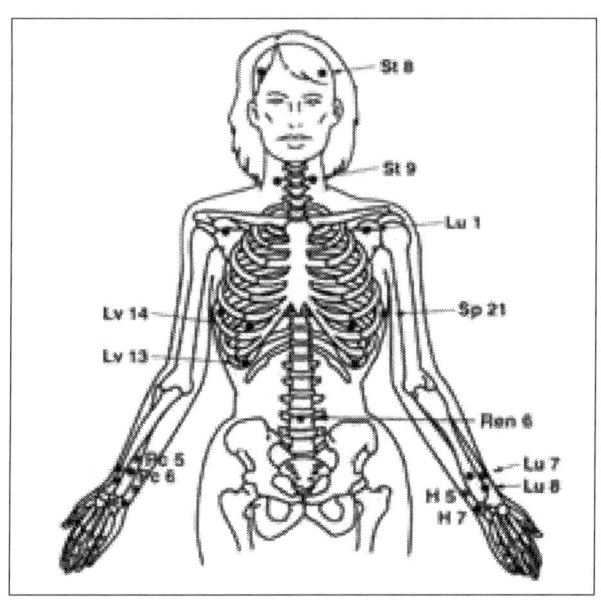
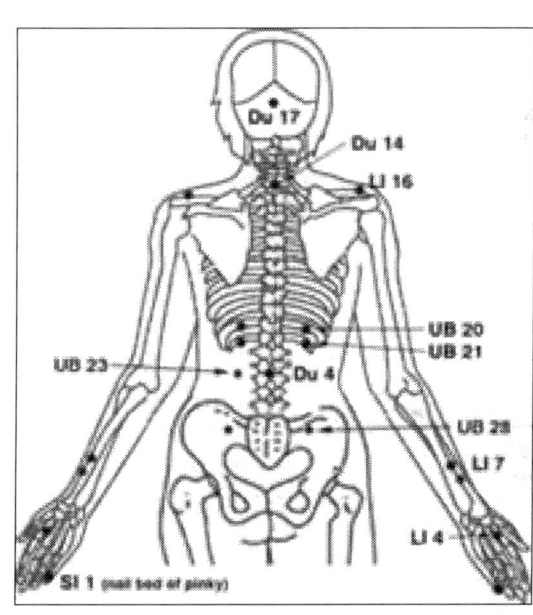
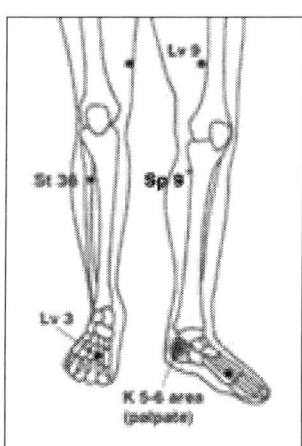
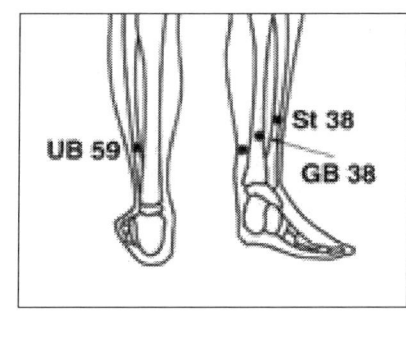
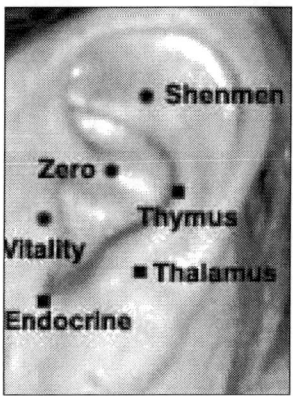

---

[247] For details about this process, see book Hands of Light by Barbara Ann Brennan, Bantam Books 1988
[248] See website http://www.hmt.com/cyp/nonprof/ecap/ about the work of Bernie Siegal, M.D. in this regard
[249] This is disturbance of human bioenergy caused by disharmonious relationship to Earth energies, such as ley lines, underground water and radiation.

CHRONIC PAIN AND DEPRESSION

Pain becomes chronic when, for a host of possible reasons, the body is not able to maintain the integrity of its bio-electric circulation and communication network during recovery from an acute injury or disease. This book offers a wealth of understandings and techniques to assist chronic pain patients. The Four-Step process detailed in Section III is ideal for this purpose. Depression is common among patients with chronic pain. In this case, if we ask the question "What came first, the chicken or the egg?" the answer can be both in many cases. Unresolved core emotional and spiritual issues, when felt as depression, can predispose individuals to chronic physical pain, which may be an outpicturing of pain of the feeling body. Yet the experience of unresolving pain over a long period of time can also cause depression. It is probably a complex mixture of both factors that accounts for most chronic pain conditions.

Consider:

Step One and Two meridian balancing
Bodywork, possibly with electro-massage to invigorate body and promote circulation of bio-electric energy
Emotional/spiritual core healing sessions, when indicated, chakra clearing
Any applicable microcurrent techniques detailed in Chapter Seven

Adjunctive Treatments: There are valuable nutritional supplements for chronic pain and depression[250]:

DLPA: This is the "d" molecular form of amino acid phenylalanine. It prevents endorphins from being broken down by bodily enzymes, thus maintaining a high level of endorphin in the system. It's effect is cumulative, taking a few weeks to reach total effect, and it does not create addiction or tolerance in the body. DLPA is also helpful for depression and relieving chronic pain. Most patients may be started with one 750 mg capsule before breakfast, and on the second day add another before lunch. Very severe pain patients may require 3 -4 capsules/day. It is available in health food stores.

DMAE (Dimethyl Amino Ethanol): A byproduct of procaine, DMAE is also available in health food stores. It is converted into acetylcholine in the brain. It is an energizer and relieves depression.
Choline with Vitamin B-5: Twinlabs makes a combination Neuro-Vite useful for increasing serotonin and dopamine levels for relieving depression.
Tyrosine: 500mg 2X/day
5-hydroxy tryptophane: this form still available, increases serotonin levels
St. John's Wort (Hypericum): 300 mg 3Xday, increase serotonin and dopamine levels in the brain
MAGNESIUM: For chronic muscular pain, useful for migraines. 450 mg 2X/day.
GINKO BILOBA: Increases circulation of blood, helpful for cold extremities (Raynaud's Syndrome), headaches, and PMS. Also well known for sharpening mental faculties.

ANTIOXIDANTS: The following antioxidants are important in reducing inflammation, tissue damage and pain:
Vitamin C- large doses have reversed many severe degenerative conditions
Vitamin E- Prevents endorphin breakdown, helpful with Alzheimer's disease to reduce brain inflammation
Selenium

---

[250] This list of supplements is largely derived from a lecture by Dr. Arnold Fox at the American Academy of Pain Management annual symposium, September 1997.

EDEMA

Swelling and bloating of the body that may be caused by poor kidney function, heart or liver disease, allergies or digestive difficulties, particularly with protein assimilation. Edema can aggravate or mimic many conditions such as carpal tunnel syndrome (swelling of the median nerve), asthma or bronchitis (fluid in the lungs) or low back pain (fluid in the spinal cord area).

TREATMENT METHODS

Milliamp or Microamp Pad Treatment:	Acu-points:
Use pads, starting with milliamp current or microamp at sensational level, then follow with lower current at lower Hz: Step 1 - Preset mA Pads #1, set Hz to 2.5. Time- 5- 10 minutes. Place electrodes over motor points of muscles in edematous area, and turn up intensity to level of gentle muscle contractions to promote pumping of pooled fluids. Use caution and observe patient carefully for any adverse reaction. Step 2- Preset µA Pads #3, set Hz to 900 Time- 5 - 10 minutes or longer Electro-massage over mildly edemateous areas @ 2.5 Hz – see Chapter 13.	Acute edema due to External causes: Lu 7, LI 4, Sp 9, UB 28, LI 6 Edema due to Internal causes: St 36, UB 20, Ren 6, Ren 9 (with moxa or – current), UB 23, Du 4, UB 39. Edema due to Heart weakness – H 5, Pc 5 or 6, Lu 1 Consider stimulating EAV Lymphatic meridian points that correspond to affected region. **Note- See Cancer Pain diagrams for locations of acu-points St 36 and Sp 9**

Adjunctive treatments: Supplement with B complex vitamins, specifically B6, free-form amino acids for better protein absorption, potassium, restrict sodium, vitamin C. Avoid caffeine, alcohol, high salt, animal proteins, simple sugars, chocolate, tobacco, eat natural, whole-foods diet.

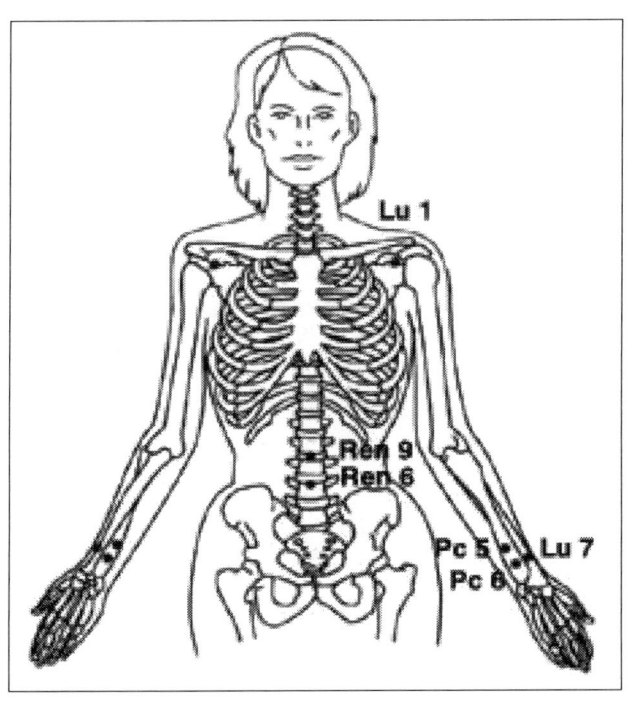
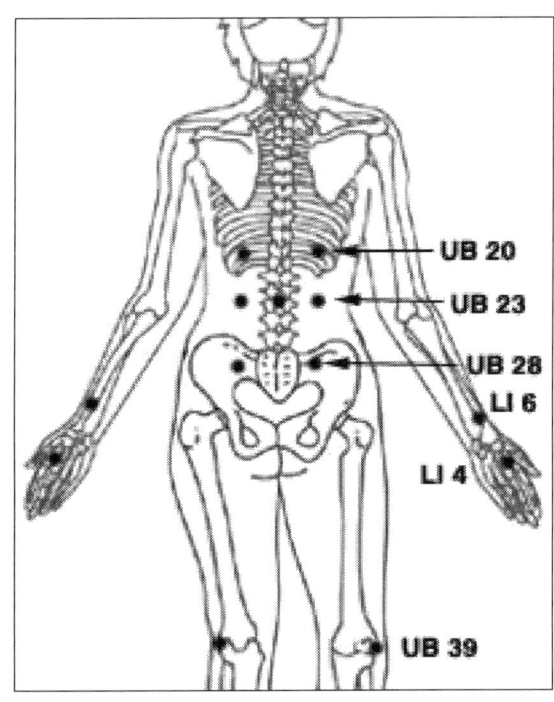

Eye Diseases

There have been many reports of successful improvements in patients with eye diseases through microcurrent treatment, specifically macular degeneration and other retinal diseases, and nearsightedness. The protocol given here may also benefit patients with glaucoma or conjunctivitis, as it is a general tonic to the nerves of the eye. This protocol must be used with caution, monitoring for any adverse effects. Many eye diseases, particularly in the elderly, are linked to side effects of pharmaceuticals. Consider alternative approaches to unnecessary drug intake to protect vision.

Treatment Methods

1. Have patient hold brass hand mass of device in hand of the side of the eye being treated. Set polarity to negative, waveform to slope, and frequency to 80 Hz. Set timer of device to 12 seconds.
2. Using trigger probe with cotton tips, treat a series of local acu-points around the orbit in direction from medial, upward and outward. This means that you start with the inner canthus, and then go to eyebrow points, then the outer canthus, and then continue around the eye until all points are stimulated for 12 seconds each. The points will often be tender when treatment is commenced. Adjust microcurrent intensity to level where the patient feels no electrical stimulation, but can see gentle flashing light in the eye from the retina being stimulated. Correct intensity level will very from person to person.
3. After all points are treated, have patient switch hand holding the hand mass, and repeat treatment on the eye of that side of the body.
4. Adjust frequency down to 8 Hz and repeat above procedure.
5. Adjust frequency down to 0.6 Hz and switch polarity to biphasic and treat each eye again. This time discontinue use of hand mass, and use two probes in combination around the eye. Use the two probe tips to treat sets of the same orbital acu-points that will pass current through the eye directly. Treat from above to below, left to right, and other diagonal placements. During this stage, place one probe on occipital hollows (GB 20) with other on eye points that remain tender and treat for 6 – 12 seconds each.

This treatment may be augmented by treating the following acu-points with needles or microcurrent: K 6, GB 37, TW 3, SI 3, LI 4. You may use kinesiology to determine the appropriateness of these points.

Adjunctive Treatments- Eliminate or reduce foods that can damage vision, such as animal fats, sugar, fried and processed foods, wheat, alcohol, tobacco and excessive coffee. There are many nutritional supplements that can support healthy vision. These include Vitamin A, E and C, zinc, selenium and other anti-oxidants and ginko biloba. Cataracts may be prevented in many cases by large doses of flavenoids, Vitamin E, N-acetylcysteine and Vitamin B2.

TREATMENT FORMULARY II: OTHER SPECIFIC CONDITIONS   279

EYE DISEASES

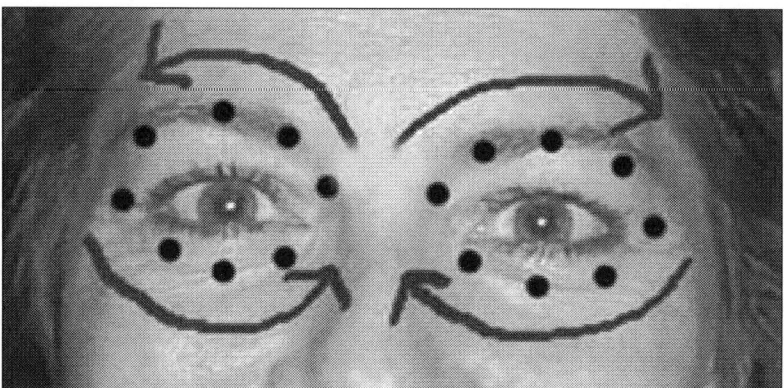
Treatment points for macular degeration probe technique – see previous page. These points can also be rubbed by patients as part of a home care regimen

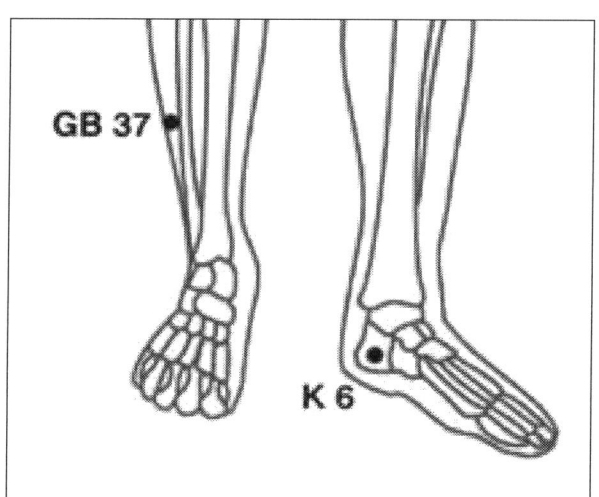

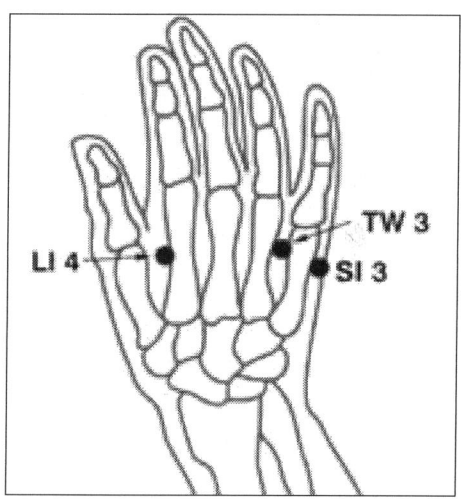

Fibromyalgia (FMS) and Chronic Fatigue Syndrome (CFS)

These conditions are listed together because they are different ways of describing the same complex of symptoms. These symptoms include diffuse pain, stiffness and aching, fatigue, poor sleeping, compromise of the immune system, hormonal imbalances and possible GI symptoms such as constipation, diarrhea and poor assimilation of nutrients. FMS patients have soreness on many of 18 characteristic tender points, most of which are on the Small Intestine, Urinary Bladder and Gall Bladder meridians. When patients complain primarily of pain, the condition is usually labeled fibromyalgia, when the primary complaint is of fatigue, CFS[251]. From a TCM perspective, these conditions arise from a combination of Qi and Yin deficiencies of the Spleen, Kidneys and Heart Blood, and stagnation or damp heat associated with the Liver and Spleen.[252] From a Western perspective, current research suggests causative factors of nutrient deficiency and various viral infections, notably hepatitis C[253]. Some practitioners have also reported significant success with fibromyalgia patients when they use the substance guaifenesin.[254] Such use of therapeutic nutrients can offer a valuable synergistic treatment agents with microcurrent electro-acupuncture.

For this condition, it is particularly important to use the entire Four-Step Protocol, as these conditions should be seen as a combination of Internal causes with myofascial stagnation. The guidelines described below are based upon the techniques outlined in Chapters 11 through 14.

Treatment Methods	Acu-Points
Step One: Vital for FMS/CFS patients. It is vital to palpate the patient's abdomen, which is likely to show several regions with pressure pain, pulsing or tension. Correctly selected Step One treatment points and polarities should be able to significantly release these abdominal signs, which is a major step toward healing. Step Two: Treatment of the tender points on the UB, SI and GB meridians, using microcurrent dermatome/distal or Mu-Shu techniques, with + on tense abdominal points and – on tense Back Shu points. Kyotoshin (needles with moxa) is also applicable. Step Three: These patients need to practice stretching, which may be difficult in the early stages of treatment. Systematic stretching and mobilization with simultaneous gentle microcurrent I.F. pad treatment will often be beneficial. They will not do well with deep massage therapies. Step Four: Take-home treatments, exercises and appropriate dietary regimens are very important for continued progress[255].	**Acu-points - Extraordinary Vessels:** Although evaluation may indicate any set of Master points, those that most commonly are indicated in the author's experience are: SI 3 → UB 62, and Manaka's Cross Syndrome treatment utilizing P 6/Lv 3 on the right and TW 5/GB 41 on the left. **Acu-Points - Ah Shi** Tender points on UB, SI and GB meridians. Other useful acu-points can be selected according to individual presentation. These points may be treated in pairs (→) or singly with patient holding hand mass and the acu-point treated with microcurrent trigger probe. *Pain associated with nervous tension:* LI 4- →Lv 3+ *Mobilize Yang through Du Mai:* Du 20+→Du 4- *Tendino-muscular reunion points very helpful:* GB 13, ST 3, GB 22, Ren 3 – treat tender pts. *Support Spleen functioning:* St 36, Sp 6, UB 20

---

[251] Donaldson, Sella and Mueller, The Neural Plasticity Model of Fibromyalgia, Practical Pain Management, May/June 2001
[252] Flaws, Bob, Curing Fibromyalgia Naturally, Blue Poppy Press, 2000, Chapter 7
[253] Vickery, Brice, Fibromyalgia Update: A New and Terrible Demon, The American Chiropractor, Vol. 23 Issue 5, 2001
[254] For details about this promising treatment see website: http://www.guaidoc.com/
[255] Flaws, Bob, Curing Fibromyalgia Naturally, Blue Poppy Press, 2000, Chapter 11

	Tonify Yin: Sp 6, K 3 *Insomnia:* P 6, H 7 *Liver Qi and Blood support:* Lv 3 + 8, Sp 10 *Open circulation of upper body:* LI 4, TW 5, LI 11 + 15, GB 20 + 21, UB 10, Du 14

Adjunctive Treatments- Proper nutrition through diet and supplementation is crucial for treating these conditions. Intake of foods and drinks based on simple sugars, alcohol caffeine or anything artificial must be curtailed. Pure water consumption must be increased. Herbal medicine has been effective – using antiviral herbs during early stages of treatments, and immune-boosting and systemic tonic herbs afterwards. Herbal information is beyond the scope of this book, however some herbs commonly used are goldenseal, echinacea and licorice during an infectious stage, and astragalus, Siberian ginseng and goldenseal during recovery phase. Chinese tonic formulas must be customized to the symptomatic presentation of individual patients. An increase in stretching and exercise is essential during the recovery process, and afterwards. CFS is frequently interconnected with abdication of aspects of personal power. Many CFS patients can resolve their symptoms through a process of reclaiming their power of personal choice and expression.

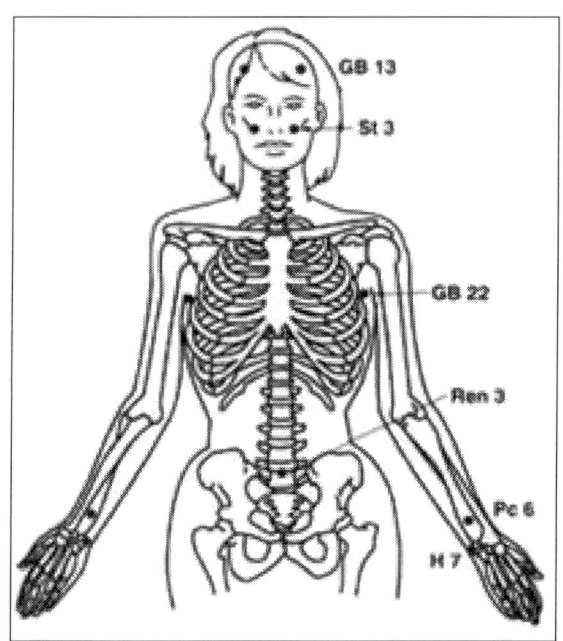
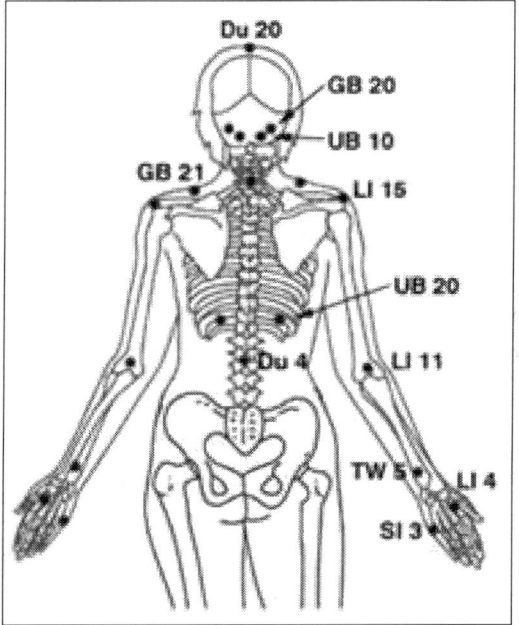
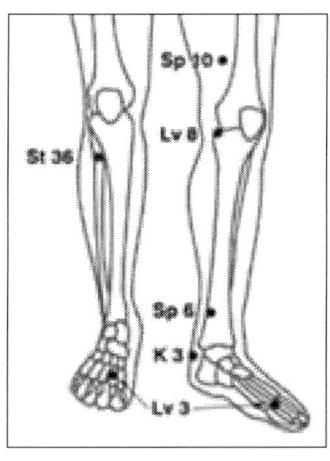

Lymph Drainage

German research into electro-acupuncture shows that lymph stasis accompanies chronic pain and inflammation, and that dispersal of this stasis is essential in resolving the painful condition. Voll and his colleagues discovered a lymphatic meridian[256] between the classical Lung and Large Intestine channels.

Treatment Methods	Acu-Points
Microcurrent Pad Treatment Use pads over shoddy nodes and lymph ducts. **Electro-massage and Pad Treatment:** Microcurrent pad treatment and electro-massage can also be used for regional lymphatic drainage, placing pads on major lymphatic ducts and distal zones. For example, use biphasic from clavicular area to Hoku point for upper extremities, and groin to sole of foot for lower extremity. Combine with very superficial lymphatic draining massage simultaneously. Patient must drink lots of pure water throughout course of treatments, or uncomfortable discharge symptoms are likely. Consider these parameters for pad treatment: *Polarity:* polarized; proximal (+), distal (-) *Frequency:* 10 + 300 Hz *Intensity:* 200 µA *Waveform:* Square *Time:* 10-15 minutes	Here are some of the most useful lymphatic vessel points, which can be treated at the EAV frequency of 2.5 Hz by placing a + probe on the local targeted region (such as tonsil) and the – probe on the LMV point: LMV.1-1: Lymph drainage of the ear LMV.1-2: Lymph drainage of the tonsils of the pharynx LMV.2/2a: Lymph drainage of the jaw and eye LMV.3: Lymph drainage of the nose and sinuses LMV.4: Lymph drainage of the lung LMV.4a: Lymph drainage of the esophagus LMV.4b: Lymph drainage of the larynx LMV.5: Lymph drainage of the heart

Peripheral Neuropathy, Nerve Regeneration

Useful for neuromas, nerve damage, or post-stroke. This method may require a long course of treatments, with frequent monitoring of progress. This treatment appears to be most effective when neuropathies are due to demyelinated peripheral nerve fibers, and is less successful for treating central nervous system lesions at our present state of knowledge.

Treatment Methods	Acu-Points
Local-Distal Polarized Probe Treatment: Local face acu-points (+), distal points (-) Lv **Polarized Pad Treatment:** Use polarized treatment with + pad over affected nerve root, and - on most distal area of pain, numbness, or tingling. *Polarity:* polarized; proximal (+), distal (-) *Frequency:* 0.6 Hz *Intensity:* 100-200 µA *Mode:* 2:1 *Time:* 20-30 minutes	**Acu-points - Local/Distal Combination** St 36 → UB 60, K 1 → Lv 3, GB 34 → UB 60, Sp 9 → Sp 6

---

[256] See next page for diagram of Voll Lymphatic Vessel

Adjunctive Treatments- Eat balanced, whole food diet, avoid stimulants, refined sugars and tobacco. The following supplements can support healthy nerve function -

Vitamin B-1: For neuritic pain, 1 gram/day recommended

Vitamin B-3: Large doses have been found effective for schizophrenia, severe depression

Vitamin B-6: Helps restore nerve receptor sites, useful in weaning off pain medications and anti-depressants. 25 - 50 mg 2 -3X/day.

Vitamin B-12: 1000 or more grams/day for neuropathic pain, such as herpes zoster, possibly trigeminal neuralgia, RSD. Give orally or by injection, up to 5000 gG/day.

Folic Acid: 5 - 10 mg 2X day

Panthothenic acid

Lecithin, calcium and magnesium

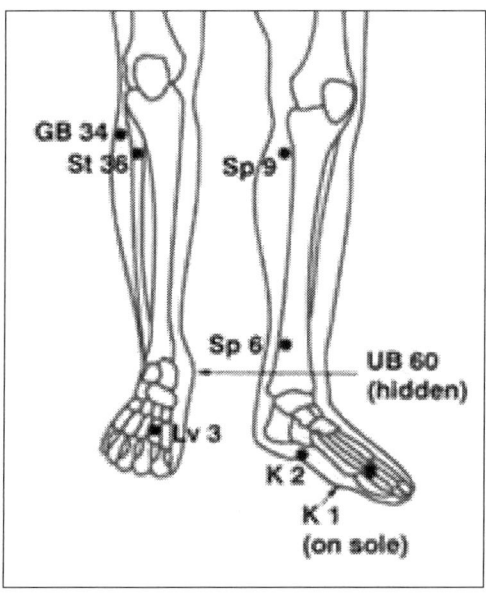

Leg acu-points for treatment of peripheral neuropathy

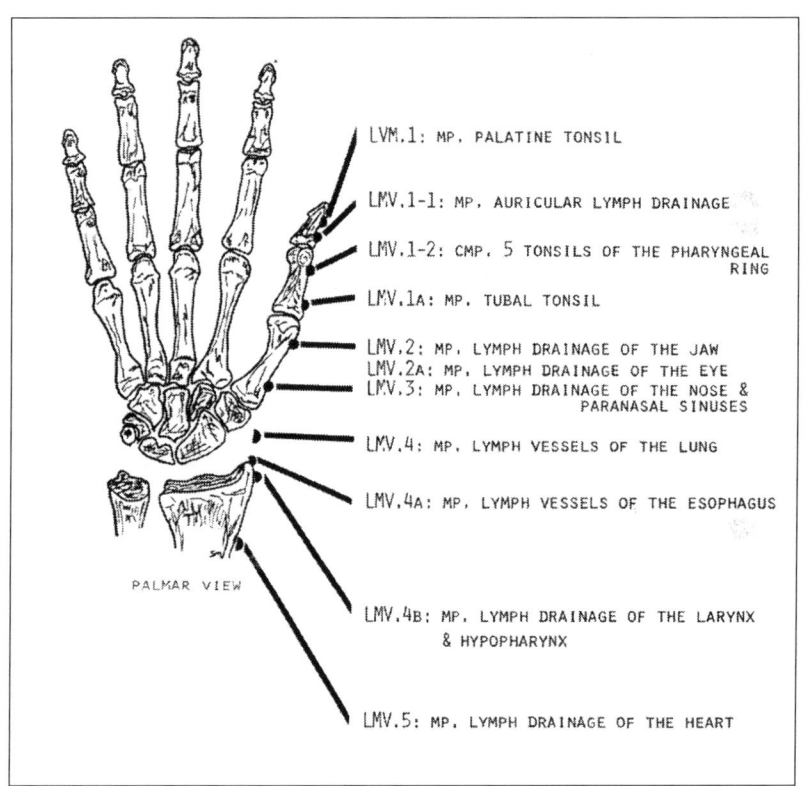

EAV Lymphatic meridian hand points. See also Treatment Formulary, Section III

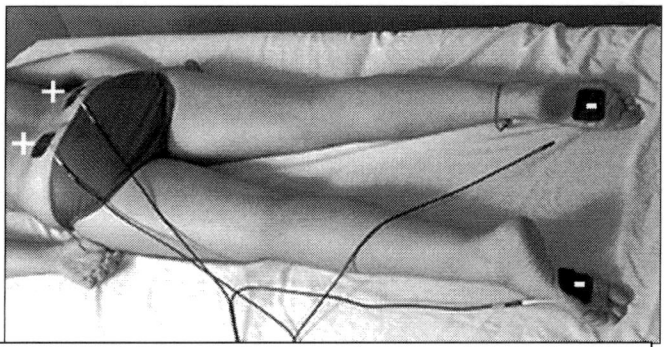

Pad placements for treatment of peripheral neuropathy, with each pad channel crossing midline of body

Reflex Sympathetic Dystrophy

Treatment Methods

Polarized Microcurrent Pad Treatment
This difficult condition may be successfully treated in many cases using the Four-Step process and Great Loops treatment.
1. Four Step Protocol - Steps One and Two
2. Use probe preset #2, with patient holding hand mass and trigger probe used to stimulate sore or tender points of <u>opposite quadrant</u> of body from affected area. For example, for RSD burning pain of right hand, search and stimulate tender points on area of left foot and ankle.
3. Once there is some pain relief from this distal technique, follow with polarized dermatome stimulation on affected arm and hand
   Acutron Mentor: Pad preset #5, modify polarity to negative
   Polarity: Polarized; neck nerve roots (+), hand (-)
   Waveform: Sloped
   Frequency: Low Hz (9.4, 9.7, 10 Hz - confirm with kinesiology
   Intensity: Low
 	
Combine this treatment with appropriate manipulation of misaligned vertebrae, paying particular attention to C7 - T1 area.

Adjunctive Treatments- See Peripheral Neuropathy, above

Restless Leg Syndrome

Restless Leg syndrome is a condition of uncontrolled movement of the legs.

Treatment Methods
Combination Probe, I.F. and Polarized Microcurrent Pad Treatment [257]: 1. Palpate to locate trigger points in longissimus muscles and rhomboids under shoulder blades. 2. Release with high Hz, high intensity microcurrent probes (Acutron Mentor- Probe preset #3). 3. Place I.F. pads to cover entire area from shoulder to buttocks, and apply milliamp-microamp combination therapy (Acutron Mentor - I.F. preset #5). 4. Complete with polarized microcurrent pads following L 4 – S 2 dermatomes of legs, with + pads proximal and – pads distal **Adjunctive Treatments-** See Peripheral Neuropathy, above

---

[257] Protocol thanks to office of Dr. Barnwell in Flagstaff, AZ

SCAR AND ADHESIONS TREATMENTS

TREATMENT METHODS
Probes, Pads or Electro-massage Treatment: The principle here is to apply microcurrent stimulation while simultaneously moving or manipulating the area of adhesion, usually with friction massage. Negative (-) current has a documented tissue softening effect, and in combination with stretching exercises and friction massage can significantly help to free up restrictive adhesions *Polarity:* Polarized; area to be softened (-), with (+) electrode at least 20 cm away *Waveform:* Square *Frequency:* 300-500 Hz *Intensity:* 100 μA *Mode:* 2:1 For post-surgical and injury scars, look at the coloration. If the color is well blended into surrounding skin, it is unlikely that there is any significant meridian blockage. If a purplish or other discoloration is present, it is important to open the flow through the scar. Using conductance measurements of your microcurrent device, measure the circumference of the scar, marking any areas with very high readings. Using the following parameters, discharge each of these "hot" points down to a reading of 50 or lower by treating in 12 second bursts and then re-measuring: *Polarity:* Polarized; (+) over hot spots; patient can hold hand mass to ground circuit *Frequency:* 0.1 Hz *Intensity:* 50 μA

RESTLESS LEG SYNDROME

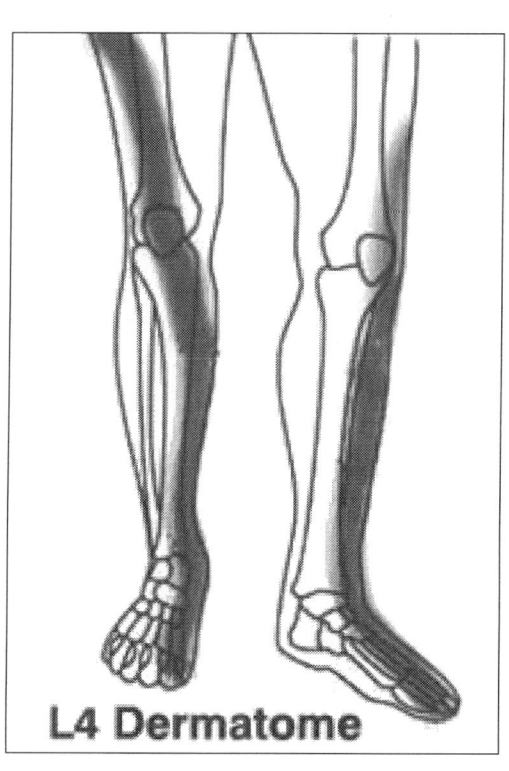

L4 Dermatome

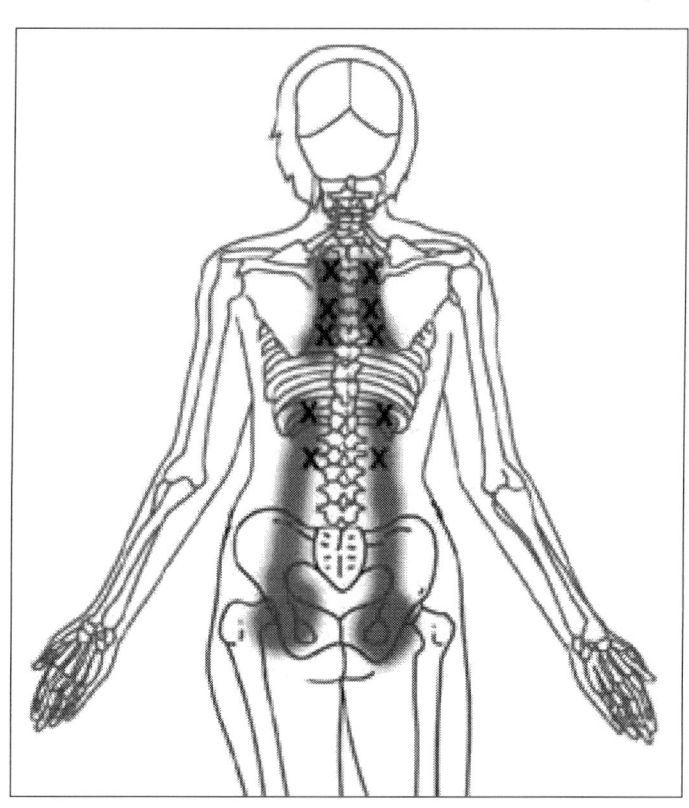

SHINGLES OR OTHER RIB PAIN

TREATMENT METHODS	ACU-POINTS
Four Step Protocol - Steps One and Two First, balance meridians with this treatment **Polarized Pad Treatment:** Use pad placements that stimulate entire course of affected nerves. Place one set from channel A with + pad on nerve root and - pad on nerve anterior to mid-axillary line. Place other set of pads from channel B with + pad over affected nerve posterior to mid-axillary line (behind other pad), and - pad over termination of nerve on front of body. DO NOT MAKE ANY PLACEMENT THAT PASSES CURRENT THROUGH THE CHEST, ESPECIALLY IN PATIENTS WITH HEART DISORDERS. *Acutron Mentor:* Probe preset #2 or #4	**Acu-points - Distal** GB 34, TW 5 + 6, distal GB meridian on dorsum of foot and corresponding ear points in acute phase. Concentrate on distal points in acute shingles pain. **Acu-points - Ear** thorax, chest, zero, Shenmen, occiput, thoracic spinal cord

Adjunctive Treatments- Remove refined carbohydrates from diet. Vitamin B12 injections have been helpful combined with adenosine monophophate (AMP). Other useful supplements – Calcium, magnesium, high doses of Vitamin C and bioflavenoids, L-lysine.

STROKE, PARALYSIS AND MAJOR HEAD INJURY

There have been many practitioners reporting successful results treating patients with these conditions using microcurrent therapeutics. This has mainly been accomplished through application of the basic and advanced techniques presented in this book over long periods of time. There have been some promising results in some studies in healing spinal cord injuries in animals using microcurrent.[258] With continued research, it is likely that these results can be applied to humans in the not too distant future. From what we know now, here are some valuable methods to consider:

TREATMENT METHODS
Scalp Acupuncture: Scalp acupuncture points may be stimulated with microcurrent, with or without needles. For best results, place hand mass or metal grounding plate under patient's bare feet connected to hand mass jack of device. Use trigger probe with – polarity to treat scalp points. The following EAV frequencies are recommended (kinesiology may be used to confirm the most resonant selection): Flaccid paralysis: 9.4, 8.3 Hz Spastic paralysis: 7.7, 5.9, 7.7 Hz **Micro-system Stimulation:** Stimulate ear, hand and foot points corresponding to affected body area **Polarized Pad Treatment Along Affected Limbs:**

---

[258] For details, see work of Richard Borgens of Purdue University at websites:
http://www.psych.purdue.edu/~punweb/faculty/borgens.htm
http://www.purdue.edu/UNS/html4ever/981112.Borgens.peg.html

see Peripheral Neuropathy protocol

Cross-body treatment:
For one-sided afflictions such as hemiplegia, treat healthy side with needles and microcurrent for several sessions and note results

Kinetic electro-therapeutics:
Place microcurrent I.F. pads over low back and pelvic region of patients in stroke rehab, and ask them to practice standing up and sitting down from walker or wheelchair, walking in place or other exercises. This has sometimes surprising results.

In the case of major head injury patients, some cannot communicate verbally to give feedback. This presents some challenges, as they cannot communicate when current is too high or uncomfortable. Yet, by observing relaxation of high tone of spastic musculature, some practitioners have been able to verify significant improvement through microcurrent treatment using basic local techniques of application.[259]

Adjunctive Treatments- Diet rich in magnesium and/or magnesium supplements, whole food diet, trace minerals, avoid simple carbohydrates. Helpful supplements – Vitamins C, B6, B3, B complex, free-form amino acids. Specifically prescribed Chinese herbal formulas frequently effective.

SHINGLES/RIB PAIN

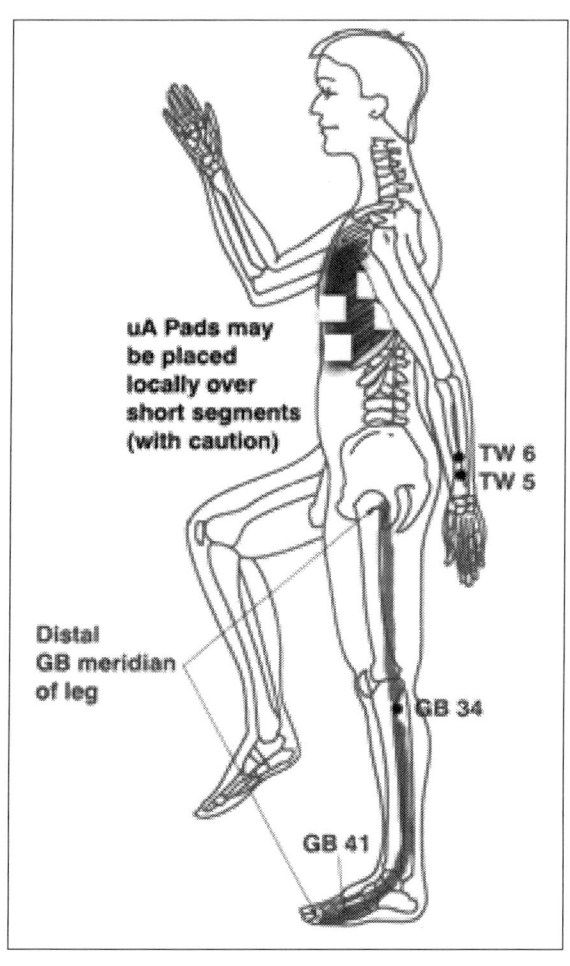
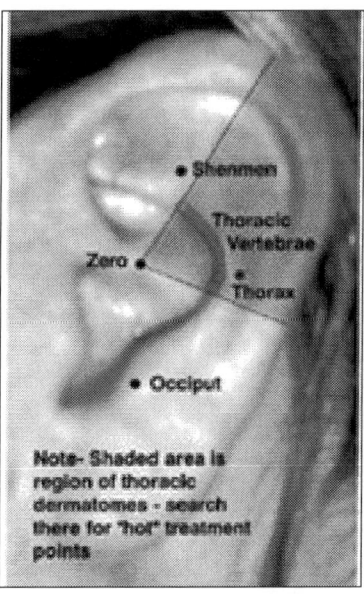

[259] For details on this see website www.eastwestmed.com and search for keyword "hightone"

TENDINITIS

Place probe on belly of muscle and treat to tendon. Use O/I probe technique and interferential μA or mA – μA combination pad placements for acute cases.

THORACIC OUTLET SYNDROME

Symptoms are pain, numbness and tingling of the arms, most commonly along the ulnar aspect, due to compression of the brachial plexus and subclavian artery and vein in the region of the first rib.

TREATMENT METHODS	ACU-POINTS
In a protocol offered by A. Katz,[260] polarized microcurrent pads are used over the affected area with + pad over the tender points of anterior scalene muscle insertion area and – pad over P 6 or SI 3, whichever is more reactive. Stimulation is applied for 20 minutes at 75μA. Katz places these pads over oblique needle insertions in the indicated regions. Lower extremity points St 41 or Lv 4 on opposite side are needled or treated with microcurrent probes to balance the treatment according to the style of Master Tong's acupuncture.	Upper Extremity: P 6 or SI 3 (tender points of anterior scalene muscle insertion area) Lower Extremity: St 41 or Lv 4 on opposite side

WHIPLASH

TREATMENT METHODS	ACU-POINTS
Use Manaka's Whiplash treatment followed by local stimulation of injured muscles using O/I technique. **Whiplash treatment**: Use needles and ion-pumping cords or polarized microcurrent probes to treat the point combinations listed in the next column *Polarity:* Polarized (check w/ kinesiology) *Frequency:* 10 Hz *Intensity:* 75 μA *Duration::* 20-30 seconds Follow with O/I stimulation of affected muscles. Use Baker formula to set Hz – length of muscle in inches X 1/10. For example, for 6" SCM muscle, set Hz to 0.6. You can use gentle microcurrent I.F. to complete treatment by flooding entire neck area.	**Acu-points - Local/Distal Combination** Manaka's Whiplash Treatment: SI 3 (+) left hand→UB 62 (-) right foot TW 5 (-) right hand→GB 41 (+) left foot

---

[260] Katz, Alejandro, <u>Thoracic Outlet Syndrome</u>, Acupuncture Today, December 2001

WHIPLASH

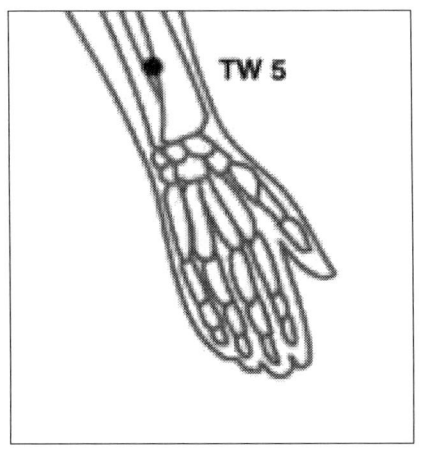

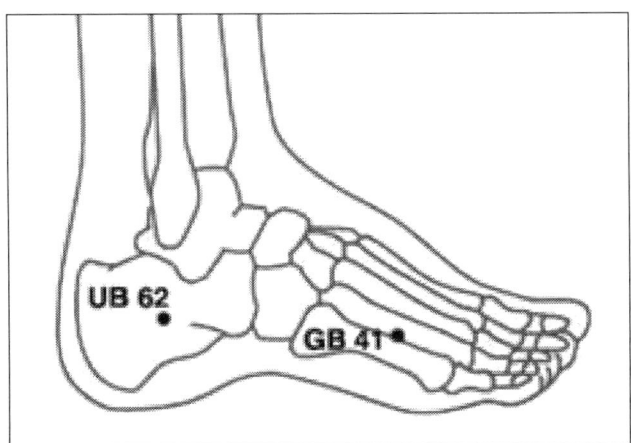

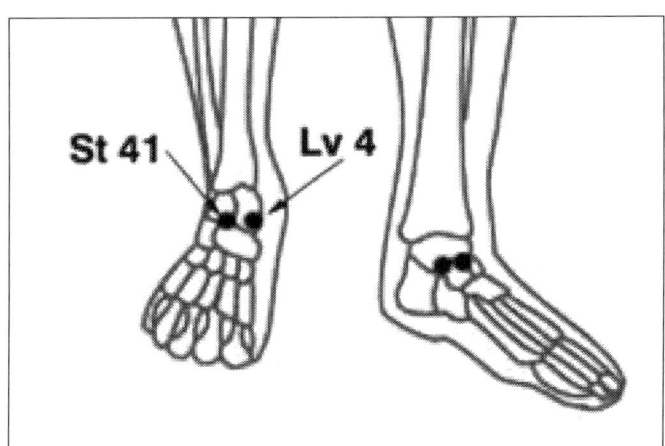

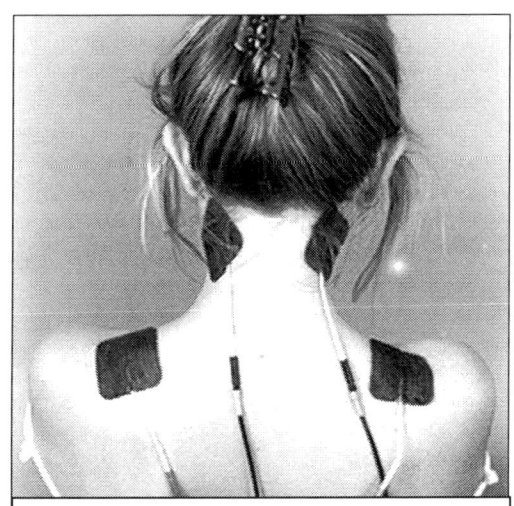

Micro-interferential treatment of whole neck following auto accident

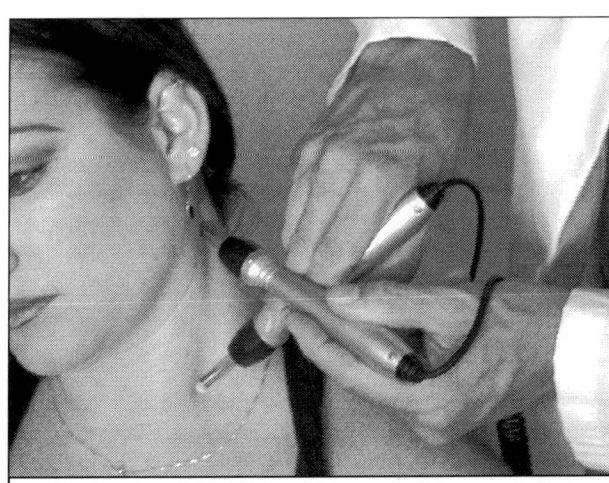

Origin-insertion probe treatment of sterno-cleido-mastoid muscle for treatment of whiplash

Treatment Formulary Section III

EAV Treatment Protocols

Chapter 17 covers methods of electronic meridian testing (EMT), including the system developed by Reinhold Voll and his colleagues. These doctors should be given a great deal of recognition for helping to initiate the modern science of energy medicine. Their tremendous contribution still has not been fully recognized or utilized in our medical and complementary healing arts, and is certainly ahead of its time. While a complete treatment of Electroacupuncture According to Voll (EAV) is beyond the scope of this book, this section of the Formulary details some valuable treatment methods and examples. Much of what is presented here is taken from Voll's writings that were translated into English and published in the American Journal of Acupuncture in the 1970's.[261] I have also derived a great deal of information from my EAV mentor Dr. Charles McWilliams. He has kindly given permission for me to reproduce some of the EAV point diagrams from his book Treatise of Acupuncture – Volume I & II[262]. The diagrams given here are by no means complete, and I highly recommend any interested student of EAV to purchase the book. Dr. McWilliams offers the finest English language home study and residency study programs in EAV that I am aware of.

Voll and his colleagues made four great contributions to the modern practice of acupuncture:

1) Development of the first commercial microcurrent stimulator, the Dermatron.[263]

2) Charting many "new" acu-points and meridians not recognized by traditional acupuncture. Many of these are referenced in this section. While they are often the same as traditional TCM acu-points, in many cases they are different in location and indication.

3) The determination of precise resonant electrical treatment frequencies which target many specific tissue systems and diseases. This is in accord with the Law of Resonance which is a basis for all healing arts.[264]

4) One of the most impactful contributions of EAV is the art of remedy testing. This is the practice of using an electronic ohmmeter to measure subtle changes in electrical conductivity over specific test acu-points, in response to the introduction of substances into the electromagnetic field of the patient. This final aspect of EAV is what has been embraced the most by modern energy medicine, and has been utilized by such devices as the Interro, Computron, Best, Vegatest and many others. Remedy testing is not covered in this book, as it is a major subject in itself. Some microcurrent devices that have a 0 – 100 scale conductivity meters may be used for this purpose.

---

[261] Most of the detailed information in this section is derived from his article 20 Years of Electroacupuncture Therapy Using Low-Frequency Current Pulses, as published in English in the American Journal of Acupuncture in 1975.
[262] Available through PanAmerican Institute – http://www.panaminstitute.com/
[263] Manufactured by Pitterling Electronic GMBH, Munich, Germany
[264] See Chapter Three of this book for more about the Law of Resonance

EAV Therapy

As you read these technique descriptions, you will see that they overlap with much of what has already been presented in Chapters 7 and 9. As stated above, although Voll's discovery of electronic remedy testing has received the most attention from modern practitioners, there is also great value in the microcurrent electro-acupuncture therapies he developed during the earlier part of his career. I hope more practitioners will pay attention to these remarkable methods.

EAV utilizes microcurrents in the low frequency range of 0.8 – 10 Hz, which resonate harmoniously with the targeted bodily tissues to be treated. Of this range, the <u>lowest values target blood and lymph, the middle frequencies the autonomic and peripheral nervous systems, and the higher values the internal organs</u>. Using a sweeping frequency modulation through these frequencies can increase therapeutic effect and decrease treatment time by up to 40%.[265]

In this system, acu-points may be measured on an ohmmeter device with a 0 – 100 conductivity scale. Readings above 65 are considered Excess, with the corresponding Organ/tissue system pathologically overactive. Readings below 50 are considered energetically deficient.

MERIDIAN BALANCING PRINCIPLES
(based on use of measuring device with 0 – 100 scale)

Treatment Parameter:	Tonification (supplement)	Sedation (drain)
Indication	"Deficient" meridian test point reading 45 or below	"Excess" meridian test point reading 65 or above
Current intensity	Higher currents of 75 – 200 µA	Lower currents of 25 – 50 µA
Frequency	Lower frequency of 0.6 – 10 Hz	Higher frequency of 80 – several hundred Hz
Waveform	Square or slope	Sawtooth
Polarity placement	Negative polarity over acu-point to be tonified, may use Source, tonification or other special points	Positive polarity over acu-point to be sedated, may use Source, sedation, entry-exit or other special points
Stimulation time	Just until meter rises to 50 – 60, then stop, usually about 20 – 60 seconds per point	Just until meter lowers to 50, then stop. Treat in short 6-second bursts, be sure not to over-stimulate

For both tonification and sedation, the practitioner should alternate between applying brief current bursts and then pausing to read the conductivity meter. This real time monitoring will

---

[265] Designated as "ramp Hz" modulation on the Acutron Mentor device

allow for precise treatment timing. When the reading is brought to "50"on the meter, the point is balanced and stimulation should be stopped. It is vital to not overdo tonification or sedation, as the desired effect may then be reversed.

EAV Basic Therapy

Voll started most treatments using what he called Basic Therapy. This is administered by balancing to "50" major distal points on all the meridians affected by a disorder, using sedation or tonification as needed. It is similar in intent to the Step One root treatment presented in this book in Chapter Eleven. Meridians are bilaterally treated that are directly affected, such as the Stomach channel for stomach problems or the Pericardium channel for circulatory disorders. Other meridians are selected for treatment according to energetic relationships such as:

- *Yin-Yang coupled function:* When treating Stomach, include Spleen. When treating Liver, include Gall Bladder. Source and Luo points are useful for this aspect of treatment.

- *Five Element relationships:* For deficiency diseases of the son, treat the mother. For example, the Large Intestine (Metal) can be treated to benefit the Urinary Bladder (Water), or the Liver (Wood) can be used to benefit the Heart (Fire). For excess diseases, treat the Control function, such as the Lungs (Metal) to calm the Liver (Wood) or the Kidney (Water) to reduce Heart Fire.[266]

- *Chinese Clock:* Functions with opposite energy peaks can be used to benefit each other. For example, the Triple Warmer can be treated to benefit the Spleen, or the Bladder for the Lungs.[267]

- *Secondary Vessels:* In some cases of energy stagnation the two microcurrent probes must be used to bridge between the terminal point of one meridian and the entry point of the next in the circulation of energy. For examples, with energy stagnation in the head, treat from SI 18→UB 1, or from LI 20→St 4. For bronchial asthma in the chest region, treat from Sp 21→H 1 and Lv 14→Lu 1.

- *Alarm points:* These can be treated when other methods do not produce desired effects. The microcurrent Mu-Shu method is an excellent method for this purpose[268].

- *Lymph vessel points:* The specific points of the EAV Lymphatic Vessel are indicated for draining the lymphatic vessels around the organs, which may be essential for relief of chronic inflammatory pain and disease. Please see the entry on Lymphatic Drainage in Section II of the Formulary. These points should be stimulated at 2.5 Hz for any non-responsive cases of chronic pain. The patient must drink large quantities of pure water during the entire treatment regimen.

In its most advanced form, EAV therapy is administered by applying a specific resonant frequency and polarity to acu-points that directly and indirectly affect the bodily function to be treated. This is a very powerful system in which is in accord with the the four Universal Laws described in Chapter 3 - Polarity, Resonance, Economy and Biasology.

---

[266] See Chapter Eleven for Five Element reference charts
[267] See Chapter Seventeen for Chinese Clock details
[268] See Chapter Nine

EAV Microcurrent Techniques

1. *Pain Point Treatment*

   This is similar to the Circling and Chasing the Dragon probe techniques, except that in EAV each local point is balanced to "50" on the meter using the above methods. If any point is resistent to correction, points above and below it on the same meridian are balanced, which will usually permit balancing of the point in question.

2. *Cross Hatching*

   A probe or roller electrode are used at high intensity to stimulate in a cross-hatched pattern over the affected area, with both electrodes close together. This may be used to relax asthmatic muscular spasms, or to treat tight neck and spinal musculature in conjunction with osseous manipulation.

3. *Rolling*

   A 8mm roller electrode may be used to release or promote lymphatic drainage of any part of the body after initial meridian balancing (Step One). The region should be rolled until the skin turns red.

4. *Electrical Moxa*

   This can be delivered through pad electrodes, with high tickling intensities delivered to the local area in brief bursts. Voll advocated 10 Hz as the ideal treatment frequency for this purpose.[269] This method can be useful for tendinitis, periostitis, calcaneal spurs and arthritis.

5. Longitudinal and Transverse Therapy

   Longitudinal therapy is the practice of passing currents along an entire extremity. Such treatment has been described in this book for the treatment of peripheral neuropathy, sciatica and many other extremity disorders. It is also valuable for edema, lymphatic swelling, hematoma, circulatory leg diseases and bone fractures. For treatment of the legs, pads can be placed from the sole of the foot to the groin or S-I joint of the lower back, depending on the desired current pathway. For the upper extremity, current can be passed from the palms of the hands to the shoulder region or neck nerve roots. Transverse therapy is passing microcurrents across joint regions and for treatment of injuries, varicosities and thrombophlebtis. As there is may be a danger of releasing a blood clot into circulation by this latter method, it is vital that the positive electrode be placed over the affected local area and the negative at some distance. Such patients must be under medical monitoring.

---

[269] The Acutron Mentor can produce this treatment by using microamp pad preset #4, Acute. Modify modulation to Burst, set comfortable on and off times and increase intensity to clearly feelable level. If results are unsatisfactory, try milliamp-microamp combination (I.F. #5).

Treatment Examples

In all listed conditions, the highest frequencies target the organs, the middle ones the nervous system, and the lowest blood and lymph. In all EAV point suggestions, Basic Treatment (Step One meridian balancing) should be done prior to treating these indicated special points. The acu-point names in **bold** are on the "new" EAV meridians, or extra points on the traditional meridians. Those in regular type are on the 14 principal meridians. Diagrams are offered for major points on the "new" EAV meridians.

Hypertension

Treatment Methods	EAV Acu-Points
Use pads to pass microcurrent from palm to palm bilaterally using the appropriate frequency. 3.3 Hz: arteriosclerosis 6.0 Hz: red (Liver or Heart Yang) hypertension 9.2 Hz: diastolic hypertension 9.4 Hz: spastic hypertension	St 36 GB 20 LI 11

Varicosities

Treatment Methods	EAV Acu-Points
Place pads on body to surround affected area. 10 Hz: phlebitis and varicose ulcers 9.4 Hz: varicosities and circulatory disorders 2.5 Hz: edema	**Circulation 8d** **Allergy 1a** *Arms:* Lu 7 *Legs:* St 32

Bronchial asthma

Treatment Methods	EAV Acu-Points
Place pads on spastic chest musculature or use probes to treat specific acu-points. <u>Caution</u>- do not pass any currents through chest on cardiac patients or with pacemakers. 2.5 Hz: sinusitis, or edema of varicose or lymphogenic origin 5.9 Hz: spastic contraction of the free branches of the bronchioles 6.0 Hz: abnormal high tone of the vagus nerve 6.3 Hz: emotional lability leading to asthmatic attacks 9.3 Hz: chronic bronchitis 9.5 Hz: laryngitis and tracheitis	See discussion of asthma in Section II for suggested acu-points

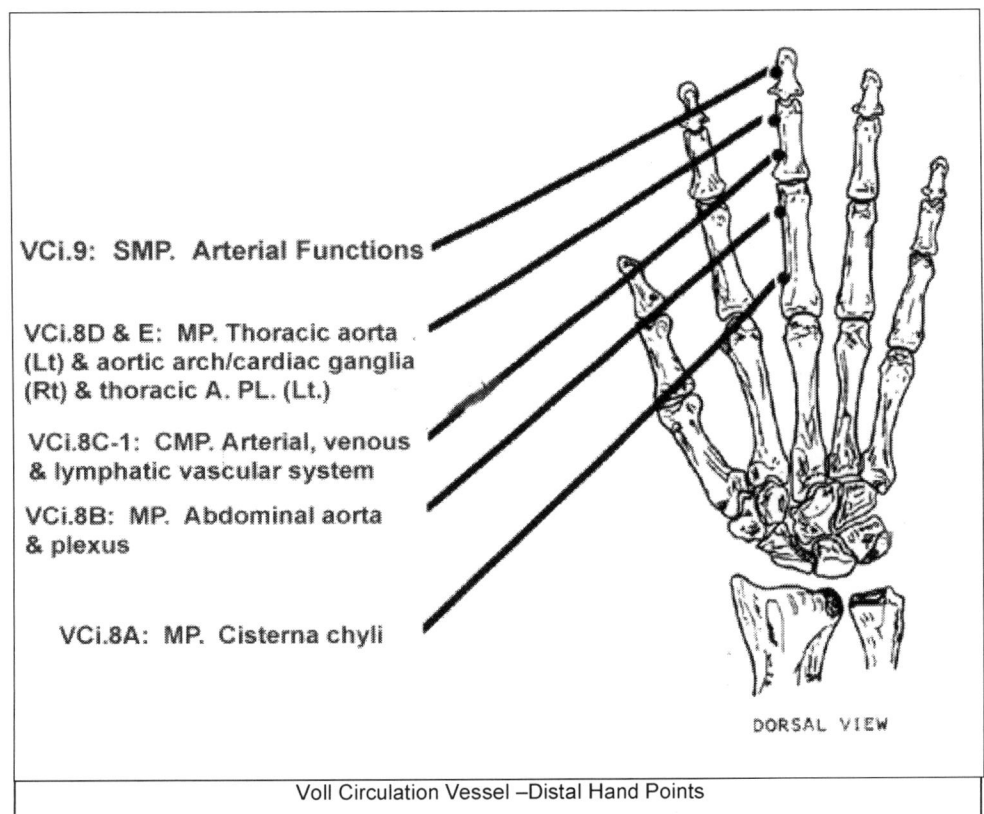

Voll Circulation Vessel – Distal Hand Points

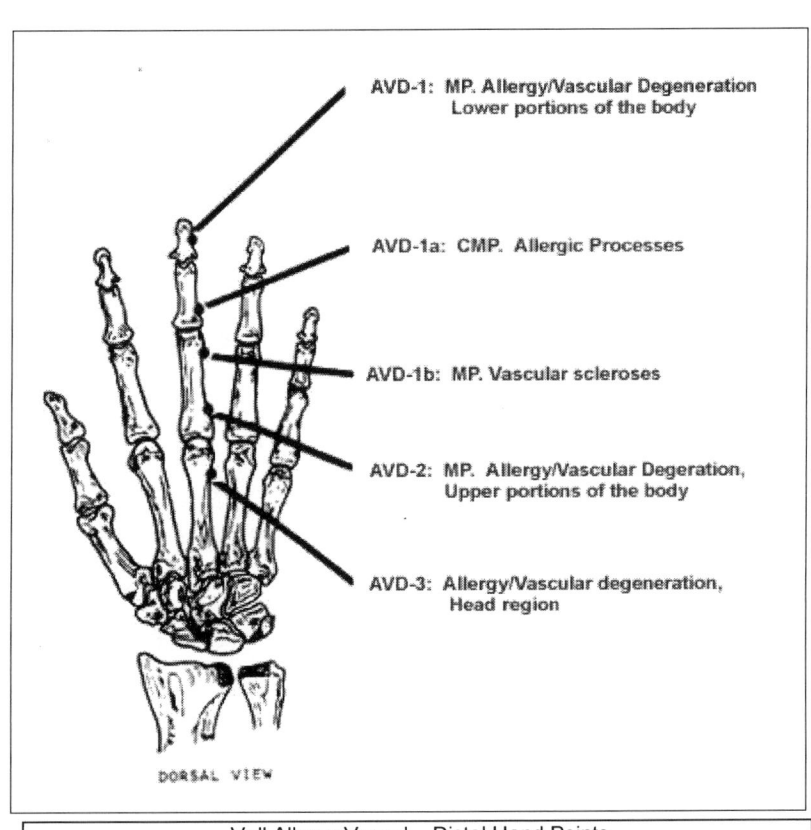

Voll Allergy Vessel – Distal Hand Points

Joint problems

TREATMENT METHODS	EAV ACU-POINTS
After meridian balancing use microcurrent I.F. four-pad placements for large joints, two-pad placement for smaller joints. 1.2 Hz: arthralgia 6.8 Hz: muscles supporting the joints 9.2 Hz: renal excretory insufficiency 9.4 Hz: gout 9.6 Hz: arthritis and arthrosis 9.7 Hz: rheumatoid complaints	Use local and distal acu-points, Great Loops point sets or other indicated points

Neuritis and Neuralgia

TREATMENT METHODS	EAV ACU-POINTS
Treat indicated points with appropriate Hz 3.9 Hz: for most neuralgias, including trigeminal 7.5 Hz: specific for trigeminal neuralgia 9.3 Hz: flaccid paralysis 9.4 Hz: paresis (partial or progressive paralysis)	*Upper extremity*: SI 7, **nerve degeneration vessel 2** *Sacral or pudendal area:* UB 60, **nerve degeneration vessel 1** *Spinal Involvement:* Du 13 *Trigeminal area*: UB 9, **nerve degeneration 3** Use roller electrode for local treatment follow-up

Bone Disease, Osteoporosis, Fractures

TREATMENT METHODS	EAV ACU-POINTS
Treat with pads or roller electrode above and below fracture or cast. This promotes rapid callus formation and prevents lymphatic stasis in area. 9.6 Hz: for arthritis, arthrosis, spinal column damage	*General:* UB 11, UB 12 *Upper extremity*: TW 15, LI 15 *Lower extremity:* GB 33, ST 30, SP 11a, GB 29, **joint degeneration vessel 1**

Hematoma and Lymphoedema of Jaw

TREATMENT METHODS	EAV ACU-POINTS
Use probes and roller electrode. 2.5 Hz: Edema, lymphatic drainage	Lymph 2, 11, 12, 13, 14 Other relevant Lymph points can be used.

Dupuytren Contracture:

TREATMENT METHODS	EAV ACU-POINTS
After Step One balancing of meridians, apply local current through pads to affected area of hand and wrist. 6.8 Hz: Dupuytren contracture	Use local treatment with pads and use probes to treat proximal points on affected meridians, including Pericardium

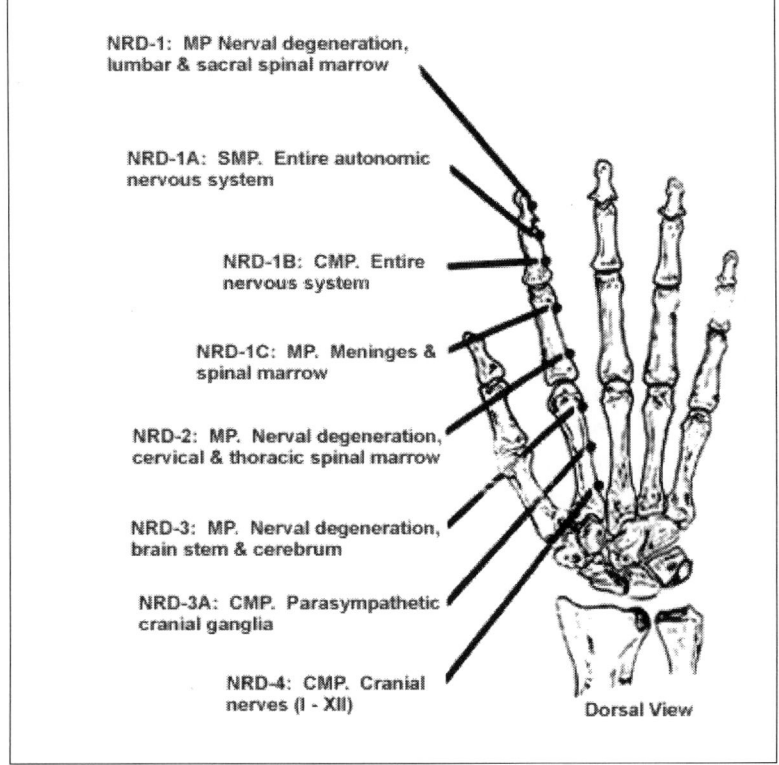

Voll Nerve Degeneration Vessel – Hand Points

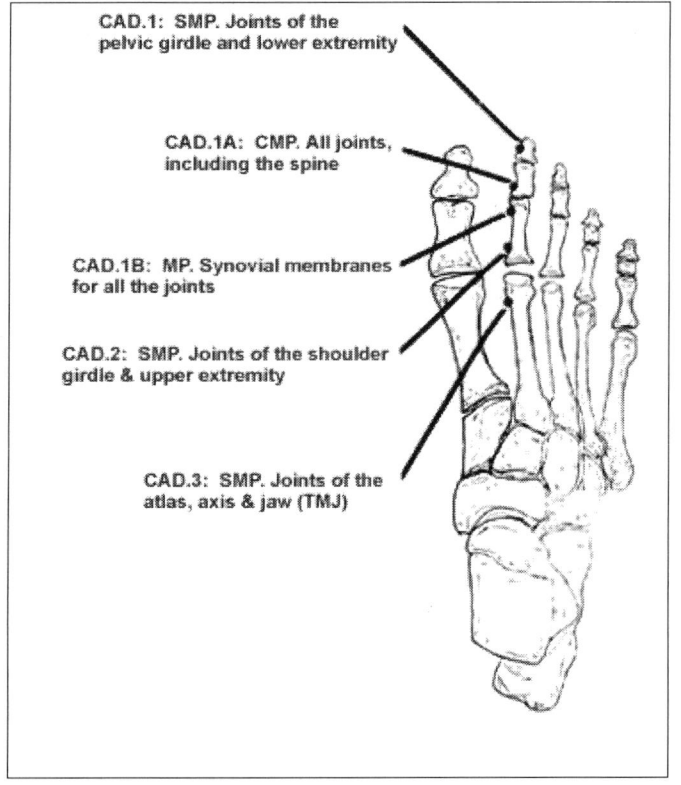

Voll Joint Degeneration Vessel

Renal Colic

TREATMENT METHODS	EAV ACU-POINTS
Use probes to treat acu-points with appropriate Hz. Longitudinal therapy from sole of foot to above alarm point of kidney or urinary bladder is applicable. 3.5 Hz: Kidney stones	EAV points (balance all points to 50) Kid 1 – 12 on affected side *If stone has reached ureter:* GB 25, Ren 3, UB 67- 50

Biliary and Pancreatic Colic

TREATMENT METHODS	EAV ACU-POINTS
Use probes to treat acu-points with appropriate Hz. Then apply pads. For biliary colic, apply pads in front and back of the gall bladder organ from GB 24 on front to corresponding back region. For pancreatic colic, apply pads from right of umbilicus to back. 3.5 Hz: Biliary / pancreatic colic	Biliary Colic: balance GB points 44 – 30, GB 24 and SI 3 to "50" on the conductivity meter Pancreatic Colic: balance spleen points 1 – 10, Lv 13 and SI 3 to "50",

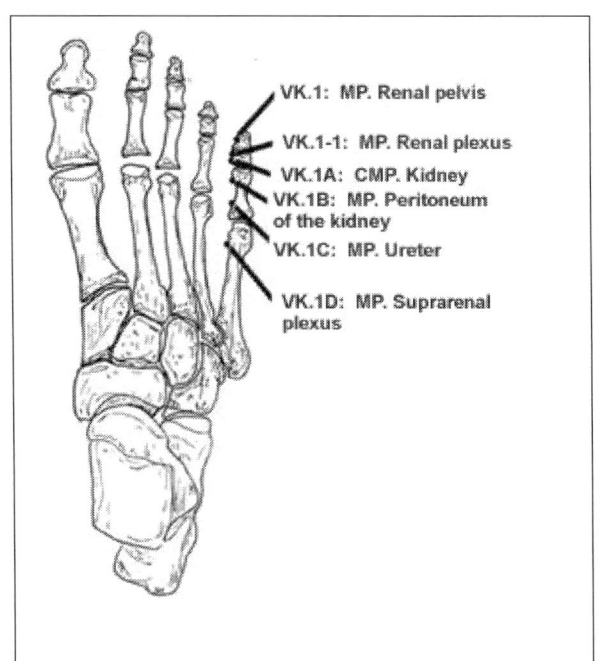

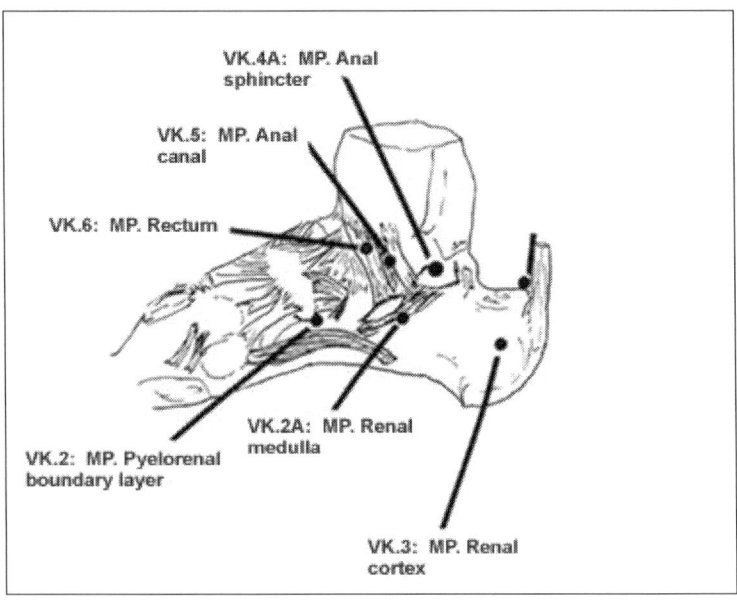

Voll Kidney Vessel – Foot Points

TREATMENT FORMULARY III: EAV PROTOCOLS

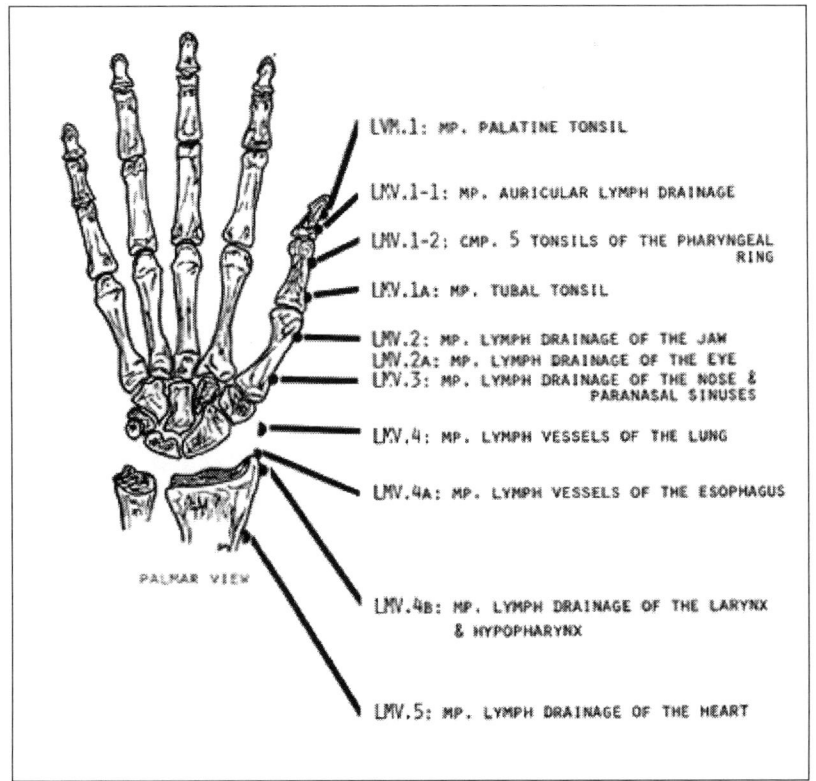

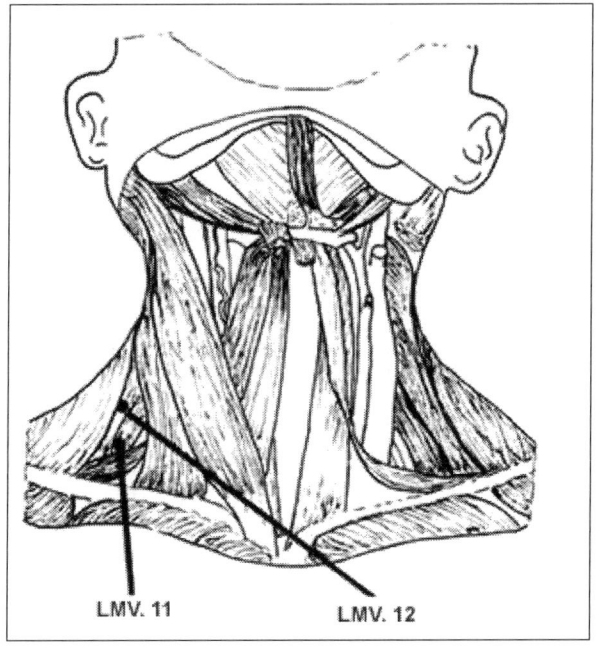

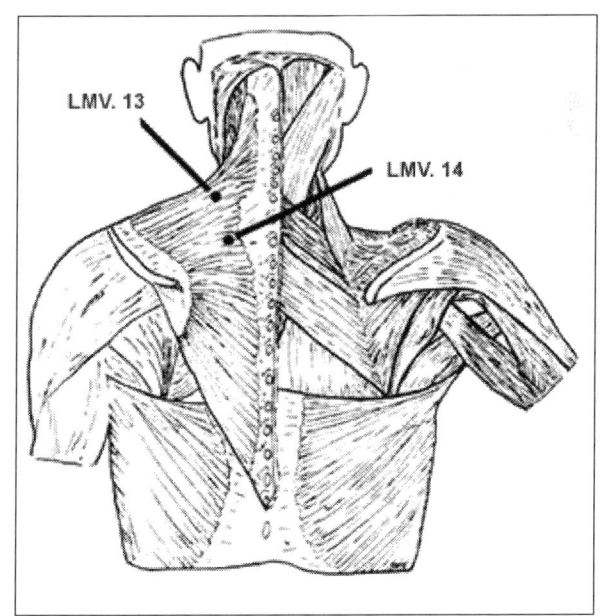

Voll Lymphatic Vessel – Of great importance for treatment of many chronic pain conditions

EAV Headache Treatments

Voll offered very detailed instructions for using points and frequencies for treating many types of headaches, as reproduced here. Treatment is carried out using microcurrent probe electrodes at sub-sensational intensities, at the indicated frequencies. Many of the frequency-point combinations may be used to treat the root conditions listed, even if there are no headache symptoms. Apparently, Voll treated these points singly, with the patient holding a grounding hand mass. A useful alternative method is to use a set of two polarized probes, with the + probe on a head point and the − probe on an appropriate distal point.

TREATMENT METHODS	EAV ACU-POINTS
Viscerally produced headaches 4.0 Hz: menorrhagia 4.9 Hz: dysmenorrhea 9.4 Hz: digestive headaches 8.5 Hz: biliary headaches 9.4 Hz: urogenitally caused headaches	*General:* Balance the 3 distal points on the UB, GB and St meridians and use probes to open secondary vessels between SI 18→UB 1, TW 21→GB 1, and LI 20→St 4. *Digestive headaches:* St 1 + 5, plus other sore frontal points *Biliary headache:* GB 1 and sore temporal points *Urogenital headaches:* **UB 49a to 51**
Vascular headaches 4.0 Hz: headache with vertigo 5.5 Hz: hormonal disturbances, angiospasms and paresthesias 6.0 Hz: hypertonic headache 9.4 Hz: migraines and other circulatory disturbances	*Carotid sinus:* St 12 *Brain vessels:* **nerve degeneration 3** *Pons:* UB 9 *Medulla:* UB 10 *Balance sympathetic nervous system:* GB 20
Endocrine-induced headaches 4.0 Hz: pituitary disturbances 4.9 Hz: ovarian disturbances 9.6 Hz: for parathyroid disturbances	*Pituitary:* SI 15, TW 16, GB 21 *Reproductive:* Lv 16, Sp 11 *Parathyroid:* St 9 *Thyroid:* St 10 *Adrenals:* UB 22
Cerebral headaches 1.2 and 6.3 Hz: headaches with elevated stimulus threshold and concussions	*Pons:* UB 9 *Medulla:* UB 10 *Mesencephalon:* GB 9 *Diencephalons* GB 7 *Entire brain :* **Nerve degeneration 3**
Meningeal headaches 4.9 Hz: meningeal headaches	*Meninges:* TW 19 also treat secondary vessels from UB 1→**Du 23a** and from LI 20→UB 1
Sinus headaches 2.5 Hz: lymph and blood stasis, sinuses	*Frontal sinuses:* UB 2 *Maxillary sinuses:* St 5 *Ethmoid sinus:* LI 20→UB 1 *Lateral Nasal sinuses:* LI 19 *Nose-head sinus vault:* Du 23 *All sinuses:* **Lymph 13 and 14**

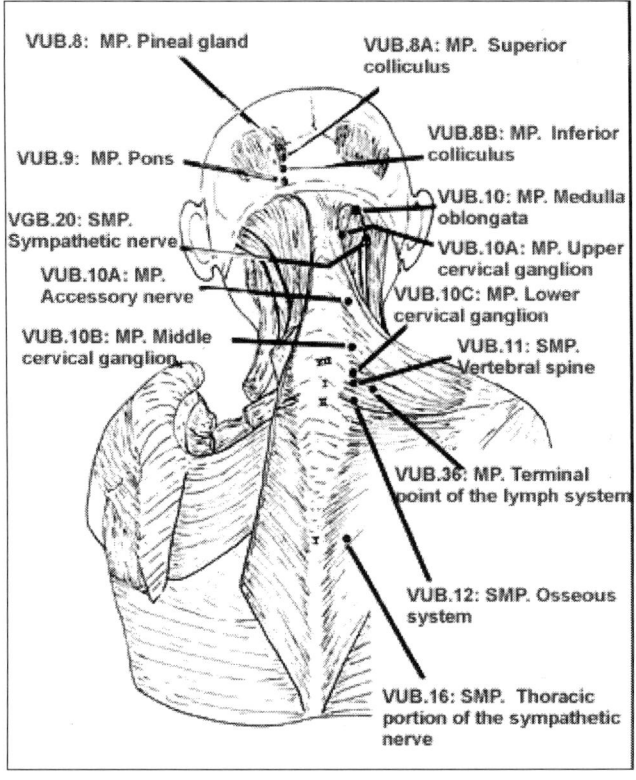

Voll Bladder Vessel – Upper Back Points

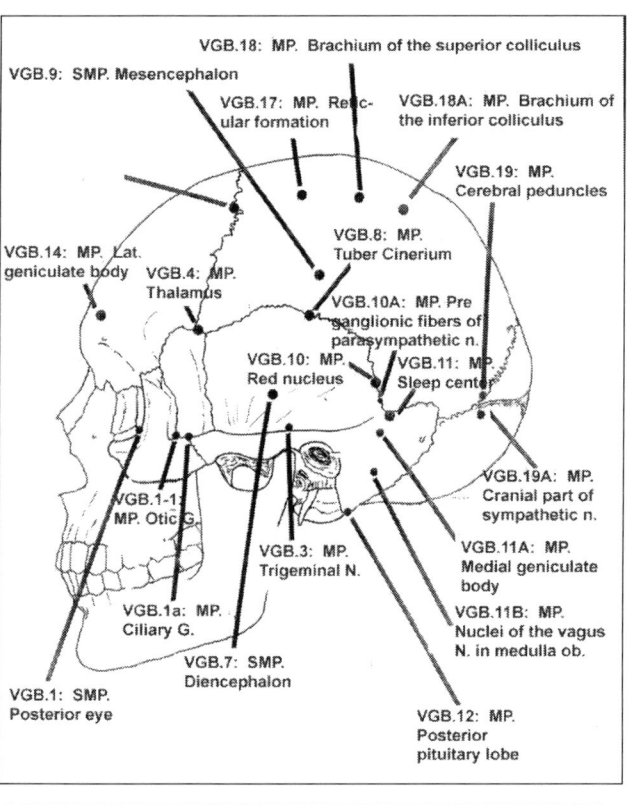

Voll Gall Bladder Vessel – Head Points

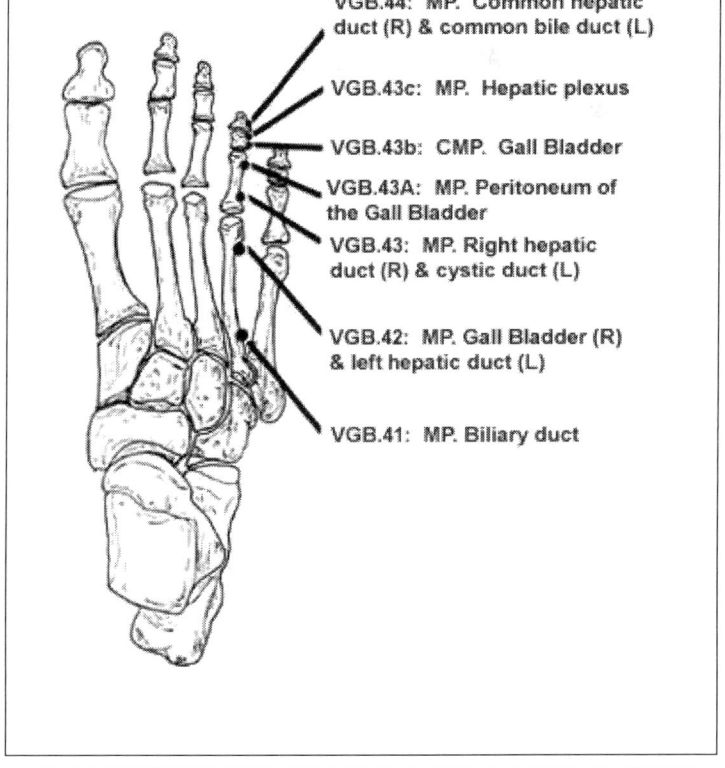

Voll Gall Bladder Vessel – Foot Points

Opthalmological headaches 3.6 and 4.9 Hz to reduce inflammation	*Anterior eye:* TW 21 *Posterior eye:* GB 1 *Sinus cavernosus:* UB 1→**Du 23a** *Ethmoid sinus:* LI 20→UB 1
Otological headaches 9.2 Hz: ear problems 5.8 Hz: if vertigo present	*Middle ear and tympanic membrane:* TW 17 *Inner ear:* TW 18 *Outer ear and auditory canal:* SI 19 outer ear *Lymph drainage of ear:* **Lymph 1-1**
Odontogenic headaches 3.6 and 4.9 Hz to reduce inflammation	*Center of Maxilla:* GV 25 *Lateral maxilla:* St 7 *Lateral mandible:* St 8 *Central mandible:* Ren 24 *Lymph drainage of jaw:* **Lymph 2**
Tonsillogenic headache 9.4 Hz: reduce inflammation of tonsils	*Palantine tonsils:* **Lymph 1** *Tubal tonsils:* **Lymph 1a** and LI 18 *Pharyngeal tonsil:* **Ren 23c** and LI 17 *Lingual tonsils:* **St 3a** *All tonsils:* **Lymph 12**
Vertebral induced headache 9.6 Hz: Spinal column damage	*Entire spinal column:* UB 11 *Cervical vertebrae:* SI 6 *Lumbar vertebrae:* UB 61 *Thoracic vertebrae:* UB 29 *Atlas-axis joint of neck:* **Joint degeneration vessel 3** *Lymph supply of spine:* **Lymph 12** *Laryngeal tonists affecting cervical vertebrae:* LI 17 *Thymus to help maintain spinal ligaments:* St 11
Allergic headaches 9.6 Hz: calcium metabolism 8.1 Hz: water, sodium and potassium balance 1.7 Hz: sympathetic nervous system	*Allergy control:* Allergy 1, 2, 3 *Parathyroid gland:* St 9 *Carotid sinus:* St 11 *Adjust sympathetic nervous system:* GB 20 *Regulate parasympathetic nervous system:* **St 10a**

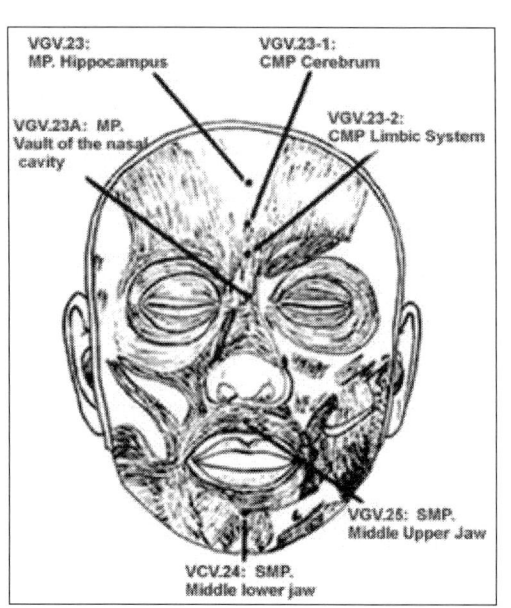

Voll Governor Vessel – Facial Points

TREATMENT FORMULARY III: EAV PROTOCOLS 303

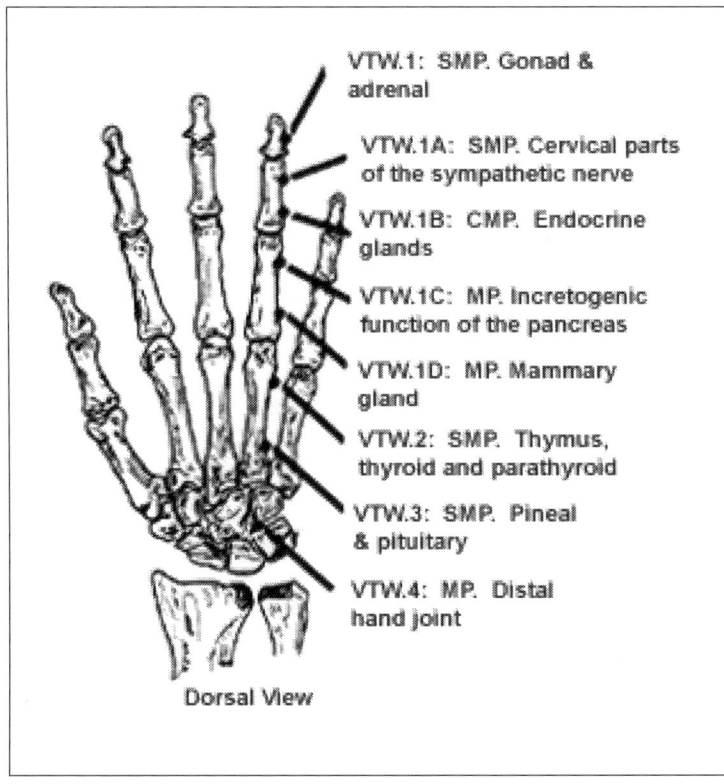

Voll Triple Warmer Vessel - These points measure the specific endocrine glands

- VTW.1: SMP. Gonad & adrenal
- VTW.1A: SMP. Cervical parts of the sympathetic nerve
- VTW.1B: CMP. Endocrine glands
- VTW.1C: MP. Incretogenic function of the pancreas
- VTW.1D: MP. Mammary gland
- VTW.2: SMP. Thymus, thyroid and parathyroid
- VTW.3: SMP. Pineal & pituitary
- VTW.4: MP. Distal hand joint

Dorsal View

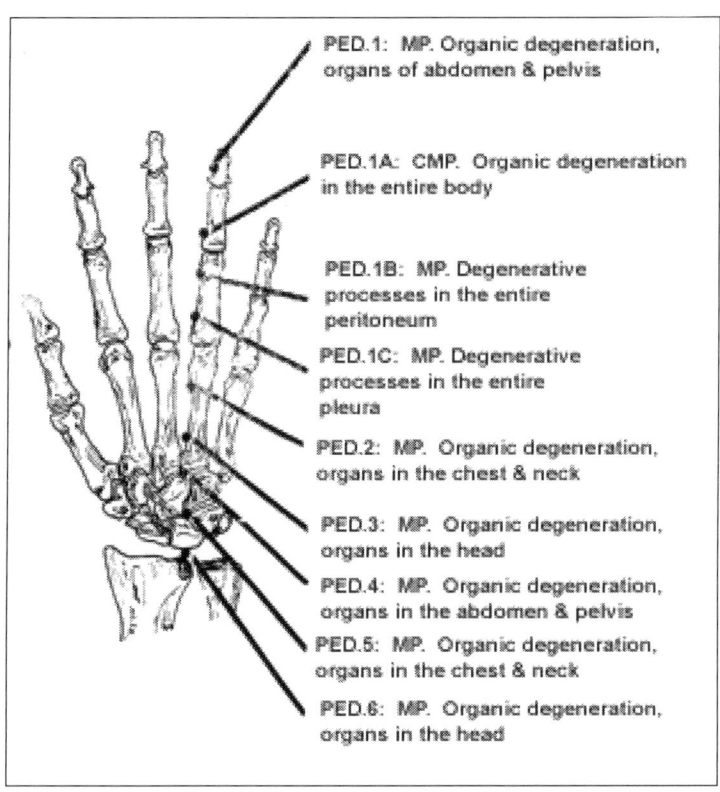

Voll Organ Degeneration Vessel – PED stands for Parenchymal and Epithelial Degeneration

- PED.1: MP. Organic degeneration, organs of abdomen & pelvis
- PED.1A: CMP. Organic degeneration in the entire body
- PED.1B: MP. Degenerative processes in the entire peritoneum
- PED.1C: MP. Degenerative processes in the entire pleura
- PED.2: MP. Organic degeneration, organs in the chest & neck
- PED.3: MP. Organic degeneration, organs in the head
- PED.4: MP. Organic degeneration, organs in the abdomen & pelvis
- PED.5: MP. Organic degeneration, organs in the chest & neck
- PED.6: MP. Organic degeneration, organs in the head

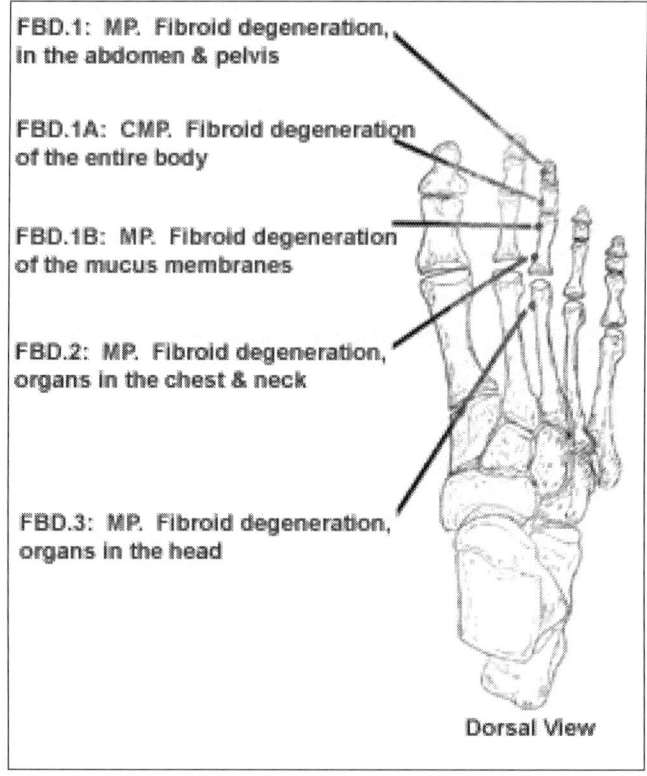

Voll Fibroid Degeneration Vessel

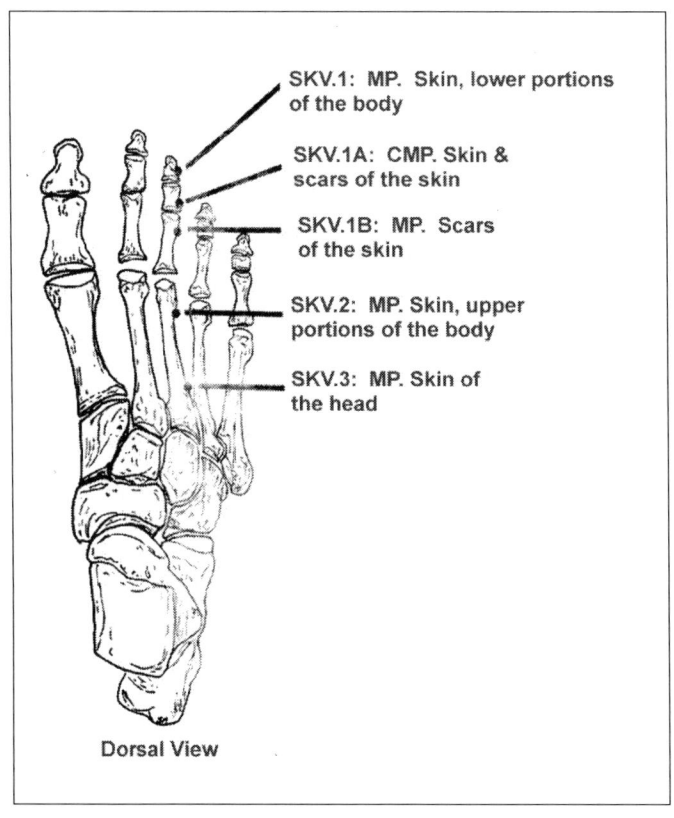

Voll Skin Vessel

Treatment Formulary III: EAV Protocols 305

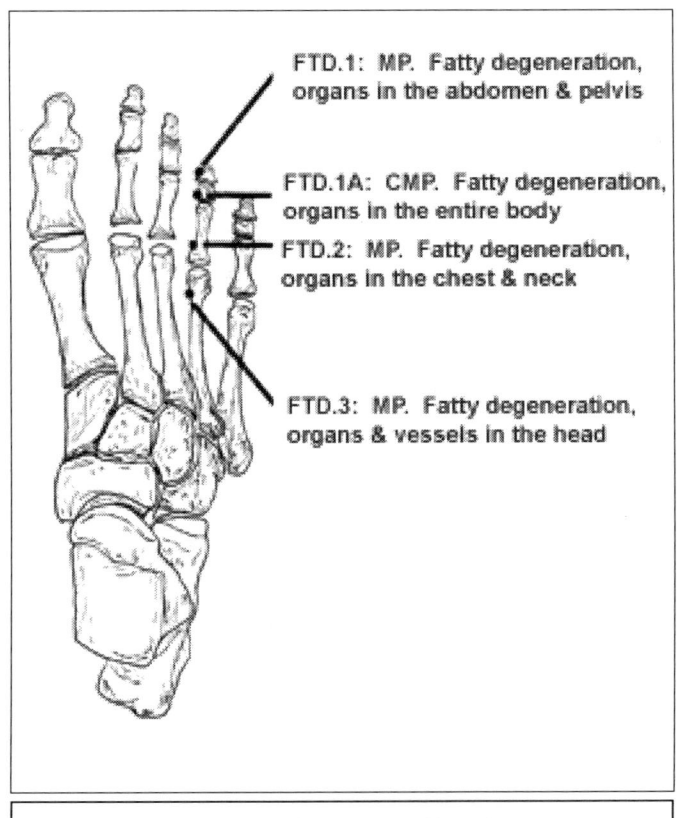

Voll Fatty Degeneration Vessel

BIBLIOGRAPHY

1. Alternative Medicine: The Definitive Guide, Burton Goldberg Group, 1995
2. Becker, Robert, Cross Currents, Jeremy P. Tarcher, 1990
3. Becker, Robert, The Body Electric, Morrow, Quill, 1985
4. Bensoussan, Alan, The Vital Meridian, Churchill Livingstone, 1991
5. Chan, Pedro, Electro-Acupuncture, Chan's Corporation, 1974
6. De-Xin, Yan, Aging and Blood Stasis, Blue Poppy Press, 1995
7. Essentials of Chinese Acupuncture, Foreign Languages Press, 1980
8. Flaws, Bob, Sticking to the Point, Blue Poppy Press, 1994
9. Kahn, Joseph, Principles and Practice of Electrotherapy, Churchill Livingstone, 1987
10. Kaptchuk, Ted, The Web That Has No Weaver, Congden and Weed, 1983
11. Lakhovsky, Georges, The Secret of Life, Noontide Press, 1992
12. Lee, Miriam, Master Tong's Acupuncture, Blue Poppy Press, 1992
13. Maciocia, Giovanni, The Foundations of Chinese Medicine, Churchill Livingstone, 1998
14. Manaka, Yoshio, Chasing the Dragon's Tail, Paradigm Publications, 1995
15. Mann, Felix, Acupuncture, The Ancient Chinese Healing Art and How It Works Scientifically, Vintage Books, 1973
16. Matsumoto and Birch, Five Elements and Ten Stems, Paradigm Publications (no date)
17. Matsumoto and Birch, Hara Diagnosis, Reflections on the Sea, Paradigm Publications, 1988
18. McWilliams, Charles, Treatise of Acupuncture, Volumes I – VIII, Health Sciences Research, 1983
19. Nelson and Currier, Clinical Electrotherapy, Appleton and Lange, 1987
20. Oda, Hirohisa, Ryodoraku Textbook, Naniwasha Publishing, 1989
21. Richard Gerber, Vibrational Medicine, Bear and Co. 1988
22. Seem, Mark, A New American Acupuncture, Blue Poppy Press 1993
23. Starwynn, Darren, Advanced Electromedicine, self published, 1999
24. Tan and Rush, Twelve and Twelve In Acupuncture, self published, 1991
25. Tan and Rush, Twenty Four More In Acupuncture, self published, 1991
26. Tortoro and Anagnostakos, Principles of Anatomy and Physiology, 3rd Edition, Harper and Row 1981
27. Various authors, American Journal of Acupuncture, 1974 – 1999. Each article quoted is referenced in a footnote in the applicable sections

RESOURCES

For correspondance with the publisher or author, or for ordering additional copies of this book:
email: info@DesertHeartPress.com

AcuLogic™ software information: Write to the author, c/o info@DesertHeartPress.com

Information on hands-on seminars on microcurrent electro-acupuncture, Vibrational Beauty™ whole-body facial treatment and other relevant subjects:
email: seminars@neta.com   web: www.east-westseminars.com

Acutron Mentor™ sales and information: Contact Microcurrent Research, Inc.
1-800-872-6789, email: microcurrent@neta.com, web: www.microcurrentresearch.com

Information on transformational Core Healing trainings and intensives:
email: info@OneHeartTeachings.com   web: www.OneHeartTeachings.com

Research studies, practitioner referral database, links: www.eastwestmed.com

To find valuable information (sometimes) about current research and resources in electromedicine on the Internet, place the following keywords into a good search engine:

electromedicine

acupuncture

electro-acupuncture

microcurrent

Royal Rife

Nordenstrom

Manaka

Organizations:

International Society For The Study Of Subtle Energies And Energy Medicine: 5800 W 6th, Topeka, Kansas 66606 (913) 273-7500, FAX: (913) 273-8625

Panamerican Institute- EAV and naturopathic residential medical instruction:
http://www.panaminstitute.com/

List of valuable website links for acupuncture resources and organizations from Acupuncture Today publication: http://www.acupuncturetoday.com/links.html

Index

A

abdominal 11, 30, 33, 68, 107, 109, 110, 144, 147, 148, 151, 159, 166, 183, 191, 200, 202, 207, 222, 224, 250, 252, 272, 280
abdominal diagnosis 68, 222
abdominal pain 159
abdominal reaction patterns 151
accelerate healing 79, 181
accommodation 43, 49, 57, 186
Acne 6, 264
action potentials 22, 34
AcuLogic Software 213
acu-points 10, 11, 25, 27, 29, 30, 31, 33, 34, 35, 36, 38, 39, 47, 48, 49, 50, 52, 54, 58, 64, 67, 68, 70, 74, 78, 79, 82, 86, 87, 90, 91, 92, 93, 95, 96, 99, 103, 107, 108, 115, 128, 136, 138, 139, 151, 153, 172, 173, 180, 183, 188, 191, 192, 196, 205, 208, 212, 218, 219, 229, 231, 234, 236, 256, 264, 268, 269, 277, 278, 280, 282, 290, 291, 292, 294, 296, 298
acupressure 67, 140, 205
acupuncture ... 3, 7, 9, 12, 13, 14, 15, 16, 19, 21, 22, 23, 25, 27, 28, 29, 30, 31, 32, 33, 34, 35, 36, 37, 38, 39, 40, 42, 43, 45, 47, 48, 49, 50, 62, 63, 64, 65, 66, 67, 69, 70, 73, 74, 78, 79, 89, 90, 95, 97, 103, 104, 108, 109, 115, 120, 123, 125, 135, 136, 137, 138, 140, 143, 144, 150, 152, 153, 156, 158, 162, 168, 170, 172, 173, 179, 181, 183, 186, 187, 188, 191, 193, 205, 206, 219, 222, 224, 229, 230, 232, 242, 250, 260, 272, 274, 286, 288, 290
acupuncture needles . 21, 33, 37, 39, 47, 79, 123, 144, 162, 230, 242
    acupuncture needle 13
acupuncture practice ... 12, 36, 50, 115, 143, 144
acute pain 21, 29, 32, 39, 55, 57, 67, 69, 80, 81, 82, 97, 112, 127, 129, 180, 181, 182, 183, 270
acute phase 81, 286
Acute probe technique 229, 230
Acutron Mentor 12, 14, 31, 49, 54, 56, 58, 86, 92, 93, 97, 100, 103, 108, 112, 128, 130, 145, 173, 174, 181, 182, 183, 211, 220, 236, 238, 256, 264, 268, 270, 272, 284, 286, 291, 293
addiction 19, 91, 276
adenosine triphosphate .... See ATP
adhesion 285
Adhesive capsulitis 244
Adrenals 300
aggravation 46, 98, 129
ah-shi points 79, 91, 97
AIDS 19
Akabane 206, 212
Alcoholism 268
alligator clips 21, 39, 136, 141, 270
allopathic medicine 20, 73, 78
alternating currents 32
anesthesia 21, 22, 49, 60, 61, 129
ankle ... 93, 96, 118, 131, 248, 258, 260, 284
anode 34, 51, 52, 53, 95
Anterior-posterior treatment 252
anxiety 12, 158, 162, 164
Arndt-Schultz lLaw 127
arteriosclerosis 294
arthritis 58, 91, 110, 196, 266, 293, 296
asthma ... 105, 110, 158, 162, 209, 221, 264, 268, 277, 292, 294
athletic injuries 65, 129
Atoms
    atom 51
ATP 22, 47, 79, 81, 99, 171, 209, 270
aura .... See also etheric
auricular 86, 87, 93, 112, 136, 138, 174, 183, 187, 205, 268, 274
autonomic nervous system ..... 103, 208. See also sympathetic, parasympathetic
Ayurveda 215

B

back ... 13, 21, 25, 31, 33, 36, 39, 46, 50, 54, 59, 60, 62, 66, 68, 74, 78, 81, 90, 91, 92, 97, 101, 103, 107, 108, 110, 111, 112, 115, 121, 123, 127, 128, 129, 131, 132, 137, 138, 144, 148, 149, 155, 158, 159, 161, 162, 163, 164, 165, 167, 173, 174, 175, 176, 180, 183, 184, 185, 186, 187, 188, 198, 199, 202, 218, 219, 221, 225, 230, 236, 240, 242, 250, 252, 254, 256, 260, 268, 272, 277, 286, 293, 298

Back Shu points..... 140, 161, 162, 163, 164, 165, 166, 167, 212, 250, 252, 280
backache 12, 159
Baker formula 101, 288
balancing the meridians system 32
Basic Therapy 292
battery 33, 77
Baxie points 123, 248
Bell's palsy 100
BFD 5, 192, 207, 211, 212, 213, 214
biases 48, 170, 224
Biliary 298, 300
biochemical 20, 27, 192
Bioelectro-magnetics 27
biofeedback 61, 64
biphasic 46, 56, 80, 82, 92, 99, 104, 125, 131, 132, 133, 172, 230, 232, 234, 236, 248, 260, 278, 282
bleeding 66, 90, 180, 181, 183, 184, 185, 250
blockage of Qi 182
Blood.. 27, 48, 62, 63, 64, 65, 66, 67, 69, 70, 90, 91, 110, 113, 156, 157, 161, 170, 171, 182, 183, 184, 185, 186, 188, 210, 218, 232, 250, 256, 264, 280, 306
Blood stagnation 67
blood stasis 181, 183, 184, 300
blood vessels 32, 35, 39, 209
body balancing 121, 152, 210, 230
bodywork 5, 19, 48, 62, 73, 90, 135, 141, 168, 169, 170, 172, 177, 244
bone 22, 23, 29, 35, 59, 60, 62, 101, 127, 196, 293

C

calcium 22, 23, 266, 270, 283, 302
cancer .. 10, 12, 19, 23, 24, 31, 32, 209, 219, 222, 250, 274, 275
cancer constitution 222
capacitance
 see also charge 29, 30, 31, 34, 53
carpal tunnel syndrome ... 54, 58, 92, 94, 96, 132, 133, 240, 277
Carpal tunnel syndrome 93, 117
cell membranes 34, 99, 127, 270
chakra 43, 91, 193, 276
charge.... 10, 30, 32, 33, 34, 38, 39, 79, 90, 95, 99, 172, 180, 188, 210, 275
Chasing the Dragon's Tail 32, 137, 158, 174, 252, 306
children 10, 37, 100, 127, 140, 141, 143, 187, 264
Chinese clock 138, 147, 148, 223, 292
Chinese Clock 292
Chinese herbal medicine 78, 185

chiropractic..... 12, 13, 15, 47, 53, 61, 73, 78, 104, 125, 126, 135, 137, 140, 177, 191, 238, 272, 293
Chong/Yinwei 150, 155
chronic fatigue syndrome 90
chronic pain.... 12, 19, 46, 50, 55, 58, 60, 61, 62, 65, 69, 78, 116, 125, 129, 144, 170, 176, 180, 184, 186, 209, 217, 270, 276, 282, 292
Circling the Dragon 4, 58, 88, 91, 92, 93, 98, 120, 172, 240, 242, 252, 254, 258
circuit...... 31, 32, 52, 53, 111, 112, 117, 119, 153, 167, 181, 210, 213, 285
circulatory system 22
Classic Interferential 126, 129, 130, 183
Cold 45, 63, 66, 67, 110, 157, 232, 268
cold feet 158
color 96, 127, 153, 158, 285
combination treatments 49
Command points 192
concussions 180, 300
conductive gel 127
conductive medium 34, 51, 52
conductivity 29, 31, 39, 40, 52, 57, 86, 87, 88, 94, 96, 112, 172, 175, 181, 206, 207, 208, 210, 236, 246, 258, 290, 291, 298
connective tissue 22, 34, 35, 36
consciousness ... 22, 42, 47, 61, 63, 64, 136, 153, 188, 195, 207, 212
contradictory information 136
cool down 130, 132
Core healing 268
correct pressure 215
correspondences 43, 67, 153
Cosmetic 100
cotton swabs ....
counter probe 56, 105, 112, 176
counter-bias 48, 185, 188, 224
counter-flow 198
Cross Fibre 101
Cross Syndrome 151, 219, 280
cupping 90, 205
current parameters 50
current penetration 126
currents of injury 32, 39
cutaneo-viscero reflex 205
cystitis 66, 158

D

Dai/Yangwei 150
dampness 256
DC 35, 219
de-differentiation 23
dehydration 32
deltoid muscle 92

demyelinated 282
Dense-Disperse.................................49, 61
depolarization 22, 127
depression ... 12, 64, 65, 110, 143, 156, 162, 164, 185, 276, 283
dermatomes..... 4, 36, 58, 79, 82, 91, 92, 93, 94, 98, 102, 103, 104, 105, 107, 118, 120, 132, 133, 230, 246, 260, 280, 284
desensitization...264
detoxification...218
Differential diagnosis 263
Direct current
  direct current 32
disease 9, 12, 20, 22, 24, 27, 28, 30, 39, 48, 62, 63, 64, 65, 78, 90, 104, 110, 111, 116, 144, 158, 162, 163, 167, 180, 185, 193, 215, 218, 219, 221, 222, 230, 232, 242, 250, 266, 268, 272, 276, 277, 292
disk degeneration 238
dispersion of Qi..21
distal acu-points..................................30, 39
distal point.. 11, 81, 87, 89, 97, 98, 105, 108, 112, 117, 120, 121, 122, 165, 172, 182, 184, 192, 230, 232, 240, 250, 252, 254, 258, 264, 274, 300
Drug Addiction 268
drugs..61, 62, 70, 136
Du/Yangchaio 150
duodenal ulcer 158
Dupuytren contracture 296
dynorphins 49, 60, 61
dysmenorrhea.................... 65, 66, 184, 300

E

ear... See auricular
EAV.. 5, 7, 44, 206, 209, 210, 212, 214, 217, 232, 272, 277, 282, 286, 290, 292, 293, 294, 296, 298, 300
edema 20, 80, 110, 125, 180, 183, 277, 293, 294
Eight Guiding Principles 45, 67
elbow . 20, 97, 112, 118, 121, 122, 131, 136, 143, 159, 166, 246
elderly 111, 121, 127, 130, 133, 167, 183, 186, 217, 256, 266, 278
Electric current..... 15, 19, 29, 51, 52, 54, 79, 111, 116, 127, 167
Electric muscle stimulator........................126
electrical current .. 10, 15, 19, 51, 52, 54, 79, 111, 116, 127, 167
electrical field...29
electrical potentials.....................22, 29, 30
electro-acupuncture 7, 10, 15, 16, 19, 20, 21, 31, 38, 39, 40, 42, 44, 46, 48, 50, 51, 53, 56, 61, 64, 66, 67, 68, 72, 73, 77, 80, 89, 115, 128, 132, 137, 139, 151, 152, 156, 172, 180, 188, 196, 209, 231, 254, 256, 258, 260, 280, 282, 291, 307
electrode .. 10, 15, 21, 31, 46, 56, 73, 80, 96, 127, 128, 132, 133, 174, 208, 210, 230, 234, 270, 272, 274, 285, 293, 296
Electrodermal screening 218
electro-diagnostic methods............. 205, 214
electroencephalograms 22
electrolysis 21, 32, 79, 82
electrolyte.. 32, 33
electromagnetic energies. 19, 20, 27, 28, 54, 116, 206, 209
electromagnetic pollution 23, 65, 275
electro-massage 5, 39, 55, 90, 120, 140, 165, 169, 171, 174, 175, 176, 177, 232, 242, 244, 246, 250, 252, 260, 276, 277, 282, 285
Electro-medicine 19
electron 51, 53, 54, 56, 82, 110, 210, 226
electronic meridian testing . 5, 12, 16, 50, 53, 68, 87, 89, 144, 145, 148, 149, 191, 192, 200, 205, 206, 207, 208, 209, 211, 212, 213, 214, 215, 216, 217, 218, 219, 220, 221, 222, 225, 290
electro-physiology 34, 36, 40, 129, 130
electro-therapeutic parameters........ 9, 51, 97
electro-therapy 13, 15, 19, 20, 38, 48, 49, 52, 56, 57, 58, 77, 78, 80, 81, 82, 83, 110, 125, 140, 173, 179, 180, 230, 231
embryonic development.................. 139, 144
emergency medical intervention............. 136
emotion 64, 153, 155, 156
emotions .. 12, 19, 43, 64, 67, 156, 157, 186, 189, 196
emphysema 209
EMT .... See Electronic Meridian Testing
endocrine glands..................................... 23
endorphins 49, 60, 276
energetic evaluation 191, 195, 199, 208, 222
energy 3, 8, 12, 15, 16, 19, 20, 21, 22, 23, 24, 28, 29, 31, 32, 33, 34, 36, 37, 38, 39, 42, 43, 44, 47, 48, 49, 50, 51, 53, 64, 65, 66, 67, 68, 70, 77, 78, 79, 81, 82, 92, 97, 99, 104, 116, 129, 136, 137, 138, 139, 140, 144, 145, 152, 153, 155, 156, 158, 161, 165, 168, 171, 172, 177, 180, 182, 185, 193, 196, 197, 198, 199, 206, 207, 209, 211, 212, 216, 218, 222, 223, 224, 226, 242, 263, 274, 275, 276, 290, 292
energy medicine..... 3, 15, 16, 19, 20, 24, 31, 42, 50, 77, 290
epileptic seizures 22
epistaxis 159
etheric 20, 196, 275

exercise 13, 36, 61, 81, 82, 90, 113, 132, 133, 140, 169, 171, 172, 173, 180, 185, 186, 188, 193, 219, 230, 242, 256, 272, 281
extraordinary vessels. 32, 47, 108, 116, 137, 138, 139, 140, 144, 145, 147, 149, 150, 151, 152, 153, 155, 161, 167, 203, 224, 236, 250, 280
Extraordinary Vessels........................47, 155
eyes 65, 158, 159, 164, 184, 256

F

fascia 22, 29, 35, 100, 205, 209
fascial network......................23, 36, 39, 172
FDA...9, 10, 52
feedback system........................81, 101, 171
fibromyalgia 69, 90, 176, 266, 280
first aid 67, 69, 181
Five Element correspondences...............153
fixed polarity...132
fluids 32, 33, 70, 80, 180, 182, 209, 277
Four-Step Protocol16, 65, 69, 111, 134, 136, 141, 161, 166, 169, 177, 191, 210, 218, 225, 266, 280
fracture healing..23
frequencies 23, 24, 25, 37, 38, 44, 49, 50, 53, 55, 58, 60, 61, 100, 103, 126, 127, 129, 206, 232, 270, 272, 286, 290, 291, 294, 300

G

Gall Bladder... 109, 110, 111, 117, 121, 144, 147, 148, 155, 157, 159, 162, 165, 167, 200, 202, 221, 222, 224, 225, 256, 280, 292
gastrocnemius ... 6, 138, 145, 147, 151, 155, 163, 165, 167, 191, 224, 225, 252, 258, 260
genitals 159, 162
geopathic stress.......................................275
Golgi tendon 101
gout..77, 296
granulation...128
Great Loops4, 73, 93, 96, 97, 115, 116, 117, 119, 120, 121, 122, 166, 174, 182, 183, 224, 230, 248, 256, 258, 274, 284, 296
gwasha...205
gynecological problems...........................158

H

hand... 31, 50, 70, 87, 93, 94, 102, 112, 113, 115, 120, 121, 133, 136, 138, 153, 155, 158, 161, 164, 166, 171, 173, 174, 175, 176, 182, 183, 186, 187, 188, 195, 196, 197, 198, 199, 202, 208, 210, 211, 213, 214, 215, 218, 219, 221, 224, 230, 236, 238, 240, 242, 244, 248, 250, 252, 260, 268, 274, 278, 280, 284, 285, 286, 288, 296, 300
hand mass 87, 153, 174, 210, 211, 213, 214, 268, 278, 280, 284, 285, 286, 300
hara...... 23, 35, 69, 136, 144, 191, 192, 193, 195, 196, 200, 208, 252, 306 See also Tantien
harmony 15, 28, 47, 63, 64, 65
hatha yoga 36, 254
headaches 58, 59, 65, 66, 69, 91, 92, 93, 104, 158, 159, 180, 184, 219, 222, 232, 234, 236, 276, 300, 302
Healing
healing..... 4, 6, 22, 79, 205, 270, 271, 306
healing mode 132, 270
healing touch.. 127
Heart .. 63, 64, 105, 109, 110, 111, 116, 121, 148, 153, 155, 157, 158, 162, 163, 164, 167, 200, 202, 219, 221, 222, 224, 225, 277, 280, 292, 294
Heat ... 63, 66, 157, 184, 218, 219, 232, 256, 268
hemorrhoids........................... 110, 158, 221
herbal formulas 45, 62, 71, 136, 266, 268, 287
herniated disks........................... 59, 62, 176
herpes zoster 158, 159, 283
high blood pressure 143, 158
high frequency 32, 61
high volt pulsed galvanic............. 20, 32, 126
High-volt pulsed galvanic stimulator 126
hips 74, 118, 159, 186, 256
holistic....... 20, 62, 67, 71, 83, 141, 179, 210
homeopathy 13, 20, 24, 25, 43, 47, 78
homeostasis... 20, 24, 47, 50, 55, 57, 62, 63, 80, 132, 145, 155
hormones22, 23, 29, 89, 208, 219, 266, 280, 300
Hua-To points 103, 107, 108, 242
Hun 63, 64, 65, 162, 164
hydration 185
hypersensitive 69, 98, 99, 132, 168, 242
hypertension 69, 294

I

Ice Electrotherapy................................... 181
imbalanced meridians............................. 148
immune system23, 28, 48, 70, 187, 211, 280
immune-boosting 281
indicator drops 207, 208, 217, 218

inflammation 55, 69, 80, 81, 82, 89, 97, 170, 180, 187, 216, 218, 266, 276, 282, 302
Infraspinatus 240
insanity 159
insomnia 110, 158, 162, 164, 219
intention 188, 193, 198, 199
intercostal neuralgia 158
interference 29, 126, 139
interferential ... 13, 20, 32, 39, 46, 55, 64, 70, 73, 74, 78, 81, 93, 123, 126, 127, 128, 129, 130, 132, 133, 171, 174, 175, 176, 183, 185, 206, 230, 238, 246, 248, 254, 256, 260, 272, 288
Interpreting Electronic Meridian Testing Patterns 5, 215
interstitial spaces 30, 32, 39
intradermal needles 140, 186, 187
intra-oral 86, 100
ion pellets 186, 187
ionic activity 30, 88
ion-pumping cords . 32, 35, 38, 47, 136, 144, 145, 147, 288
iontophoresis 20

J

jiaohui points 151
joint pain 159

K

key imbalance 145, 148, 149, 203, 220
Kidney 62, 109, 111, 116, 121, 122, 123, 145, 147, 148, 149, 153, 155, 162, 163, 164, 167, 188, 193, 200, 202, 208, 218, 219, 221, 222, 224, 225, 232, 250, 260, 266, 268, 292, 298
Kidney Yin deficiency 62, 145
kinesiology ... 3, 5, 16, 35, 43, 50, 54, 81, 96, 99, 101, 108, 109, 110, 121, 138, 145, 148, 166, 168, 191, 195, 196, 199, 202, 207, 208, 220, 222, 224, 225, 231, 232, 250, 252, 260, 266, 278, 284, 286, 288
kinetic 52, 64, 73, 82, 127, 131, 132, 133, 172, 231, 256
knee pain 158
knees ... 74, 87, 89, 118, 184, 192, 198, 202, 225, 236, 256, 272
Korean hand points 70, 93, 186
kori 90
kyutoshin 162, 163, 166

L

laser 30
lateral epicondylitis 20
Lateral knee injury 256
latissimus dorsi 244
left-right imbalances 140, 211, 215
leg length differences 161
levator scapula 236, 240, 244
Liao points 250
life functions 21
light 7, 21, 28, 31, 33, 127, 161, 164, 202, 210, 220, 278
Ling Ku combination 230, 252
liver 48, 65, 158, 264, 266, 277
Liver ... 3, 33, 53, 62, 63, 64, 65, 68, 99, 105, 109, 110, 111, 121, 129, 138, 145, 147, 148, 149, 155, 157, 162, 164, 167, 200, 202, 205, 215, 217, 218, 219, 221, 222, 224, 225, 232, 256, 268, 274, 280, 292, 294
Liver Fire 62, 145
Low-volt stimulator 125
Lumbo-sacral 252
Lungs ... 29, 63, 64, 105, 109, 110, 153, 155, 157, 164, 200, 226, 242, 268, 292
Luo-Connecting 137, 144, 158
lupus 90, 219, 266
lymphatic system . 80, 90, 99, 125, 170, 174, 180, 209, 218, 282, 291, 292, 293, 294, 296, 300

M

macular degeneration 65, 278
Magnetism .... See magnets
magnets 35, 45, 47, 54, 95, 137
Manaka 7, 12, 16, 32, 35, 38, 47, 48, 50, 109, 111, 136, 137, 138, 139, 140, 141, 144, 145, 150, 151, 152, 155, 162, 163, 167, 172, 174, 187, 188, 191, 192, 193, 195, 199, 200, 202, 219, 224, 226, 236, 244, 258, 280, 288, 306
manipulation 5, 19, 30, 33, 38, 48, 62, 70, 73, 74, 90, 104, 120, 135, 140, 141, 169, 172, 177, 179, 232, 238, 284, 293
masseter 101, 234
Master and Coupled points 138, 145, 151
Master points 32, 47, 95, 151, 152, 164, 192, 220, 230, 280
Medial knee injury 256
meditation 43, 47, 61, 156
Meniere's syndrome 158, 159
mental illness 23, 164, 219

meridian... 4, 5, 6, 19, 21, 23, 25, 29, 31, 34, 35, 36, 38, 39, 40, 48, 50, 53, 57, 64, 65, 66, 68, 70, 73, 74, 78, 79, 81, 83, 86, 87, 89, 93, 95, 97, 99, 107, 111, 115, 116, 117, 119, 120, 121, 122, 125, 127, 129, 132, 136, 137, 138, 139, 140, 141, 143, 144, 145, 146, 148, 149, 151, 152, 153, 155, 156, 158, 161, 162, 163, 164, 166, 172, 173, 177, 181, 182, 183, 184, 188, 191, 192, 193, 195, 200, 203, 205, 206, 207, 208, 209, 210, 212, 214, 215, 216, 217, 219, 222, 223, 224, 225, 226, 230, 240, 246, 274, 276, 277, 282, 285, 286, 290, 291, 292, 293, 294, 296

meridian balancing ... 93, 144, 161, 177, 215

meridian system 19, 34, 36, 73, 87, 122, 139, 143, 144, 161, 205, 214

metabolism 29, 269, 302

microcurrent 4, 5, 7, 9, 10, 12, 13, 14, 15, 16, 17, 19, 20, 21, 25, 31, 32, 33, 35, 37, 38, 39, 40, 42, 46, 47, 50, 51, 54, 64, 68, 69, 70, 73, 74, 77, 78, 79, 80, 81, 82, 86, 87, 88, 89, 90, 93, 95, 96, 97, 98, 99, 101, 104, 105, 108, 111, 112, 115, 116, 117, 122, 123, 125, 127, 129, 130, 131, 132, 133, 137, 139, 140, 141, 143, 144, 145, 148, 151, 152, 153, 156, 163, 165, 166, 167, 170, 171, 172, 173, 174, 175, 176, 177, 179, 180, 181, 182, 184, 185, 186, 188, 206, 209, 210, 211, 229, 230, 232, 234, 238, 242, 244, 246, 248, 252, 254, 256, 260, 264, 268, 270, 272, 274, 276, 278, 280, 284, 285, 286, 288, 290, 291, 292, 293, 294, 296, 300, 307

microcurrent device . 12, 31, 73, 96, 98, 101, 122, 123, 172, 175, 181, 182, 230, 285

microcurrent electro-acupuncture.............. 19

Microcurrent electro-acupuncture.............. 19

microcurrent therapy.. 7, 12, 33, 73, 74, 104, 209

micro-system 6, 93, 112, 113, 138, 141, 158, 182, 196, 224, 286

Migraine prevention 232

migraines 65, 68, 143

milliamp.... 19, 21, 32, 39, 55, 70, 73, 74, 79, 80, 98, 125, 127, 128, 129, 130, 132, 133, 170, 180, 181, 182, 183, 206, 272, 277, 284, 293

Milliamp-Microamp combination 129

mineral deficiencies 186

motion 81, 82, 88, 90, 93, 127, 131, 132, 133, 170, 171, 172, 173, 256

motor actions 22

motor fibers 103

motor points 129, 182, 277

moxibustion 68, 137, 140, 162, 163, 166, 167, 170, 173, 184, 185, 219, 229, 277, 280

MRI 43, 62, 205, 254

muscle cells 22

muscle stimulators 20

muscle tension 20, 69, 128, 209

muscles.... 22, 29, 35, 50, 53, 70, 80, 81, 82, 90, 91, 100, 101, 102, 103, 104, 107, 126, 129, 138, 152, 163, 165, 171, 172, 174, 180, 182, 183, 186, 188, 191, 195, 196, 202, 209, 224, 234, 236, 238, 240, 242, 244, 252, 254, 260, 272, 277, 284, 288, 296

musculoskeletal problems 159

Mu-Shu technique..... 91, 110, 111, 158, 166

Mussat 29, 33, 34

myofascial 13, 16, 23, 37, 58, 65, 67, 79, 90, 91, 97, 112, 131, 132, 135, 140, 170, 172, 174, 176, 192, 205, 212, 214, 229, 238, 254, 280

Myofascial release 70, 169

N

Nakatani... 5, 12, 25, 29, 191, 208, 212, 216, 220, 221, 222

nanoamps 34, 79

naturopathic 53

neck 10, 22, 65, 68, 70, 80, 91, 92, 102, 103, 104, 108, 110, 121, 123, 129, 132, 133, 159, 173, 176, 180, 186, 196, 221, 232, 236, 238, 240, 242, 246, 248, 272, 284, 288, 293, 302

needle insertion.. 30

negative probe ... 81, 93, 94, 96, 97, 98, 105, 107, 108, 112, 118, 120, 152, 153, 156, 173, 174, 182

negatively charged........................... 21, 110

Nei Jing 36, 90, 115

nerve block........................... 21, 68, 132, 180

nerve bundle 22

nerve fibers 60, 282

nervous system 9, 22, 27, 34, 36, 60, 61, 62, 63, 81, 91, 99, 100, 101, 102, 103, 108, 110, 121, 138, 161, 170, 180, 188, 192, 205, 208, 236, 274, 282, 294, 300, 302

nervousness.................................... 208, 219

neuralgia 221, 272

neuromuscular imbalances..................... 170

Neuromuscular re-education 170

neurosis 158

non-needle 7, 37, 38, 40, 90, 122, 139

Nordenstrom 31, 32, 274

nutrition 144, 185, 281

O

O Ring testing 50, 195, 202, 203
octahedron 138, 139, 140, 150, 152
octaves 43
Ohm's Law 52, 53, 206
ohmmeter 25, 52, 86, 87, 208, 212, 290, 291
organs 12, 22, 29, 32, 35, 48, 50, 53, 60, 62, 74, 77, 101, 103, 104, 105, 108, 110, 186, 191, 192, 205, 209, 221, 250, 291, 292, 294
Organs 29, 35, 43, 52, 53, 65, 67, 70, 91, 108, 110, 153, 156, 161, 166, 167, 191, 192, 193, 199, 206, 208, 211, 212, 218, 219
origin-insertion 101, 102, 238
oscilloscope 57
Osseous manipulation 177
Osteoarthritis 266
osteoporosis 23

P

pacemaker 22, 104, 242
pad electrodes ... 10, 39, 125, 127, 133, 181, 182, 211, 274, 293
pad longevity 128
pad stimulation 123, 125, 127, 131, 133, 184, 238, 256
pain 3, 7, 9, 10, 12, 15, 16, 19, 20, 21, 23, 24, 29, 30, 31, 32, 33, 35, 37, 38, 39, 45, 46, 48, 49, 50, 54, 55, 58, 59, 60, 61, 62, 63, 64, 65, 66, 67, 68, 69, 71, 73, 74, 77, 78, 79, 80, 81, 82, 87, 89, 90, 91, 92, 93, 94, 95, 96, 97, 98, 99, 100, 102, 103, 104, 107, 108, 110, 112, 115, 116, 117, 118, 120, 121, 122, 123, 125, 127, 128, 129, 130, 131, 132, 133, 135, 136, 137, 138, 139, 141, 143, 144, 149, 152, 156, 158, 159, 162, 164, 165, 166, 170, 171, 172, 173, 174, 176, 177, 179, 180, 182, 183, 184, 185, 186, 187, 188, 192, 196, 212, 214, 216, 217, 218, 219, 224, 229, 230, 232, 234, 236, 238, 240, 244, 246, 248, 250, 252, 254, 256, 258, 260, 266, 270, 274, 276, 277, 280, 282, 283, 284, 286, 288, 292
pain management 3, 9, 15, 16, 19, 23, 54, 55, 61, 62, 63, 65, 67, 68, 74, 89, 116, 143, 164, 179, 212, 224
pain relief 10, 20, 68, 77, 78, 80, 81, 102, 128, 183, 234, 258, 284
palpation .. 89, 110, 119, 121, 137, 138, 147, 148, 150, 151, 155, 163, 164, 165, 166, 174, 191, 192, 193, 202, 207, 208, 224, 225, 229, 246, 252
pancreatic colic 298
paralysis 272, 286, 296
Parathyroid 300, 302
paresthesia 94
patterns of disharmony 62, 67, 68, 144
pectoralis major 244
Pediatric
  pediatric 99
Pericardium 109, 110, 111, 121, 147, 148, 149, 153, 155, 157, 162, 163, 164, 167, 200, 202, 219, 221, 222, 224, 225, 292, 296
Peripheral neuropathy 93, 103, 117
phantom limb pain 29
pharmaceutical 22, 27, 61, 78
Phlegm 62, 66, 268
physical therapy 62, 68, 70, 73, 81, 172, 176
physicians ... 12, 36, 125, 135, 137, 166, 177
physics 28, 43
physiology 3, 59, 60, 62, 103, 108, 125, 127, 138
piezoelectricity 23, 34, 35, 36, 39, 172
pinched nerve 93, 94, 118, 132
piriformis muscle 254
pituitary 23, 300
placebo 27
plum blossom needle 205
Po 63, 64, 162, 164
polar meridian 6, 122, 138, 140, 144, 145, 146, 149, 151, 152, 153, 155, 167, 203, 223, 224, 225, 226
Polarity
  polarity 3, 5, 20, 30, 43, 44, 45, 46, 47, 56, 58, 80, 81, 92, 93, 95, 98, 100, 103, 107, 108, 112, 116, 118, 124, 147, 151, 175, 218, 219, 232, 234, 250, 260, 268, 270, 272, 282, 284, 285, 288, 291, 292
polarization 22, 33, 34, 40, 209
polarized treatment .. 21, 35, 73, 95, 97, 122, 123, 145, 163, 166, 167, 184, 230, 248, 274, 284, 288
positive and negative . 32, 38, 39, 50, 52, 93, 99, 132, 138
positively charged 21, 51
post-herpetic neuralgia 158, 159
preset ... 49, 54, 55, 57, 58, 73, 88, 123, 128, 145, 173, 174, 182, 183, 220, 236, 244, 246, 256, 264, 268, 270, 272, 284, 286, 293
pressure sore treatment 270
principal meridians ... 70, 138, 144, 151, 182, 192, 294
probe electrodes 21, 35, 73, 86, 95, 127, 146, 171, 230, 300

Prolapsed anus..221
propagated sensations 30
proprioception....... 5, 81, 101, 113, 170, 171, 172, 188
proprioceptive techniques.........................169
prostaglandins 180
psychosomatic..63
psychotherapy 156
pulse diagnosis.. 35, 50, 144, 145, 166, 191, 207, 208, 220
pulse duration 58, 125, 126, 128, 182

Q

Qi . 12, 22, 27, 28, 29, 33, 47, 48, 61, 62, 63, 64, 65, 66, 67, 68, 69, 70, 79, 81, 89, 91, 96, 99, 110, 112, 113, 116, 122, 123, 127, 129, 140, 141, 153, 154, 155, 156, 158, 161, 162, 170, 171, 182, 183, 184, 185, 186, 188, 193, 196, 197, 198, 199, 210, 211, 212, 217, 218, 219, 226, 230, 250, 256, 274, 280
Qigong 22, 23, 29, 32, 42, 70, 274
Q-tips 88, 94, 98
quadrant measurements...........................211
quadratus lumborum................................244
quantum physics..................................27, 28
Quick Key 88, 92

R

radiculopathies..... 4, 46, 80, 81, 82, 91, 93, 132
range of motion.... 31, 74, 81, 82, 91, 92, 96, 120, 133, 137, 171, 173, 236, 244, 246, 256, 258
receptor site..22
reflex sympathetic dystrophy........46, 69, 100
regeneration..................... 22, 23, 34, 35, 189
rehabilitation 13, 15, 19, 23, 61, 70, 81, 133, 170, 242
reimbursement..83
Reinhold Voll..... 7, 25, 44, 55, 137, 208, 290
remedy testing 209, 290, 291
Ren/Yinchaio 150, 155
Reproductive...300
research studies 23, 74, 266, 270
resistance 25, 29, 30, 31, 52, 53, 82, 86, 87, 88, 104, 171, 172, 173, 205, 206, 207, 212, 222, 238
Resonance
 resonance 3, 20, 24, 37, 43, 52, 53, 55, 96, 100, 116, 193, 195, 212, 213, 290, 292
resonant frequencies 24

Restless Leg syndrome 284
results 10, 12, 15, 20, 21, 27, 37, 39, 46, 48, 50, 53, 56, 58, 62, 67, 73, 74, 77, 78, 81, 82, 83, 88, 92, 96, 97, 101, 122, 125, 141, 143, 145, 171, 172, 196, 198, 202, 203, 207, 208, 215, 216, 222, 252, 260, 263, 272, 274, 286, 293
rheumatoid arthritis 66, 69, 82, 97, 266
rhomboids 242, 244, 284
Robert Becker 21, 22, 34, 45, 77, 274
Root and Branch 3, 68, 69, 70, 71, 136, 140, 141
Root treatment 122, 136, 140, 143, 170, 191, 250
rotator cuff... 87, 240
Royal Rife 24
Russian stimulation.......... 55, 70, 73, 78, 127
Ryodoraku...... 5, 25, 29, 144, 191, 206, 208, 209, 212, 215, 220, 222, 306

S

Sacro-iliac joint............................... 258, 260
scar tissue... 59, 174
sciatica 46, 58, 91, 93, 94, 96, 132, 158, 179, 221, 230, 252, 254, 293
sclerolytic 32
scoliosis 62, 139
search mode 86, 87, 89, 92, 210
sedation ... 97, 138, 145, 208, 210, 224, 226, 291, 292
semiconduction............................. 34, 35, 39
serotonin 49, 61, 276
Shaoyang............... 117, 121, 144, 145, 232
Shaoyin 111, 116, 117, 121, 167
Shen...................... 63, 64, 70, 162, 164, 268
Shiatsu 169
shortness of breath 158
shoulder 69, 77, 87, 92, 93, 97, 100, 112, 118, 121, 129, 132, 133, 158, 159, 171, 173, 183, 196, 221, 230, 232, 236, 240, 242, 244, 256, 284, 293
S-I joint............................. 133, 258, 260, 293
side effects........................... 21, 48, 62, 278
Sinus Headache..................................... 234
skin..... 10, 29, 31, 35, 52, 57, 60, 67, 79, 86, 87, 88, 94, 110, 127, 128, 131, 141, 153, 163, 174, 187, 192, 205, 206, 208, 212, 214, 215, 285, 293
Skin preparation...................................... 128
SLE .... See also lupus
Slope...................... 100, 103, 108, 175, 211
Smoking 268
sotai ... 5, 140, 170, 172, 173, 174, 229, 238, 244, 252, 254

Source points..... 36, 97, 153, 192, 193, 211, 212, 213
spasm ... 29, 80, 82, 125, 128, 180, 183, 260
specific frequencies..... See also frequencies
spinal cord 49, 60, 61, 103, 205, 277, 286
spinal ganglia..161
spinal nerves..103
spinal pain and injuries............................159
Spirit.................. 8, 21, 28, 64, 162, 189, 213
spiritual 7, 14, 21, 23, 28, 43, 47, 63, 64, 65, 70, 153, 164, 207, 219, 275, 276
Spleen 29, 64, 105, 109, 110, 111, 115, 120, 121, 147, 148, 149, 151, 153, 155, 156, 157, 158, 162, 164, 167, 188, 200, 202, 218, 219, 221, 223, 224, 225, 226, 232, 280, 292
stagnant blood......................................181
stagnation 65, 66, 67, 242, 264, 274, 275, 280, 292
stasis....... 113, 174, 183, 209, 218, 282, 296
Step One treatments 151, 152, 153, 155, 224, 230, 263
stiff neck..121, 179, 236
stomach disorders.....................................158
stress management.....................................19
stress reactions..23
stretching . 90, 176, 188, 229, 230, 240, 242, 274, 280, 281, 285
stroke 100, 102, 219, 282, 286
structural distortion and alignment......48, 69, 139, 141, 144, 161, 177
Subscapularis..242
subsensationsal..54
supplements 50, 186, 266, 276, 278, 283, 286, 287
Supraspinatus..240
surgery.. 21, 31, 48, 60, 61, 62, 70, 136, 176
swelling...................... 91, 181, 182, 277, 293
symptomatic treatment 9, 16, 31, 61, 62, 67, 68, 69, 70, 136, 137, 139, 140, 143, 168, 179, 180, 188, 232

T

Taiyang... 116, 117, 119, 121, 159, 184, 232
Tantien
  tantien 69
Tao..63, 64, 65
TCM .... 3, 12, 27, 29, 33, 61, 62, 63, 65, 67, 68, 71, 103, 108, 109, 111, 136, 145, 150, 167, 191, 192, 200, 202, 206, 208, 212, 215, 226, 232, 250, 280, 290. See also Traditional Chinese
Te Chi 30
Tendinitis
  tendinitis 6, 65, 288

tendino-muscular meridians............... 97, 173
tendon 82, 288
tennis elbow. 20, 92, 93, 117, 121, 132, 136, 174, 240
TENS 9, 10, 20, 70, 74, 78, 125, 270
thalamus 60
The Body Electric. 21, 23, 24, 27, 34, 45, 54, 77, 80, 306
The Three P's 118
therapeutic exercises............................ 186
thermocouple 33, 39
Thoracic Outlet Syndrome 6, 272, 288
thyroid 108, 300
timer................................... 87, 88, 176, 278
tinnitis................................... 110, 158, 159
tissue healing.............. 22, 55, 139, 181, 270
TMJ........................... 12, 100, 159, 234
tone.... 48, 81, 100, 101, 102, 104, 105, 170, 186, 236, 286, 294
tonification 97, 138, 145, 157, 166, 208, 209, 210, 218, 224, 226, 291, 292
toothache 158
torpedo fish 77
Traditional Chinese Medicine .. 3, 14, 27, 62, 136
Transcutaneous Electric Nerve Stimulator
  .... See TENS
trauma.................. 32, 62, 90, 116, 183, 186
trigeminal neuralgia......... 159, 221, 283, 296
trigger points 7, 8, 13, 58, 61, 70, 74, 79, 90, 91, 97, 98, 125, 131, 172, 173, 205, 229, 230, 244, 284
trigger probe. 56, 87, 88, 105, 112, 122, 123, 176, 210, 211, 214, 220, 234, 268, 278, 280, 284, 286
Triple Warmer.. 29, 110, 111, 117, 121, 144, 147, 148, 151, 153, 157, 162, 165, 167, 202, 219, 221, 222, 223, 224, 225, 244, 292
tumors..................... 10, 32, 250, 274

U

Unified Field................................ 42
universal laws 3, 20
Universe........................... 21, 28, 47, 51, 64
Urinary Bladder channel 97, 140, 161

V

vertigo 66, 221, 300, 302
vibration 21, 24, 63
viral infections 19, 68, 280
viscera......... 29, 91, 102, 103, 108, 205, 206
viscero-cutaneous reflex................. 205, 206

W

waveform 55, 57, 58, 98, 126, 127, 132, 182, 191, 211, 278
Wedensky inhibition..................................127
Western medicine.. 20, 60, 62, 65, 108, 136, 181, 192, 215
whiplash 6, 91, 100, 102, 152, 158, 159, 174, 236, 238, 240, 288, 289
whole food diet................................283, 287
Wind.......................... 63, 110, 157, 232, 268
wind-cold invasion 159
wound healing................................126, 128

X

X-signal system . 35, 47, 137, 138, 139, 143, 150

Y

Yi.....64, 162, 164
Yin 5, 30, 44, 45, 50, 62, 65, 68, 69, 91, 108, 110, 115, 117, 139, 140, 145, 152, 153, 157, 158, 161, 162, 166, 184, 198, 212, 218, 219, 232, 250, 256, 258, 280, 292
Yin and Yang 5, 30, 44, 50, 108, 140, 161

Z

Zhi.. 64, 162, 164
Zip up – zip down test............................ 197

Made in United States
Troutdale, OR
09/25/2023